The Role of Inflammatory Processes in Airway Hyperresponsiveness

EDITED BY

S. T. Holgate (*Co-ordinator*),
J. B. L. Howell, P. G. J. Burney, J. M. Drazen,
F. E. Hargreave, A. B. Kay, K. F. Kerrebijn &
L. M. Reid

BLACKWELL SCIENTIFIC PUBLICATIONS

OXFORD LONDON

EDINBURGH BOSTON MELBOURNE

© 1989 by
Blackwell Scientific Publications
Editorial Offices:
Osney Mead, Oxford OX2 0EL
8 John Street, London WC1N 2ES
23 Ainslie Place, Edinburgh EH3 6AJ
3 Cambridge Center, Suite 208
  Cambridge, Massachusetts 02142,
  USA
107 Barry Street, Carlton
  Victoria 3053, Australia

First published 1989

Set by Associated Publishing
Services Ltd, Petersfield, Hampshire;
printed and bound in Great Britain by
Billing & Sons Ltd, Worcester

DISTRIBUTORS

Marston Book Services Ltd
PO Box 87
Oxford OX2 0DT
(*Orders*: Tel: 0865 791155
    Fax: 0865 791927
    Telex: 837515)

USA
  Year Book Medical Publishers
  200 North LaSalle Street
  Chicago, Illinois 60601
  (*Orders*: Tel: (312) 726-9733)

Canada
  The C.V. Mosby Company
  5240 Finch Avenue East
  Scarborough, Ontario
  (*Orders*: Tel: (416) 298-1588)

Australia
  Blackwell Scientific Publications
  (Australia) Pty Ltd
  107 Barry Street
  Carlton, Victoria 3053
  (*Orders*: Tel: (03) 347-0300)

British Library
Cataloguing in Publication Data

The role of inflammatory processes in
  airway hyperresponsiveness
  1. Man. Bronchi. Asthma
  I. Holgate, Stephen T.
  616.2′38

ISBN 0-632-02618-9

Contents

List of Participants

W. M. ABRAHAM, *Associate Director, Mount Sinai Medical Center, 4300 Alton Road, Miami Beach, Florida 33140, USA*

H. R. ANDERSON, *Chairman and Head of Department of Clinical Epidemiology and Social Medicine, St George's Hospital Medical School, Jenner Wing, Level 0, Cranmer Terrace, London SW17 0RE, UK*

P. J. BARNES, *Professor and Chairman of Thoracic Medicine, National Heart and Lung Institute, Brompton Hospital, London SW3 6HP, UK*

P. G. J. BURNEY, *Senior Lecturer, Department of Community Medicine, United Medical and Dental Schools of Guy's and St Thomas's Hospitals, St Thomas's Campus, London SE1 7EH, UK*

B. BURROWS, *Professor of Internal Medicine, Director, Division of Respiratory Sciences, University of Arizona College of Medicine, Tucson, Arizona 85724, USA*

M. CHAN-YEUNG, *Department of Medicine, Chief, Pulmonary Division, Beth Israel Hospital, 330 Brookline Avenue, Boston, Massachusetts 02115, USA*

J. M. DRAZEN, *Associate Professor of Medicine, Chief, Pulmonary Division, Beth Israel Hospital, 330 Brookline Avenue, Boston, Massachusetts 02115, USA*

G. J. GLEICH, *Department of Immunology, Mayo Clinic, 200 First Street SW, Rochester, Minnesota 55905, USA*

F. E. HARGREAVE, *Firestone Regional Chest and Allergy Unit, St Joseph's Hospital, McMaster University, 50 Charlton Avenue East, Hamilton, Ontario L8N 4A6, Canada*

P. M. HENSON, *Department of Pediatrics, National Jewish Center for Immunology and Respiratory Medicine, 1400 Jackson Street, Denver, Colorado 80206, USA*

C. HIRSCHMANN, *Department of Anesthesiology Critical Care Medicine, Blalock Wing 1414, Johns Hopkins Hospital, 600 Wolfe, Baltimore, Maryland 21205, USA*

List of
Participants

J. HOGG, *University of British Columbia, Director, Pulmonary Research Laboratory, St Paul's Hospital, Vancouver, British Columbia V6Z 1Y6, Canada*

S. T. HOLGATE, *University of Southampton, Faculty of Medicine, Medicine 1, Level D, Centre Block, Southampton General Hospital, Tremona Road, Southampton SO9 4XY, UK*

J. B. L. HOWELL, *University of Southampton, Faculty of Medicine, Medicine 1, Level D, Centre Block, Southampton General Hospital, Tremona Road, Southampton SO9 4XY, UK*

G. W. HUNNINGHAKE, *Director, Pulmonary Division, Department of Internal Medicine, University of Iowa Hospitals, Iowa City, Iowa 52242, USA*

C. IRVIN, *National Jewish Center for Immunology and Respiratory Medicine, 1400 Jackson Street, Denver, Colorado 80206, USA*

R. C. JONGEJAN, *Department of Respiratory Disease, Sophia Children's Hospital, University Hospital Rotterdam, Gordelweg 160, PO Box 70029, 3000L Rotterdam, The Netherlands*

A. B. KAY, *Professor and Director, Department of Allergy and Clinical Immunology, National Heart and Lung Institute, Dovehouse Street, London SW3 6LY, UK*

K. F. KERREBIJN, *Professor of Paediatric Respiratory Disease, Department of Respiratory Diseases, Sophia Children's Hospital, University Hospital Rotterdam, Gordelweg 160, PO Box 70029, 3000L Rotterdam, The Netherlands*

J. KLEINERMAN, *Director, Department of Pathology, Cleveland Metropolitan General Hospital, 3395 Scranton Road, Cleveland, Ohio 44109, USA*

L. A. LAITINEN, *Director of Research Institute of Military Medicine, Department of Clinical Physiology, Central Military Hospital, Mannerheimintie 164, SF-00300 Helsinki, Finland*

T. H. LEE, *Department of Allergy and Allied Respiratory Disorders, United Medical and Dental Schools of Guy's and St Thomas's Hospitals, 4th Floor, Hunt's House, London SE1 9RT, UK*

L. M. LICHTENSTEIN, *Professor of Medicine, Johns Hopkins University School of Medicine, The Good Samaritan Hospital, 5601 Loch Raven Boulevard, Baltimore, Maryland 21239, USA*

P. T. MACKLEM, *Department of Medicine, Montreal Chest Hospital Center, 3650 Saint Urbain Street, Montreal H2X 2P4, Canada*

G. MARONE, *Division of Clinical Immunology, Department of Medicine, University of Naples, 2nd School of Medicine, Via Sergio Pansini, 5-08131 Napoli, Italy*

J. A. NADEL, *University of California, School of Medicine, Cardiovascular Research Institute, San Francisco, California 94143-0130, USA*

R. PAUWELS, *Department of Respiratory Diseases, University Hospital, De Pintelaan 185, B9000, Ghent, Belgium*

S. PERMUTT, *Department of Anesthesiology Critical Care Medicine, Johns Hopkins Hospital, 600 Wolfe, Baltimore, Maryland 21205, USA*

C. PERSSON, *Department of Clinical Pharmacology, University Hospital Lund, S221-85 Lund, Sweden*

T. PLATTS-MILLS, *Head, Division of Allergy and Clinical Immunology, University of Virginia, School of Medicine, Charlottesville, Virginia 22908, USA*

D. S. POSTMA, *Academic Hospital, Respiratory Diseases, Oostersingel 59, 9700RB Groningen, The Netherlands*

N. B. PRIDE, *Consultant Physician, Respiratory Division, Royal Postgraduate Medical School, Hammersmith Hospital, Ducane Road, London W12 0HS, UK*

L. M. REID, *Wolback Professor of Pathology, Harvard Medical School, Pathologist in Chief, The Children's Hospital, 300 Longwood Avenue, Boston, Massachusetts 02115, USA*

M. R. SEARS, *Associate Professor of Medicine, Department of Medicine, University of Otago Medical School, PO Box 913, Dunedin, New Zealand*

F. E. SPEIZER, *Professor in Medicine, Harvard Medical School, Co-Director, Channing Laboratory, Brigham and Women's Hospital, 180 Longwood Avenue, Boston, Massachusetts 02119, USA*

A. J. WOOLCOCK, *Professor of Respiratory Medicine, University of Sydney, New South Wales 2006, Australia*

Introduction and Historical Perspective

J. B. L. Howell

The conference which led to the publication of this book arose from discussions between Professor Stephen Holgate and Fisons Pharmaceuticals plc. I suspect that in their discussions, Professor Holgate and Fisons had similar objectives, but probably arrived at them from different directions.

Each topic section of this book has been drawn together by a section editor (shown in **bold** type at the beginning of each chapter). The text of the book was accepted by all the contributors at a meeting held in Florida during November 1988 under my chairmanship.

Professor Holgate, aware of the extraordinarily rapid growth of knowledge in so many aspects of what we call asthma—epidemiology, immunology, pathology, therapy, and even clinical presentation—recognised the potential benefit of bringing together individuals at the forefront of research in each field, to review and integrate current knowledge from the individual areas. By attempting to reach agreement on models of the mechanisms underlying the disorder, it was hoped to point the way to further advances in understanding. For their part, Fisons were also keen to see the development of models of the mechanisms underlying asthma that would enable the use of drugs for treatment, including their own, on a more rational basis than at present.

We have, at present, essentially only two types of drugs capable of modifying the underlying process of asthma—sodium cromoglycate and nedocromil sodium, and corticosteroids. The development of sodium cromoglycate as a treatment for asthma followed recognition of its striking property of inhibiting the immediate asthmatic reaction to inhaled allergen. In contrast, corticosteroids have no effect in preventing this response, but like sodium cromoglycate, can prevent the late reactions to inhaled allergen. Across the range of asthmatics, the majority respond in differing degrees to both drugs, with corticosteroids having the wider spectrum of action.

From my experience, I have no doubt that while there is considerable overlap between the clinical responses to these drugs, this is not total and frequently they may complement each other. After all, when sodium cromoglycate was first discovered, its clinical effectiveness in asthma was demonstrated in individuals already receiving high dose corticosteroids.[1] Equally, we are aware of many patients, poorly controlled with sodium cromoglycate who benefit from the addition of corticosteroids in asthma. Based on our early clinical experience, Roger Altounyan and I concluded that there were two types of underlying processes in asthma—sodium cromoglycate responsive and corticosteroid responsive—with varying degrees of overlap between the two.[2]

There is a danger, of which the organisers were well aware, that any conference in which asthma is discussed may become deflected from its main objectives by attempts to find an operational definition of asthma. When little was known of bronchial pathology and pulmonary physiology, there were few problems in recognising patients with chronic bronchitis and emphysema and distinguishing them from 'asthma'. In the former, symptoms and clinical evidence of airflow obstruction were chronic and irreversible; in the latter they were reversible and episodic. The introduction of simple means of measuring airflow obstruction, using timed spirometry or peak expiratory flow rates, raised the reasonable expectation that it might be possible to distinguish between these disorders by observing the reversibility of airway obstruction. This expectation was reflected in the definition of asthma agreed at the Ciba Symposium (1959).[3] Thus 'asthma refers to the condition of subjects with widespread narrowing of the bronchial airways, which changes its severity over short periods of time, either spontaneously or under treatment, and is not due to cardiovascular disease'. In 1963, The American Thoracic Society (ATS) introduced an additional clause stating that asthma can be characterised by 'increased responsiveness' of the airways.[4]

Neither of these 'definitions', which are remarkably similar to the description of asthma by Floyer in the 17th century, meet the needs of clinicians and clinical investigators wishing to identify distinct groups of subjects with airway obstruction as either asthmatic or non-asthmatic. Patients diagnosed as one or the other on clinical grounds do not separate into two corresponding groups on the basis of airway obstruction and its reversibility. Some patients labelled 'asthma' have little reversibility of their airway obstruction, particularly those with so-called 'chronic' asthma, which is, in itself, a contradiction in terms of the Ciba and ATS definitions.

So what does lead to a diagnosis of asthma? There are several possible factors: for some patients, it is the clinical presentation of discrete episodes of severe, but reversible airway obstruction, often associated with known allergic precipitants. For others with more chronic symptoms, it is the unexpected response to sodium cromoglycate or corticosteroids that infers an 'asthmatic' component. Until recently, response to these drugs has been the main evidence that specific bronchial inflammatory processes underlie 'asthma'.

With our increased knowledge of the disease, more complex models of asthma have been constructed in which two areas currently seem to be of prime importance: bronchial hyperresponsiveness and inflammation of the airways.

The increasing use of bronchoscopy with bronchoalveolar lavage (BAL) or bronchial biopsy in the investigation of bronchial diseases has enabled not only the presence of inflammation to be recognised, but also the direct study of its cellular components. *Pari passu*, standardisation of measurements of bronchial reactivity to histamine or methacholine has allowed it to be quantified and compared between subjects and clinical conditions, and in response to treatment.

It is widely believed that the inflammatory processes are in some way responsible for bronchial hyperresponsiveness, although other factors such as genetic influences are also recognised to be important. Furthermore, it is believed that effective long-term therapy in asthma acts by influencing the underlying pathophysiological processes.

This conference was designed not to address the contentious, and perhaps irrelevant, problem of whether we can agree an operational definition of asthma. Rather, its aim was to bring together the wide range of disciplines reflected in the interests of the participants, and hopefully to advance our understanding of the nature of, and interaction between, bronchial inflammation and bronchial reactivity, and to consider these in relation to the underlying mechanisms of what we choose to call asthma. A further major objective was to review the mode of action of drugs upon these processes, with the aim of offering practical guidance to clinicians on the most rational way to include these drugs in their overall management of asthma.

REFERENCES

1 Howell JBL, Altounyan REC. A double-blind trial of disodium cromoglycate in the treatment of allergic bronchial asthma. *Lancet* 1967;2:539–42.
2 Altounyan REC, Howell JBL. Treatment of asthma with disodium cromoglycate (FPL 670, Intal). *Respiration* 1969;26(Suppl.):131–40.
3 Ciba Foundation Guest Symposium. *Thorax* 1959;44:286–99.
4 American Thoracic Society. *Am Rev Respir Dis* 1962;85:762–8.

1: Clinical Presentation

**K. F. Kerrebijn, J. B. L. Howell, R. C. Jongejan,
D. S. Postma, M. R. Sears & A. J. Woolcock**

DEFINITIONS (CLINICAL DESCRIPTIONS)

Asthma, chronic airway obstruction

Consensus has not yet been reached on a working definition of the term asthma. The 'definition' agreed at the Ciba Symposium of 1959 differed little from the description given by Floyer some 300 years earlier, which describes characteristic features in qualitative rather than quantitative terms. A similar inability to arrive at a working definition of asthma occurred at the Ciba Symposium of 1971, which had been specifically organised to address this very issue.[1] It was therefore recommended that whenever studies were reported a comprehensive description of the patients should be included. While this broadens the range of patients who may be included in studies on asthma it does not solve the problem of defining a clinically cohesive group.

Despite the difficulties of defining asthma, clinicians usually have no difficulty in knowing what they mean by the term. Firstly, there are patients who have episodes of severe wheezy breathlessness, which are consistent with the descriptions given by Floyer and Ciba, and which might be termed classic asthma attacks. Such patients may be atopic or non-atopic: in atopic patients the antigen precipitating an attack is not always known. In both types of patient it is usual for attacks of varying severity to be triggered by inhaled irritants, and it is now accepted that airway hyperresponsiveness (BHR) is characteristic of these patients. Secondly, there are patients who are never free of symptoms but may have varying degrees of wheezy breathlessness, or the need for continuing anti-asthmatic treatment. Some of these patients can still manage substantial bronchodilatation in response to β-agonists, while others seem to have largely irreversible airflow obstruction with any drug. Some patients with asthma go on to develop chronic symptoms, especially those who are non-atopic. Others may have no previous history of asthma but are recognised as being of similar type because of the presence of eosinophils in the sputum and a substantial clinical response to anti-asthma treatment. This group, often with concomitant poorly reversible airflow obstruction, does not match the Ciba or Floyer description, so why should the term asthma be applied to them?

Chronic airway obstruction (CAO) is defined as a disorder characterised by decreased expiratory flow that does not change substantially over long periods of time. Specific causes such as localised disease of the upper airways, bronchiectasis, and cystic fibrosis are excluded from the definition.

According to the recent guidelines of the American Thoracic Society,[2] CAO comprises three disorders: emphysema, peripheral airways disease, and chronic bronchitis. In any patient one or all of these may be present, as may BHR.

Asthma and CAO are often regarded as two distinct entities with different aetiologies and pathogeneses.[3] Patients with CAO, however, may attain clinically important reversibility after treatment; those with asthma may develop CAO with little or no reversibility. The differentiation between these two groups is often arbitrary and difficult. Orie and co-workers have hypothesised (subsequently termed the Dutch hypothesis) that asthma and chronic airflow obstruction are two aspects of the same basic process, and that patients share a common allergic constitution and BHR.[4,5] Asthma and CAO could indeed be regarded as two separate entities if BHR was the distinguishing feature. If this is not the case, this may suggest a more general disease, but is nevertheless not full proof of the Dutch hypothesis.

The terms asthma, bronchitis, and CAO, are widely used without qualification. By defining patients or patient groups by 'definite' data such as age, gender, the type of symptoms and improvement after treatment, airflow limitation, degree of bronchodilatation after inhaled β-agonist, allergy and BHR to various stimuli, these terms become less confusing.

Airway hyperresponsiveness

BHR can be quantified by measuring the effects of inhaling methacholine (acetylcholine) or histamine. Hyperventilation with cold air, hypotonic aerosols, sulphur dioxide (SO_2) and propranolol can be used as provoking stimuli to define further characteristics. Histamine and methacholine dose–response curves (DRCs) from patients with asthma or CAO differ from those in normals by their position, slope and maximal response. The presence of a plateau was recognised as a characteristic feature of DRCs in non-asthmatics.[6] The reason for its absence in asthma remains uncertain and warrants further study. Generally only the position of the DRC is used as the indicator of BHR. Although the relationship between the position and the slope is poor,[6,7] the slope may be important in pathophysiological research.

As provocation tests have been well standardised, results in patients with asthma and CAO from all over the world can be accurately compared.[8,9] Interpretation of the results does, however, have pitfalls namely the confusion caused by the blanket diagnostic label of the patients under study.

A diagnosis of asthma is taken by some as being synonymous with the demonstration of BHR by bronchial provocation. Indeed, when a patient presents with symptoms consistent with asthma and with normal spirometry, properly performed inhalation tests with methacholine or histamine are still the most sensitive tests to support the diagnosis. An increase in airway responsiveness occurs in almost all young allergic patients with shorter or longer attacks of reversible airflow obstruction ('asthma') or years during which attacks have been occurring.

Cross-sectional studies have shown good correlations between airway responsiveness, variable airflow obstruction as measured by serial peak expiratory flow rates, and clinical symptoms. However, in recent longitudinal studies, the correlation between clinical asthma and changes in airway responsiveness is not clear, and more data are required to elucidate the relationship between symptoms and changing airway responsiveness. At the present time, while the measurements used to detect BHR give an indication of its severity, the degree of BHR does not necessarily measure the severity of clinical asthma.

The responsiveness of the airways to inhaled bronchodilator is not a useful measurement of BHR to other stimuli. A marked response to a bronchodilator may occur in subjects with mild asthma who have been exposed to a large stimulus causing severe airflow obstruction (e.g. exercise-induced asthma) but who have little increase in airway responsiveness to methacholine or histamine, or equally may occur in a patient with severe asthma with markedly increased BHR to methacholine or histamine. The severity of BHR to constrictor agents can, however, be assessed after reversal of airflow obstruction, e.g. by a short course of systemic steroids, which will not alter BHR unless given in high dosage over a prolonged period. Responsiveness to an inhaled bronchodilator should be specified as such, e.g. 'β_2-agonist responsiveness', but it must be recognised that this is not an equivalent measurement to BHR induced by bronchoconstrictor agents.

BHR also seems to be present in 60% to 80% of older, nonallergic patients with persistent airflow limitation:[10] this is never fully reversible but may vary in intensity. The finding that not all patients with CAO show BHR suggests that differences do exist in this respect between asthma and CAO.

3

SIMILARITIES AND DIFFERENCES BETWEEN DISEASE ENTITIES

Airway hyperresponsiveness in asthma and CAO

The airway responsiveness to methacholine or acetylcholine and histamine is increased in most patients with asthma and CAO. Other 'indirect' stimuli, however, produce different responses. In one study only 11% of patients with CAO showed bronchoconstriction after hyperventilation with cold air, but 96% of asthmatics reacted.[11] Table 1.1 shows the incidence of BHR to different stimuli in patients with asthma or CAO. Asthmatics have a higher incidence of BHR to methacholine, histamine, propranolol, SO_2, and isocapnic hyperventilation in cold air; the incidence of BHR to fog is higher in patients with CAO.[11-13] These differences suggest

Table 1.1 Airway hyperresponsiveness to different stimuli in patients with asthma and CAO

Stimulus	Asthma (%)	CAO (%)
Methacholine (acetylcholine)	75	64
Histamine	82	36
Propranolol	67	21
Sulphur dioxide	95	30
Hyperventilation	96	11
Fog	30	81

that different hyperresponsiveness profiles exist in these two groups of patients. Patients with asthma and CAO also differ in their susceptibility to different stimuli (Table 1.2). Asthmatics tend to be equally responsive to histamine and methacholine (acetylcholine);[11,14] patients with CAO may be more responsive to histamine than to methacholine and acetylcholine.[15] Moreover, the correlation of the methacholine responsiveness with the response to hyperventilation in cold air is very good in asthmatics but non-existent in patients with CAO.[11,16,17] In most patients with CAO the DRC to inhaled methacholine reaches a plateau at a

Table 1.2 Airway responsiveness to different stimuli in patients with asthma and CAO

Stimulus	Asthma	CAO
Histamine	+ + + +	+ + +
Methacholine (acetylcholine)	+ + + +	+ +
Propranolol	+ + +	±
SO_2	+ + +	±
Fog/hypotonic aerosol	+ (adults)	+ +
	− (children)	
Hyperventilation/cold air	+ + +	±

relatively mild degree of airway narrowing; in asthmatics a plateau cannot usually be reached.[18-20] This suggests that more than one mechanism may be responsible for the expression of BHR. Morphological differences between asthma and CAO which may relate to BHR are discussed in the section on chronic inflammation and BHR (see p. 7).

Airway calibre

Asthmatics as a group show greater airway responsiveness than non-asthmatics, whether or not baseline forced expiratory volume (FEV_1) is normal. Although subjects with moderate to severe CAO may have BHR to histamine within the range found in asthmatics, their responsiveness is often less pronounced.[10,21,22] There is, however, debate as to whether the mechanisms underlying BHR in patients with CAO are the same as those for subjects with asthma, in particular with respect to the effects of airway geometry.

What constitutes the normal range of BHR in a population with bronchial obstruction before provocation? If the FEV_1 is reduced, responsiveness is almost invariably increased: the lower the FEV_1, the higher the degree of hyperresponsiveness to inhaled histamine or methacholine. This is the consequence of the way in which BHR is generally expressed, i.e. the percentage fall from baseline FEV_1 on provocation. Any given decrease in airway radius however, causes a proportionally greater increase in measured resistance when the initial size of the airway is smaller—for example, a bronchus of 4 mm in diameter which constricts by 1 mm reduces its calibre by 44%; a bronchus of 2 mm reduces its calibre by 75% when it constricts by 1 mm. Moreover, the distribution, deposition, and retention of the inhaled aerosolised methacholine or histamine change with variations in airway obstruction, and this may amplify their effect.

In patients with asthma, Yan et al. found that the provoking dose of histamine which caused a 20% fall in FEV_1 from baseline (PC_{20} histamine) did not correlate with baseline FEV_1.[10] In patients with CAO however, PC_{20} histamine correlated significantly with the FEV_1:FVC ratio. On the other hand when the initial FEV_1 value in patients with CAO in the study by Yan was greater than 70% of the predicted value, no correlation with the percentage change in FEV_1 was found after histamine challenge. Furthermore the fall in FEV_1 with a fixed dose of histamine (39 μmol) was related to initial FEV_1 in these patients. Ramsdale et al. found a correlation between PC_{20} methacholine and FEV_1 both in 'asthmatic' and 'bronchitic' subjects.[23] In keeping with the observations of Yan et al.,[10] they also found that the airway obstruction in the patients with bronchitis explained about 75%

of the response to methacholine, but only 35% in the asthmatics. Also, when individual changes in pulmonary function have been analysed in patients with asthma after airway provocation, no correlation with degree of BHR has been observed.[14,24,25]

Patients with 'chronic bronchitis', defined by chronic sputum and cough, may have BHR even when no airway obstruction is present.[15] This may imply that the expression of BHR in patients with CAO does not depend solely on airway calibre before challenge. This is also supported by the finding that some subjects with CAO have abnormal FEV_1:FVC ratios but do not show a fall in FEV_1 after the highest challenge dose of histamine.

Yan *et al.* also showed that in 11 subjects with CAO and no increase in FEV_1 after the administration of fenoterol, a significant decrease in BHR occurred after fenoterol pretreatment.[10] Taken together, the data discussed above suggest that initial airway calibre is not the only factor determining the degree of BHR in patients with CAO.

Differences in characteristics of BHR in asthma and CAO can thus be summarised as follows:

1 In patients with CAO the severity of BHR is related to the starting airway calibre; this is less pronounced in asthmatics.[10]

2 In patients with CAO the responsiveness to methacholine is less than to equimolar doses of histamine,[15] whereas the responsiveness in patients with asthma is similar.

3 In contrast to patients with asthma, those with CAO do not bronchoconstrict in response to hyperventilation with cold dry air.[11,16,17]

4 In most patients with CAO the DRC to inhaled methacholine reaches a plateau at a relatively mild degree of airway narrowing; in asthmatics a plateau can not usually be reached.[18-20]

It remains open to question whether these differences can be explained by different characteristics of inflammation in asthma and CAO.

AIRWAY HYPERRESPONSIVENESS AND INFLAMMATION

Studies of biopsy specimens indicate that in patients with stable asthma a low grade chronic inflammation of the airway wall may exist.[26-28] More data are, however, needed to confirm and extend these observations. In patients with CAO chronic inflammation of the airway wall is a prominent feature.[29] In patients with cystic fibrosis the airways are also chronically inflamed, but unlike asthma and CAO, inflammatory cells in cystic fibrosis are mainly present in the airway lumen and not in the airway wall or epithelium.[30,31] There are differences between asthma, CAO, and cystic fibrosis in the cellular profiles of the inflammatory reaction.

In asthma eosinophils and mast cells predominate; in CAO and
cystic fibrosis neutrophils are more important. The differences
may be related to the incidence and characteristics of BHR in
these diseases.

CHAPTER I
*Clinical
Presentation*

Airway hyperresponsiveness and chronic inflammation

In patients with stable mild atopic asthma, who have not been
exposed to allergens for over six weeks, BAL and biopsy specimens
show evidence of airway inflammation. A highly significant
correlation has been shown between the responsiveness to methacholine and the number of metachromatic cells, as well as the
number of eosinophils in BAL.[32] In this study the BAL concentration of major basic protein (MBP), which might be regarded as an
indicator of eosinophilic activation, was not different in asthmatics and non-asthmatics. Another study showed that mean eosinophil counts in a group of mild symptomatic asthmatics with
hyperresponsive airways were significantly higher than those in a
group of non-symptomatic asthmatics, a group of hay fever
patients, and a group of healthy volunteers.[33] This difference was,
however, caused by two or three symptomatic asthmatics. In
most symptomatic asthmatics there was no difference in eosinophil counts between them and subjects in the other groups. In
contrast to the findings of Kirby *et al.*,[32] these investigators found
that the concentrations of MBP in BAL were increased in symptomatic patients, with a highly significant difference between the
normal and hyperreactive groups. This indicates that eosinophils
in hyperreactive asthmatics were activated. In the asthmatics and
controls there was a weak inverse correlation between the degree
of hyperresponsiveness on the one hand and the percentage of
mast cells, eosinophils, epithelial cells, and the amount of MBP in
BAL on the other. The authors concluded that their results
supported one of the current hypotheses that BHR in asthma is
secondary to epithelial cell damage mediated through products
derived from eosinophils.

A recent study[34] reported an increase in eosinophil and lymphocyte counts in BAL of patients with stable asthma as compared
to controls. The number of macrophages was only increased in
smokers but did not differ between the patients and the controls.
PD_{20} methacholine was negatively correlated with percentage
neutrophil counts but not with neutrophil activation. However,
macrophage activation was inversely correlated with PD_{20}.

Other groups have reported increased numbers of mast cells
and histamine in the BAL fluid of stable chronic asthmatics,
which could point towards an ongoing activation of mast cells.[35]
Cutz *et al.* described ultrastructural changes in epithelial cells and
the mast cells scattered between them, a thickened subepithelial

hyaline layer (basement membrane), submucosal infiltration by a mixture of inflammatory cells with only moderate numbers of eosinophils, and smooth muscle hypertrophy but no detachment of the epithelial lining in two 12 year old children with bronchial asthma who had been in remission for at least three months.[36] Holgate *et al.* reported fragile epithelial cells, epithelial shedding, thickening of the basal membrane and increased numbers of eosinophils, T-lymphocytes, monocytes and fibroblasts in the submucosa in eight mild atopic asthmatics receiving intermittent β-agonist treatment, but not in four healthy controls.[28] Lozewicz *et al.*, however, found no significant changes with regard to bronchial epithelium in similar patients with stable mild asthma, but significantly more mast cells and slightly more eosinophils in the airway wall than in controls.[27] Laitinen *et al.* and Konradova *et al.* reported evidence of destruction of the epithelium in their biopsy study of stable mild asthmatics.[26,37]

An increased responsiveness of peripheral leucocytes[38–40] as well as an increased hypodensity of eosinophils,[41] which probably both indicate cell activation, have been described in patients with asthma.

The few data published so far have shown that the number of eosinophils in BAL is increased in some but not all patients with mild symptomatic asthma. Eosinophils in BAL were not found to be increased in patients with non-symptomatic asthma whose airways are likely to be hyperresponsive. Few data exist on biopsy specimens in mild stable asthmatics, and data on the association between biopsy findings and bronchial responsiveness are lacking. In one study BHR, and an increased amount of MBP—indicating the presence of activated eosinophils in the airways of these patients—correlated.[33] If this observation can be confirmed, it strongly suggests that cell activation may be as important as the presence of inflammatory cells.

In CAO infiltration of membranous airways and respiratory bronchioles with inflammatory cells, mainly neutrophils and mononuclear cells, as well as smooth muscle hypertrophy, goblet cell metaplasia, metaplasia of the epithelium, fibrosis and thickening of the basal membrane are prominent features.[29,42] Typically, this inflammation differs from that in stable mild asthmatics in that no increased numbers of mast cells and eosinophils, or epithelial destruction are present.[43] Chronic exposure of the airways to irritants like cigarette smoke is a major risk factor in the development of CAO, although only about 25% of the smokers and ex-smokers develop chronic airflow limitation.[44] The association between smoking and BHR becomes stronger with increasing age.[45,46] The severity of BHR in smokers or in patients with CAO is strongly related to baseline airway calibre as has been described previously. In a recent study in a random population sample a significantly negative effect of cigarette smoking on baseline lung function in men over 21 years of age was found, but there was no significant correlation between smoking and BHR.[47] Cigarette consumption in the study population was however low. In another study the baseline lung function of smoking non-atopic subjects with CAO was reported to decline much faster than that in a group of non-smoking atopic asthmatics after correction for confounding variables.[48] This difference could be due to better treatment of the atopic group, but could also reflect the differences between the outcome of the inflammatory process in non-atopic smokers with CAO and atopic asthmatics. A recent study reported that in individual smokers the rate of annual decline in FEV_1, and the extent of decline in PC_{20} histamine were associated.[49]

Also, in animal models there is evidence that chronic exposure of airways to irritants can induce changes in responsiveness as a result of inflammation. Chronic exposure to SO_2 in a dog model of chronic bronchitis leads to hyporesponsiveness to inhaled, but not to intravenously administered, methacholine.[50,51] In mongrel dogs chronic exposure to nitric acid (1%) leads first to hypo-responsiveness and then to hyperresponsiveness after several months.[52] In this model there was a significant correlation between smooth muscle hypertrophy and inflammatory scores in the small airways and the total respiratory resistance and FEV_1:FVC ratio. Bronchial responsiveness was not significantly related to the pre-existing obstruction, but only five dogs were studied.

Superoxide anion production of polymorphonuclear leucocytes from peripheral blood of patients with CAO has been reported to be increased, indicating that also in this condition inflammatory cells may be activated.[53]

It has been suggested that products released by neutrophils during airway inflammation induce BHR.[54,55] Studies by de Jongste et al. indicate that the degree of inflammation of airways from patients with CAO does not correlate with the responsiveness of smooth muscle to different agonists in vitro.[56,57] This does not exclude the fact that, in vivo, neutrophils might interfere with airway reactivity at a neuronal level.

In patients with CAO, BHR might be caused by changes in the extent of shortening of the airway smooth muscle and by geometric factors such as thickness of airway walls, the amount of smooth muscle, a decreased tethering effect of lung parenchyma, or other factors that decrease the load which the muscle must overcome during shortening, such as destruction of the peribronchial support.[58] In normal subjects lowering the initial lung volume before inhalation of methacholine considerably increased the maximal bronchoconstriction to methacholine.[59,60] This

Clinical
Presentation

9

indicates that changes in lung volume, probably as a result of changes in elastic load, combine to change the forces of interdependence between airways and parenchyma that oppose airway smooth muscle contraction. Thus it is attractive to hypothesise that chronic inflammation, which causes changes in airway geometry and mechanics, without or together with a diminished elastic recoil, leads to BHR. Experimental data to support this hypothesis are, however, scanty.

Further studies are needed to elucidate the role of the chronic presence of various types of inflammatory cells and their activation state in the mechanisms underlying BHR in diseases with airway obstruction.

Airway hyperresponsiveness and acute inflammation

In patients with asthma, many exacerbations are accompanied by an acute inflammatory response. Acute inflammation is defined as a transient influx of inflammatory cells. The increased eosinophil cationic protein:albumin ratio and the high amount of MBP in BAL fluid from asthmatic patients indicate that these cells are probably activated,[33,61] but more studies are needed before we can appreciate the role of cell activation in the acute inflammatory process.

Vaccination with live, but not with killed, influenza virus induces a temporary increase of BHR in children with asthma but not in normal control subjects, irrespective of respiratory symptoms.[62–64] These observations suggest that actively replicating virus may be needed to induce an increase in BHR. It has been suggested that replication of the virus in epithelial cells leads to damage of the epithelium, thereby loosening tight junctions, and increasing mucosal permeability.[62,65] Epithelial damage could also expose afferent nerve endings to inflammatory mediators.[26] This may induce BHR as a result of increased reflex bronchoconstriction through cholinergic and non-cholinergic excitatory nerves. Host factors must also play a part, because epithelial destruction during viral infections occurs both in asthmatics and non-asthmatics; but airway responsiveness increases only in asthmatics. Other factors related to viral infections may also have a role. Infection with respiratory syncytial virus (RSV) and parainfluenza virus leads to specific IgE production and an increase in the histamine content of nasopharyngeal secretions in children with various forms of respiratory illness.[66,67] In the same study the authors proposed that dysregulation of T-cells might lead to increased production of IgE, followed by an IgE-mediated release of mast cell products, bronchoconstriction, and BHR. Changes in airway responsiveness, however, were not monitored in these studies.

The late reaction after exposure to allergens is characterised by an influx of inflammatory cells into the airway wall. Increases in the number of eosinophils, neutrophils, pulmonary macrophages and lymphocytes have been described in bronchial lavage obtained six to 48 hours after allergen challenge.[61,68,69] The magnitude of late allergic responses is related to the length and severity of the subsequent development of BHR, which may worsen for a period of several days to weeks.[70] In dual responders airway responsiveness has been reported to increase shortly or at the most some hours after the resolution of the early reaction, but well before the clinical appearance of the late response. Reports, however, are conflicting.[71-73] This indicates that there may already be changes in the lung which lead to increased BHR and precede the clinical appearance of the late response.

Sensitised subjects may develop early or late bronchoconstrictor reactions, or both, to toluene diisocyanate (TDI).[74-77] In dual responders or in single late responders, but not in single early responders, there is often an increased sensitivity to methacholine which resolves in one to four weeks.[78] Eight hours after exposure to TDI a mild eosinophilia in BAL can be found, whereas after three and eight hours there is a large increase in the number of neutrophils in BAL.[79,80] As with inhalation of antigen, BHR is increased well before the appearance of the late response.[81] Influx of neutrophils and eosinophils and extravasation of albumin, indicating enhanced vascular permeability, are all prevented by glucocorticosteroids, but not by theophylline, cromolyn, or verapamil.[75,82,83] The same is true for the increase in BHR. These findings indicate that inflammatory cells and an increase in vascular permeability are associated with the development of increased bronchial responsiveness.

Challenge with plicatic acid, which is the component of red cedar dust responsible for red cedar asthma, causes vascular permeability, influx of eosinophils and neutrophils, and sloughing of bronchial epithelial cells in sensitive subjects.[74,84,85] Biopsy specimens, taken 24 to 48 hours after challenge, indicate denudation of the bronchial epithelium, a thickened basement membrane, and infiltration of eosinophils in the bronchial epithelium and submucosa.[85] In subjects sensitive to both TDI and plicatic acid a relation exists between the development of the late inflammatory reaction and the increase in bronchial responsiveness, but this increase seems to occur before the late reaction is clinically apparent.

In BAL fluid obtained three hours after exposure of normal subjects to ozone (0.4–0.6 ppm, two hours), a significant increase in the number of neutrophils was found as well as increased amounts of PGE_2, $PGF_{2\alpha}$, and thromboxane B_2.[86] Exposure to ozone (0.4 ppm, two hours) has also been reported to change the epithelial permeability in healthy subjects but ozone has no effect in asthmatic patients.[87] Whether a causal relation exists between mediator production, cell influx, increased epithelial permeability and increased bronchial responsiveness has been studied in more detail in animal models. The results are contradictory. In a dog model increased numbers of neutrophils and shedded epithelial cells were found in BAL and epithelial biopsy specimens after exposure to ozone (2.1–3.0 ppm, two hours).[88,89] The time course of the appearance and disappearance of neutrophils also resembled that of the changes in bronchial responsiveness.[90] Furthermore, neutrophil depletion with hydroxyurea prevented the increase in bronchial responsiveness in dogs after exposure to ozone, but this might have been due to other effects of this compound as has been shown in guinea-pigs. In rats, however, exposure to 4 ppm ozone for two hours resulted in airway hyperresponsiveness without detectable neutrophil influx or increased vascular permeability in the trachea.[91] After exposure to TDI cyclophosphamide inhibited BHR but not cell influx, and hydroxyurea inhibited both.[92,93] Depletion of neutrophils by cyclophosphamide or steroids, however, did not prevent BHR after ozone (3.0 ppm, two hours).[94] Other studies conducted on the peripheral airways of dogs indicate that exposure to ozone (1.0 ppm, two hours) does not lead to an influx of inflammatory cells, but causes a prolonged increase in bronchial responsiveness.[95] In dogs indomethacin inhibits BHR but not an influx of neutrophils induced by ozone (3.0 ppm, two hours).[96] The stable thromboxane analogue U46619 can increase bronchial responsiveness, whereas the inhibitor of thromboxane synthesis, OKY-046, can prevent bronchial responsiveness induced by ozone (3.0 ppm, two hours).[97] These findings implicate cyclooxygenase products in BHR induced by ozone in dogs.

In guinea-pigs exposed to cigarette smoke the increase of bronchial responsiveness preceded the influx of neutrophils and was associated with the exudative phase before extravasation of inflammatory cells.[98] Histological examination showed increased numbers of mucosal mast cells two hours after exposure to ozone (3.0 ppm, two hours) when the increase in bronchial responsiveness was maximal.[99] Neutrophil infiltration occurred later and lasted longer than mast cell infiltration.

Although these studies may suggest that neutrophils have no (or only a minor) role in the development of BHR, inhaled supernatants of stimulated human neutrophils were able to induce BHR in dogs and rabbits.[100,101] These findings show that it is hard to know how exactly cellular influx, mediator production, and vascular or epithelial permeability increase bronchial responsiveness after challenge. It is also difficult to know in which order these events occur.

The problem with these animal studies is, however, that animals do not develop asthma and animal models may be inappropriate for the study of inflammatory processes as one of the underlying mechanisms in asthma.

Activation of human pulmonary mast cells and macrophages, which leads to release of inflammatory mediators, is likely to be a central event in the initiation of the early response after exposure to antigens and those occupational agents acting as an antigen.[74,102] These mediators not only constrict bronchial smooth muscle, increase the epithelial permeability, stimulate afferent nerve endings and act as chemoattractants, but they can also vasodilate and increase micro-vascular permeability leading to oedema of the airway wall and a change in the mechanics of the airway wall.[65] These changes in the airway wall might contribute to an increase in bronchial responsiveness.[58] An ongoing release of inflammatory mediators during the sustained reaction, characterised by an influx of activated inflammatory cells, could probably maintain the increased BHR. Substances released by these activated inflammatory cells could also lead to ongoing activation of resident cells in the airways. Studies of bronchial lavage suggest that during the late reaction eosinophils remain longer (more than 24 hours) in the airway wall than neutrophils (less than four hours).[69] This suggests that eosinophils are more important than neutrophils in maintaining the increased bronchial responsiveness after a sustained reaction induced by an allergen. This, however, seems to depend on the stimulus used, because in late phase reactions induced by TDI neutrophils are more prominent than eosinophils.

MODULATION OF AIRWAY HYPERRESPONSIVENESS

Factors which modulate the characteristics of airway hyperresponsiveness

Little is known about the environmental factors that modulate the characteristics (shape of the DRC, responses to different provoking stimuli) of BHR. In most published studies, increased and decreased levels of BHR refer to changes in the position of the DRCs to histamine or methacholine, after the airways have been exposed to the modulating factor.

Increased severity of BHR

The following factors may (transiently) increase the severity of BHR in asthmatic subjects.

Viral infections

Although viral infections have been associated with attacks of asthma,[103,104] few studies have reported on the severity of BHR either during or after viral infections in subjects with asthma. Exacerbations of BHR during experimental rhinovirus infections were shown in one study;[105] another showed no shift in the DRCs.[106] There is a small shift in DRCs following vaccination with live but not killed virus.[62,63] Viral infections were found to affect histamine release from mediator-releasing cells in one study,[107] but not in another.[63] Therefore infections probably cause a transient increase in BHR, but the time course of the increase is unknown.

Allergens and occupational sensitisers

Allergens and occupational sensitisers have been shown to shift the DRCs to the left by two or more doubling doses and this effect lasts for several hours or days in asthmatic subjects.

Allergens: the effects of allergens on BHR have been well reviewed.[108] There is some evidence to suggest that asthma may be induced by pollens,[109,110] but high doses of pollen extracts have to be given in the laboratory, and usually a 'late' reaction obtained, before an increase in BHR is observed in asthmatic subjects.[24,70] Many people are allergic to pollen but relatively few get asthma and 'pollen asthma' is described only in the northern hemisphere. After a single early response there is no increase in BHR, but there is after a dual response.[108]

Occupational sensitisers: most work has been done with TDI and western red cedar dust, and there is clear evidence that these induce asthma and that they increase the severity of BHR in sensitised subjects,[74,75,77,111,112] BHR may persist for several months after removal from occupational exposure.[76]

Air pollution

Ozone: although it has been shown that ozone increases BHR in normal subjects and in animals,[113,114] there is no evidence to suggest that it increases the severity of BHR in patients with asthma.[115] Furthermore, its effects in normal subjects seem to be transient.[116]

Sulphur dioxide (SO_2): there have been few studies on the effects of SO_2 on the severity of BHR in subjects with asthma, although in one report BHR was increased in normal subjects.[117] Accidental exposure to a high concentration of the gas has been reported to result in BHR which lasted for years.[118] Inhalation of metabisulphite—sufficient to cause airway narrowing—did not exacerbate BHR in subjects with asthma in a recent study.[119]

Nitrogen dioxide: this has been shown to potentiate the effects of exercise in asthmatic subjects,[120] but its effects on BHR, as measured by histamine and methacholine, are largely unknown. One study showed it to cause a slight increase in the severity of BHR.[121]

Fog: this is not an air pollutant, but in the laboratory ultrasonically nebulised water (fog) causes a small, transient increase in BHR in asthmatic subjects for a short time.[122] The effect is potentiated by acidity.[123]

Passive smoking: exposure to passive cigarette smoke is associated with increased asthmatic symptoms in children.[124] Passive smoking does not seem to have a pronounced effect on BHR in subjects with asthma: in adults one study showed a small increase in responses to histamine for four hours;[125] another showed a small decrease in response to methacholine.[126] Recently it was shown that parental smoking enhances BHR in school children.[127]

Allergic rhinitis

It is difficult to be sure about the role of rhinitis. Some subjects with allergic rhinitis have asymptomatic BHR[128] and some subsequently develop asthma.[129] There have been no specific studies on the severity of BHR after the onset of acute symptoms (spontaneous or induced) of rhinitis in subjects with asthma. Treatment of rhinitis, however, tends to produce an improvement in the clinical severity of asthma.[130]

Inhaled substances

In the laboratory BHR was found to be slightly increased after inhalation of benzylkonium chloride.[131] This may be relevant because benzylkonium chloride is used as a preservative in drugs. There is evidence that BHR is induced in normal subjects with platelet activating factor (PAF),[132] but this seems not to be the case in patients with asthma.[133]

Ingested agents

Ice,[134] cola drinks,[135] and tartrazine,[136] have been reported to increase the severity of BHR transiently in some subjects.

Drugs

Inhaled β-antagonists (propranolol) can increase BHR transiently.[137] In addition, some drug treatments have been shown to be associated with increases in BHR. Thus, β-agonists administered over a period of weeks or months without anti-inflammatory agents have been found to increase the severity of BHR slightly.[138-140] In a study in which theophylline was compared with inhaled beclomethasone, the improvement produced by the latter was followed by increased severity of BHR after crossover to treatment with theophylline.[141]

Exercise

The situation is obscure. Most studies have found no change in BHR to histamine or methacholine but two studies have found some increase in BHR.[142,143]

Factors which do not modulate bronchial hyperresponsiveness

Some factors have been shown not to increase the severity of BHR. These include metabisulphite,[119] allergen exposure causing only an early response,[24] repeated exposure to histamine,[144] and probably hypoxia. Direct studies of effects of hypoxia on BHR do not seem to have been carried out, but histamine challenges lead to hypoxia,[145] and histamine challenges do not exacerbate BHR.[144]

Drugs

Analysis of the protective effects of drugs on BHR provides information about the influence of different mechanisms in BHR in different disease entities.

Acute protection

In patients with asthma inhaled β-agonists in therapeutic doses protect, in a dose-dependent way, against airway narrowing caused by provoking stimuli.[146] The effect of anticholinergics is variable. The magnitude of the change in BHR seems to be related to dose.[146] The increase in FEV_1 and the reduction of BHR are therefore dose-related. When the protective effects of sympathomimetics and anticholinergics are compared in the same asthmatic patient, the change in the position of the dose–response curve for a given degree of bronchodilatation seems to be greater after the sympathomimetic (± 3 doubling doses) than after the anticholinergic drug (± 1.5 doubling doses).[147-149] This observation suggests that the effect of a β-agonist on the position of the dose–response curve is not mainly due to bronchodilatation alone, which is further supported by the fact that oral β-agonists are not protective in spite of bronchodilatation.[146]

One study has investigated the effects of a sympathomimetic and anticholinergic drug both in patients with asthma and those with CAO.[11] It compared the merits of 2 mg of the anticholinergic drug oxyfenonium bromide intramuscularly with that of 0.08 mg of the β-adrenergic drug fenoterol intramuscularly. In asthmatic subjects the sympathomimetic drug had a twofold greater protective effect against histamine provocation than the anticholinergic. The same effect was observed for SO_2 provocation. In the group with CAO, however, the anticholinergic agent had about a threefold greater effect against histamine than the sympathomimetic. As in asthmatics the effect on SO_2 was the same. These results could not simply be explained by the effects on FEV_1 before provocation. Thus the β-adrenergic drug provides the greatest protective effect in asthmatics and the anticholinergic in patients with CAO. This is in accordance with the theory of a higher cholinergic activity in patients with CAO compared with those with asthma.

One study indicates that an acute protective effect of inhaled corticosteroids on BHR to histamine is unlikely.[150] Sodium cromoglycate and nedocromil sodium acutely protect against many provoking stimuli including allergen, exercise, SO_2 and fog.[151]

Long-term effects

It has been shown that inhaled corticosteroids can progressively change BHR in asthmatic patients.[138,139,152,153] This occurs independently of change in the FEV_1 during the course of treatment. The effects also appear to be dependent on dose. Results for patients with CAO have as yet not been published, but preliminary reports do not suggest as great an effect after the same period of follow up as in asthmatics. Sodium cromoglycate[154] and nedocromil sodium[155] have also been shown to reduce the severity of BHR or to inhibit the increase that may occur during the pollen season.

Removal of patients sensitive to house dust mites from the allergen source has been shown to lead to an improvement in BHR.[156,157] It is well known that many patients with occupational asthma improve when they are removed from the sensitising agents and one study has shown that hypnosis can be beneficial in the long term.[158]

DISEASE OUTCOME

Disease outcome can be studied by looking at the general well-being of a patient, the decline in lung function, or, ultimately, the mortality. Peat *et al.* recently found that in subjects with asthma a significant correlation existed between the rate of decline of FEV_1 and BHR.[159] The more responsive the patients, the more rapid the decline. Many subjects had their BHR measured only once. As the severity of BHR may vary over time in individual asthmatics, the correlation ($r = 0.30$) was surprisingly good. Kelly *et al.* reported in 247 subjects who had had asthma as children and who were studied at the age of 28 years, that no association was found between airway responsiveness to methacholine and loss of ventilatory capacity since 21 years of age.[160] This was found in the group as a whole as well as in the subjects with a FEV_1 of less than 86% predicted at 21 years of age. Gerritsen *et al.* found that the outcome of childhood asthma in adults aged between 21–29 years could be predicted from the severity of bronchial obstruction and the degree of BHR in childhood.[161]

BHR seems to be associated with, and may itself be, an important risk factor which can predict the insidious and progressive loss of pulmonary function, which may ultimately lead to CAO.[162] In this respect much has been written on patients with CAO and moderate to severe airflow obstruction.[163-170] It is accepted that survival in patients with CAO is generally shorter than in an age- and sex-matched healthy population. Clinical and population-based studies of CAO show that initial FEV_1 value is the single best predictor of survival.[164-170] The lower the FEV_1, the worse the survival. Age is the second most important predictor, increasing age being associated with an increased risk of mortality. Other variables, such as diffusion capacity and heart rate, have only minor predictive value after adjusting for age and FEV_1. The rate of decline in FEV_1 varies from 40 to 100 ml per year depending on the study population,[163-168] which is two to three times the rate of decline in a normal non-smoking population.

Some studies have shown that, independent of age and FEV_1 value, reversibility of airflow obstruction is an important determinant of disease outcome.[164-170] But results are conflicting: is reversibility a good[164-168] or a bad[169,170] prognostic sign? Overall, the results may be interpreted as suggesting strongly that treatment has a beneficial effect on disease outcome by influencing the reversible part of airflow obstruction.[167,168]

Several longitudinal investigations have associated BHR with disease outcome. Although no investigation has studied the association between BHR and mortality, the latter seems to be related to the decline in pulmonary function in subjects with CAO.[167,169] In a study by Postma *et al.* a PC_{20} histamine concentration of less than or equal to 2 mg/ml was associated with a mean fall of 127 ml/year while a PC_{20} histamine concentration of more than 4 mg/ml was associated with a mean fall of 47 ml/year.[167] In all subjects the degree of BHR at the start of follow up was significantly correlated with pack years of smoking. As the degree of BHR was related to the decline in FEV_1 in smokers, but not in ex-smokers, a causal relation between smoking and BHR would be expected. This, however, was not found, and BHR and smoking independently influenced decline in lung function.

That BHR seems to exacerbate both the development of airflow obstruction and progressive loss of lung function in patients with CAO, especially in smokers, may have important implications for management. Of paramount importance is the categoric advice to stop smoking. A multicentre study on the effect of stopping smoking and its association with a modification of BHR in patients with CAO has been started in the USA.[171] Early detection of BHR in those at risk of airflow obstruction should also result in prompt drug treatment to prevent the consequences of this disorder.

ASTHMA MORTALITY

Fatal asthma represents the extreme end of the spectrum of severity of airway inflammation and hyperresponsiveness, culminating in asphyxiating airway obstruction. It is disconcerting that, despite the increasing availability of effective drugs for the treatment of asthma, including potent bronchodilators and agents such as cromoglycate and corticosteroids which modulate airway responsiveness, there has not been a parallel decrease in morbidity and mortality from asthma. On the contrary, hospital admissions for asthma continue to rise, especially in children,[172] and mortality from asthma seems presently to be increasing in many countries.[173,174]

Despite intensive study of asthma mortality over two decades, many uncertainties persist with regard to alleged associations between fatalities and drug therapy. Recent studies raise the further question as to whether the effects of drugs in modulating airway responsiveness could be related to mortality.

Reported asthma mortality rose significantly in young people in England and Wales, Australia, and New Zealand in the mid 1960s.[175] Although several bronchodilator drugs, including orciprenaline, adrenaline, and atropine, as well as isoprenaline in standard and high doses were used by patients dying of asthma,[176] adverse effects of high dose isoprenaline were regarded by many as 'the cause' of that epidemic.[177] The epidemiological evidence was twofold: firstly, the increase in asthma deaths occurred as high dose isoprenaline aerosol sales increased;[175] and secondly, 'excess' deaths occurred only in those countries where high dose isoprenaline was marketed.[178] The fact that some patients were found dead with their bronchodilator aerosol in their hand, and that many deaths were said to be sudden and unexpected, together with some experimental animal evidence, lent credibility to the hypothesis that death was due to cardiotoxicity of isoprenaline,[179] or the freon propellant.[180] An alternative interpretation, however, was that use of a symptom-relieving medication in a severe attack led to a false sense of security and lack of further appropriate treatment. The association with high strength isoprenaline was disputed in Australia, where mortality fell substantially after 1966 while sales of high strength isoprenaline continued to increase.[181] Furthermore, there was no regional correlation in various Australian states between fatalities and sales of aerosols for asthmatics.

Recent reviews have suggested that the 'epidemic' of the mid 1960s could have been largely or totally spurious. This viewpoint requires that the availability of more effective bronchodilator treatment enabled asthma to be diagnosed more readily resulting in the increase in certified deaths due to asthma.[182] While this might be conceivable in older patients, it seems unlikely in younger people, in whom the diagnosis of asthma is usually straightforward and not complicated by other diseases.

The second increase in asthma mortality in New Zealand from 1977 onwards[183] was investigated by detailed review of all patients certified as having died from asthma during the two years between 1981 to 1983.[184-191] In young people accuracy of certification was high, but accuracy decreased in those older than 35.[185]

The initial speculation of Wilson et al. that the combination of oral theophylline with inhaled β-sympathomimetic was a factor in asthma mortality, was based on a study of 22 deaths in young people in Auckland.[192] Despite the small numbers involved and the lack of information about patterns of drug treatment in asthmatics not dying of their disease, the hypothesis gained almost the same credibility as the association between isoprenaline and the mortalities of the mid 1960s epidemic in England and elsewhere. Wilson et al. did suggest, however, that the increase in deaths from asthma could be an indirect result of increasing use of theophylline and β-agonists if these agents replaced anti-inflammatory asthma treatments such as cromoglycate and inhaled corticosteroids.

Sales of anti-asthma drugs in New Zealand, Australia, and England and Wales between 1975 and 1981 showed substantial increases in all four categories (β-sympathomimetics, theophyllines, cromoglycate and inhaled corticosteroids) in each country.[193] The greatest annual increase in sales in New Zealand occurred three years after the rise in mortality in young people. This suggested that the increased drug use was a secondary response related to a greater prevalence or severity of asthma, rather than there being a direct causal relation between increasing drug treatment and mortality.

Detailed review of the circumstances of 271 deaths from asthma in New Zealand between 1981 and 1983 identified a few patients in whom excessive doses of β-sympathomimetics alone or with theophylline may possibly have contributed to death from direct toxicity,[185] and others for whom frequent use of bronchodilators caused a delay in obtaining more appropriate help for a severe attack.[189] The overwhelming evidence from that study, however, pointed to undertreatment of severe asthma, both long and short term, especially with disease-modifying drugs.[187-190]

The epidemiological evidence for a direct association between increasing use of β-agonists or theophylline with mortality rates therefore remains open to considerable doubt, but there may be an indirect association.

Pharmacological evidence for association between bronchodilators and mortality

The beneficial action of β-sympathomimetic drugs on airway smooth muscle is accompanied by effects on heart rate and skeletal muscle function, with tachycardia and tremor being clinically important but usually not serious side effects of treatment.[194] Arrhythmias have been shown in hypoxic animals given β-agonists,[179] and these may be aggravated by concomitant administration of theophylline. Such evidence is sparse in studies in man. Of 40 patients admitted to hospital with self-poisoning with salbutamol, 26 had a sinus tachycardia, six had symptomatic palpitations, two had a serum potassium concentration below 2.6 mmol/l, but none had ventricular arrhythmias despite very high doses of salbutamol.[195] Serum potassium has been noted to decrease significantly in healthy subjects given inhalations of fenoterol,[196] and in another study theophylline increased hypokalaemia and tachycardia induced by salbutamol in normal subjects.[197] The addition of theophylline to salbutamol, while increasing heart rate and supraventricular extrasystoles, did not greatly increase ventricular arrhythmias in patients with CAO.[198] Likewise, no evidence for ventricular arrhythmias was found in asthmatic children treated with theophylline who had been given either subcutaneous epinephrine or metaproterenol.[199] Thus, the data in human studies do not strongly support an association between administration of β-sympathomimetics and death from cardiac arrhythmia.

Patients hospitalised with acute severe asthma almost invariably have subtherapeutic serum theophylline concentrations on admission. Overdosage of theophylline is uncommon, perhaps because the adverse effects of nausea and vomiting reduce intake. While intravenous aminophylline can induce arrhythmias, these are rare in clinical practice except in massive overdosage.[200] It is therefore unlikely that theophylline alone could account for mortality from asthma by its arrhythmogenic potential.

The recent work of Beasley et al.,[201] who showed bronchoconstrictor effects from preservatives in bronchodilator solutions, is disturbing; the possibility that fatal bronchoconstriction could result from such agents during nebulisation of bronchodilators must be considered.

Evidence for tachyphylaxis to β-agonists

Several studies have suggested that the frequent administration of β-sympathomimetics could lead to down-regulation of airway β-receptors. A reduced response to salbutamol, as measured by specific airway conductance, was found in normal subjects after four weeks of regular treatment; asthmatics, however, showed no such loss of efficacy.[202] In another study a decrease in central airway bronchodilator responsiveness to acutely inhaled salbutamol and subcutaneous terbutaline, as measured by airway conductance, was found after four weeks of treatment with inhaled salbutamol, but small airway bronchodilator responsiveness, as measured by the partial expiratory flow curve, was not affected.[203] This was interpreted as indicating selective 'subsensitisation' of β-receptors in the large central airways where a proportionately greater amount of inhaled β-agonist aerosol would necessarily be deposited. Svedmyr et al. found no evidence for reduced airway responses to β-adrenergic drugs during prolonged treatment with β-sympathomimetics, although there was a reduction in tremor and tachycardiac responses.[204]

The clinical relevance of airway β-receptor desensitisation, if indeed it does occur, is that the β-receptors may be poorly responsive to β-agonists during an attack because of previous excess use of β-sympathomimetics. In a study of patients with acute severe asthma admitted to a Boston emergency room, however, the response of FEV_1 during the first hour of treatment with β-sympathomimetics alone was not significantly different among patients who had used β-sympathomimetics before admission compared with those who had not.[205] No corticosteroids or theophylline was used during this observation period. Corticosteroids resolve the mild tachyphylaxis which does occur in normal subjects.[206]

Evidence that β-agonists cause airway instability

Some studies have suggested that the regular use of a β-agonist may be associated with an increase in airway lability. Kraan et al.

compared airway responsiveness in patients treated with bude-sonide and terbutaline using a crossover study design, and showed a significant increase in histamine PC_{20} during treatment with budesonide compared with a slight decrease in PC_{20}, indicating worsening airway responsiveness during terbutaline treatment.[138] This increase in airway responsiveness was suggested as possibly due to β-receptor desensitisation. Similar results were obtained in children by Kerrebijn *et al.*[139] Van Metre reported that 30 patients with severe asthma, who were resistant to all usual forms of treatment including corticosteroids, showed improvement when nebulised isoproterenol was discontinued.[207] They suggested that regular use of this agent had caused intractable asthma. More recently, Vathenen *et al.* found a rebound increase in airway responsiveness following cessation of bronchodilator treatment,[140] (though their interpretation of the data has been challenged).[208] These studies suggest that treatment of asthmatics with β-sympathomimetics alone, without corticosteroid or other disease-modifying treatment may, in fact, be deleterious. The relief of symptoms by bronchodilator, without treatment of the underlying airway inflammation, may allow the inflammation to proceed unchecked and perhaps even to be aggravated by allowing the patient to continue exposure to inciting agents. The clinical relevance of these observations remains to be determined.

Evidence for inappropriate treatment of asthma; overreliance on bronchodilators and underuse of corticosteroids

Studies of asthma mortality in the United Kingdom[209-214] and more recently in New Zealand[185-191] have identified a consistent pattern of treatment associated with mortality. In addition to lack of appreciation of the severity of asthma both by the patient and the doctor, bronchodilators were often used in high dosage, frequently as sole treatment, and corticosteroid treatment greatly underused.

In the British Thoracic Association study[213] corticosteroids were given to less than 50% of those patients who could have received such treatment during their final episode. Similarly, in New Zealand 46% of those treated during the fatal attack were given little or no corticosteroid even when the opportunity existed. Rather, emphasis was placed on increased use of bronchodilators—usually inhaled β-sympathomimetics by pressurised aerosol—and in New Zealand these were also administered by nebuliser. The availability of a domiciliary nebuliser, which had been prescribed for 75 of the 271 New Zealand patients under study, accounted for a delay in seeking medical attention for asthma in up to 8% of all patients dying from acute asthma; delay associated with continued ineffective use of a metered dose inhaler was much more common. While some patients died during the administration of nebulised β-agonist, in each case the patient was *in extremis* when the nebulisation was started. There were no cases detected among the fatalities where the patient had only a mild or moderate asthma attack before nebuliser treatment was given. In all cases the reviewing panel concluded that death had occurred despite, rather than because of, β-agonist treatment.

In the Auckland case control study conducted at the same time as the New Zealand national mortality study,[215,216] drugs used by hospital-based and community-based control subjects were compared with those used by asthmatics suffering fatal attacks. When matched for severity, patients with fatal asthma tended to be less well treated, to have had less adequate use of corticosteroids, and to be receiving more complicated drug regimens with a multiplicity of drugs than those who survived.

At the time of the New Zealand national mortality study, no reliable information was available as to patterns of drug treatment for asthma in the community. Whether the underuse of corticosteroids seen in fatal asthma was characteristic only of that group, or part of a national trend, was quite unknown. More recently, a community study of anti-asthma drug usage has been conducted.[217] Subjects for whom a prescription for salbutamol was written during a specified period were identified at randomly selected pharmacies and the patient subsequently interviewed regarding their condition, treatment, and understanding of their asthma management. Of patients with persistent daily symptoms due to asthma, only 42% received inhaled corticosteroids, and 16% oral corticosteroids. Cromoglycate was used by 20% of patients with persistent symptoms, while 33% of this group used only bronchodilators. These data indicate widespread underusage of disease-modifying treatment in the community as well as in those who die of their disease.

The beneficial effect of inhaled corticosteroids seems to be of relatively short duration, being lost in most patients within 1–3 weeks after cessation of therapy.[141] It is therefore conceivable that withdrawal of or non-compliance with agents which have modified the severity of BHR could possibly increase the risk of death from asthma.

Evidence for reduction in mortality by use of appropriate drugs

This is a difficult area in which to obtain convincing evidence. Mortality from asthma declined in England and Wales in the late 1960s after considerable publicity was given to the hypothesis that excessive use of β-agonists was linked to the fatalities. Whether this association was one of cause and effect is conjectural; emphasis on adequate assessment of severity and use of corticosteroids may have produced the decline as much as caution in use of β-agonists. Similarly, in New Zealand mortality from asthma in young people declined from 1983 to 1985 as publicity regarding asthma deaths increased but before the results of the national study were known, or the study even completed. Awareness that asthma can be a fatal disease and that it should be taken seriously may have had as great an effect on mortality as promotion of more appropriate drugs for use in the management of chronic and acute asthma. In New Zealand use of inhaled and oral corticosteroids has continued to increase. Despite this, fatalities in young people again increased in 1986 to a level near that pertaining in the early 1980s. This could be due to a complacency that the 'epidemic' was over—or be due to the same or different unknown factors which led to the 'epidemic' in the late 1970s, despite more appropriate drug treatments being available. Provisional 1987 figures show resumption of the downward trend in mortality rate.

That corticosteroids are effective in the management of acute severe asthma is seldom disputed; recent studies have again shown benefit from early intervention with corticosteroids in both children[218] and adults.[219] Our present understanding of asthma as an inflammatory disease of the airways suggests that the rational approach to management—reducing morbidity and preventing mortality—is the continuing use of anti-inflammatory, disease-modifying drugs as the fundamental treatment, with use of bronchodilators as additional palliative treatment to be used intermittently to relieve symptomatic obstruction. Much longer term epidemiological studies are required to show whether this approach will significantly reduce asthma mortality.

REFERENCES

1 Ciba Foundation Study Group No. 38. *The identification of asthma.* Edinburgh and London: Churchill Livingstone 1971.

2 American Thoracic Society. Standards for the diagnosis and care of patients with chronic obstructive pulmonary disease (COPD) and asthma. *Am Rev Respir Dis* 1987;136:225–43.

3 Pride N. Smoking, allergy and airways obstruction: revival of the Dutch hypothesis. *Clin Allergy* 1986;16:3–6.

4 Orie NGM, Sluiter HJ, De Vries K, Tammeling GJ, Witkop J. The host factor in bronchitis. In: *Bronchitis: an international symposium, 27–29 April 1960,* Groningen. Assen: Royal Van Gorcum 1961:43–59.

5 Van der Lende R, De Kroon JPM, Van der Meulen GG *et al.* Possible indicators of endogeneous factors in the development of CNSLD. In: Orie NGM, Van der Lende R, eds. *Bronchitis III. Proceedings of the 3rd international symposium on bronchitis,* 23–26 September 1969, Groningen. Assen: Royal Van Gorcum 1970:52–70.

6 Woolcock AJ, Salome CM, Yan K. The shape of the dose–response curve to histamine in asthmatic and normal subjects. *Am Rev Respir Dis* 1984;130:71–5.

7 Malo JL, Cartier A, Pineau L, Gagnon G, Martin RR. Slope of the dose-response curve to inhaled histamine and methacholine and PC_{20} in subjects with symptoms of hyperexcitability and in normal subjects. *Am Rev Respir Dis* 1985;**132**:644–7.

8 Cockcroft DW. Bronchial inhalation tests I. Measurements of non-allergic bronchial responsiveness to methacholine. *Ann Allergy* 1985;**55**:527–34.

9 Eiser NM, Kerrebijn KF, Quanjer PH. Guidelines for standardization of bronchial challenges with non-specific, bronchoconstricting agents. *Bull Eur Physiopathol Respir* 1983;**19**:459–514.

10 Yan K, Salome CM, Woolcock AJ. Prevalence and nature of bronchial hyperresponsiveness in subjects with chronic obstructive pulmonary disease. *Am Rev Respir Dis* 1985;**132**:25–9.

11 De Vries K. Clinical significance of bronchial hyperreactivity. In: Nadel J, Pauwels R, Snashell PD, eds. *Bronchial hyperresponsiveness, normal and abnormal control, assessment and therapy.* Oxford: Blackwell Scientific Publications 1988:359–71.

12 De Vries K, Gökemeyer JDM, Koeter GH *et al.* Cholinergic and adrenergic mechanisms in bronchial hyperreactivity. In: Morley J, ed. *Perspectives in asthma. I Bronchial hyperreactivity.* New York: Academic Press 1982:107–21.

13 Postma DS, De Vries K, Sluiter HJ. Bronchial hyperreactivity, an overview. *Neth J Med* 1986;**29**:334–41.

14 Juniper EF, Frith PA, Hargreave FE. Airway responsiveness to histamine and metacholine; relationship of minimum treatment to control symptoms of asthma. *Thorax* 1981;**36**:575–9.

15 Du Toit JI, Woolcock AJ, Salome CM *et al.* Characteristics of bronchial hyperresponsiveness in smokers with chronic airflow limitation. *Am Rev Respir Dis* 1986;**134**:498–501.

16 Salome CF, Schoeffel RE, Woolcock AJ. Comparison of bronchial reactivity to histamine and methacholine in asthmatics. *Clin Allergy* 1980;**10**:541–6.

17 Ramsdale EH, Morris MM, Roberts RR, Hargreave FE. Bronchial responsiveness to methacholine in chronic bronchitis: relationship to airflow obstruction and cold air responsiveness. *Thorax* 1984;**39**:912–8.

18 Michoud MC, Lelorier J, Amyot R. Factors modulating the interindividual variability of airway responsiveness to histamine. The influence of H_1 and H_2 receptors. *Bull Eur Physiopathol Respir* 1981;**17**:807–21.

19 Woolcock AJ, Salome CM, Yan K. The shape of the dose-response curve to histamine in asthmatic and normal subjects. *Am Rev Respir Dis* 1984;**130**:171–5.

20 Sterk PJ, Daniel EE, Zamel N, Hargreave FE. Limited bronchoconstriction to methacholine using partial flow–volume curves in nonasthmatic subjects. *Am Rev Respir Dis* 1985;**132**:272–7.

21 Bahous J, Cartier A, Ouimet G, Pineau L, Malo JL. Non-allergic bronchial hyperexcitability in chronic bronchitis. *Am Rev Respir Dis* 1985;**129**:216–20.

22 Klein RC, Salvaggio JE. Non-specificity of the bronchoconstricting effect of histamine and acetyl-methylcholine in patients with obstructive airway disease. *J Allergy* 1966;**37**:158–68.

23 Ramsdale EH, Roberts RS, Morris MM, Hargreave FE. Differences in responsiveness to hyperventilation and methacholine in asthma and chronic bronchitis. *Thorax* 1985;**40**:422–6.

24 Cockcroft DW, Ruffin RE, Dolovich J, Hargreave FE. Allergen-induced increase in non-allergic bronchial reactivity. *Clin Allergy* 1977;**7**:503–13.

25 Holtzman MJ, Cunningham JH, Sheller JH, Irsigler GN, Nadel JA, Boushey KA. Effect of ozone on bronchial reactivity in atopic and non-atopic subjects. *Am Rev Respir Dis* 1979;**120**:1059–67.

26 Laitinen LA, Heino M, Laitinen A, Kava T, Haahtela T. Damage of the airway epithelium and bronchial reactivity in patients with asthma. *Am Rev Respir Dis* 1985;**131**:599–606.

27 Lozewicz S, Gomez E, Ferguson H, Davies RJ. Inflammatory cells in the airways in mild asthma. *Br Med J* 1988;**297**:1515–6.

28 Holgate ST, Roche W, Roberts A, Beasly RC. Inflammation as the basis of asthma. In: Sluiter HJ, Vander Lende R, eds. *Bronchitis VI.* Assen: Royal Van Gorcum 1989:163–74.

29 Cosio MG, Hale KA, Niewoehner DE. Morphologic and morphometric effects of prolonged cigarette smoking in the small airways. *Am Rev Respir Dis* 1980;**122**:265–71.

30 Gilljam H, Motakefi A, Robertson B, Strandvik B. Ultrastructure of the bronchial epithelium in adult patients with cystic fibrosis. *Eur J Respir Dis* 1987;**71**:187–94.

31 Jefferey PK, Brain ARP, Nelson F. Electron microscopic studies of airway epithelium in patients with cystic fibrosis (abstract). *10th International Cystic Fibrosis Congress,* Sydney 1988:51.

32 Kirby JG, Hargreave FE, Gleich GJ, O'Byrne PM. Bronchoalveolar cell profiles of asthmatic and non-asthmatic subjects. *Am Rev Respir Dis* 1987;**136**:379–83.

33 Wardlaw AJ, Dunnette S, Gleich GJ, Collins JV, Kay AB. Eosinophils and mast cells in bronchoalveolar lavage in subjects with mild asthma. *Am Rev Respir Dis* 1988;**137**:62–9.

34 Kelly C, Ward C, Stenton CS, Bird G, Hendrick DJ, Walters EH. Number and activity of inflammatory cells in bronchoalveolar lavage fluid in asthma and their relation to airway responsiveness. *Thorax* 1988;**43**:684–92.

35 Casale TB, Wood D, Richardson HB, Trapp S, Metzker WJ, Zavala D, Hunninghake GW. Elevated bronchoalveolar lavage fluid histamine levels in allergic asthmatics are associated with methacholine bronchial hyperresponsiveness. *J Clin Invest* 1987;**79**:1197–1203.

36 Cutz E, Levison H, Cooper DM. Ultrastructure of airways in children with asthma. *Histopathology* 1978;**2**:407–21.

37 Konradova V, Copova C, Sukova B, Houstek J. Ultrastructure of the bronchial epithelium in three children with asthma. *Pediatr Pulmonol* 1985;**1**:182–7.

38 Findlay SR, Lichtenstein LM. Basophil 'releasability' in patients with asthma. *Am Rev Respir Dis* 1986;**122**:53–60.

39 Neijens HJ, Raatgeep RE, Degenhart HJ, Duiverman EJ, Kerrebijn KF. Altered leukocyte response in relation to the basic abnormality in children with asthma and bronchial hyperresponsiveness. *Am Rev Respir Dis* 1984;**130**:744–7.

40 Placet M, Kazimierezak W, Lichtenstein LM. Abnormalities of basophil 'releasability' in atopic and asthmatic individuals. *J Allergy Clin Immunol* 1986;**78**:968–73.

41 Shult PA, Cega M, Jadidi S, Virtis R, Warner T, Graziano FM, Busse WW. The presence of hypodense eosinophils and diminished chemiluminescence response in asthma. *J Allergy Clin Immunol* 1988;**81**:429–37.

42 Hunninghake GW, Crystal RG. Cigarette smoking and lung destruction. *Am Rev Respir Dis* 1983;**128**:833–8.

43 Mullen JBM, Wiggs B, Wright JL, Hogg JC, Pare PD. Nonspecific airway reactivity in cigarette smokers. *Am Rev Respir Dis* 1986;**133**:120–5.

44 Taylor RG, Joyce H, Gross E, Holland F, Pride NB. Bronchial reactivity to inhaled histamine and annual rate of decline in FEV_1 in male smokers and ex-smokers. *Thorax* 1984;**40**:9–16.

45 Burney PGJ, Britton JR, Chinn S. Descriptive epidemiology of bronchial reactivity in an adult population; results from a community study. *Thorax* 1987;**42**:38–44.

46 Pride NB, Taylor RG, Lim TK, Joyce H, Watson A. Bronchial hyperresponsiveness as a risk factor for progressive airflow obstruction in smokers. *Bull Eur Physiopathol Respir* 1987;**23**:369–75.

47 Rijcken B, Schouten JP, Weiss ST, Speizer FE, Van der Lende R. The relationship between airway responsiveness to histamine and pulmonary

function level in a random population sample. *Am Rev Respir Dis* 1988;**137**:826–32.

48 Burrows B, Bloom JW, Traver GA, Cline MS. The course and prognosis of different forms of chronic airways obstruction in a sample from the general population. *N Engl J Med* 1987;**317**:1309–14.

49 Lim TK, Taylor RG, Watson A, Joyce H, Pride NB. Changes in bronchial responsiveness to inhaled histamine over four years in middle aged male smokers and ex-smokers. *Thorax* 1988;**43**:599–604.

50 Seltzer J, Scanlon PD, Drazen JM, Ingram RH, Reid L. Morphologic correlation of physiologic changes caused by sulfur dioxide induced bronchitis in dogs. *Am Rev Respir Dis* 1984;**129**:790–7.

51 Scanlon PD, Seltzer J, Ingram RH, Reid L, Drazen JM. Chronic exposure to sulfur dioxide (physiologic and histologic evaluation of dogs exposed to 50 or 15 ppm). *Am Rev Respir Dis* 1987;**135**:831–9.

52 Fujita M, Schroeder MA, Hyatt RE. Canine model of chronic bronchial injury. *Am Rev Respir Dis* 1988;**137**:429–34.

53 Postma DS, Renkema TEJ, Noordhoek JA, Faber H, Sluiter JH, Kauffman H. Association between non-specific bronchial hyperreactivity and superoxide anion production by polymorphonuclear leukocytes in chronic airflow obstruction. *Am Rev Respir Dis* 1988;**137**:57–61.

54 Snapper JR, Brigham KL. Inflammation and airway reactivity. *Exp Lung Res* 1984;**6**:83–9.

55 O'Byrne PM, Hargreave FE, Kirby JG. Airway inflammation and hyperresponsiveness. *Am Rev Respir Dis* 1987;**136**:S35–7.

56 de Jongste JC, Mons H, van Strik R, Bontá IL, Kerrebijn KF. Comparison of human bronchiolar smooth muscle responsiveness *in vitro* with histological signs of inflammation. *Thorax* 1987;**42**:870–6.

57 de Jongste JC, Sterk PJ, Willems LNA, Mons H, Timmers MC, Kerrebijn KF. Comparison of maximal bronchoconstriction *in vivo* and airway smooth muscle responses *in vitro* in nonasthmatic humans. *Am Rev Respir Dis* 1988;**138**:321–6.

58 Moreno RH, Hogg JC, Pare PD. Mechanics of airway narrowing. *Am Rev Respir Dis* 1986;**133**:1171–80.

59 Ding DJ, Martin JG, Macklem PT. Effects of lung volume on maximal methacholine induced bronchoconstriction in normal humans. *J Appl Physiol* 1987;**62**:1324–30.

60 Gayrard P, Badier M, Vervloet D, Orehek J. Different bronchoconstrictor effects of carbachol boluses inhaled near residual volume or total lung capacity. *Respiration* 1987;**51**:81–5.

61 de Monchy JGR, Kauffman HF, Venge P *et al.* Bronchoalveolar eosinophilia during allergen-induced late asthmatic reactions. *Am Rev Respir Dis* 1985;**131**:373–6.

62 Kava T. Acute respiratory infections, influenza vaccination and airway reactivity in asthma. *Eur J Respir Dis* 1987;**70**(Suppl. 150):7–38.

63 de Jongste JC, Degenhart HJ, Neijens HJ, Duiverman EJ, Raatgeep HC, Kerrebijn KF. Bronchial responsiveness and leucocyte reactivity after influenza vaccine in asthmatic patients. *Eur J Respir Dis* 1984;**65**:196–200.

64 Laitinen LA, Kava T. Bronchial reactivity following uncomplicated influenza A infection in healthy subjects and asthmatic patients. *Eur J Respir Dis* 1980;**61**(Suppl. 106):51–8.

65 Hogg JC. Bronchial mucosal permeability and its relationship to airways hyperreactivity. *J Allergy Clin Immunol* 1981;**61**:421–5.

66 Welliver RC, Kaul TN, Ogra PL. The appearance of cell-bound IgE in respiratory tract epithelium after respiratory-syncytial virus infection. *N Engl J Med* 1980;**303**:1198–202.

67 Welliver RC, Wong DT, Sun M, Middleton E, Vaughan RS, Ogra PL. The development of respiratory syncytial virus-specific IgE and the release of histamine in nasopharyngeal secretions after infection. *N Engl J Med*

1981;**305**:841-6.

68 Metzger WJ, Zavala D, Richerson HB *et al.* Local allergen challenge and bronchoalveolar lavage of allergic asthmatic lungs. *Am Rev Respir Dis* 1987;**135**:433-40.

69 Fick RB, Richardson HB, Zavala DC, Hunninghake GW. Bronchoalveolar lavage in allergic asthmatics. *Am Rev Respir Dis* 1987;**135**:1204-9.

70 Cartier A, Thomson NC, Frith PA, Roberts R, Hargreave FE. Allergen-induced increase in bronchial responsiveness to histamine: relationship to the late asthmatic response and change in airway calibre. *J Allergy Clin Immunol* 1982;**70**:170-7.

71 Cockcroft DW, Murdock KY. Changes in bronchial responsiveness to histamine at intervals after allergen challenge. *Thorax* 1987;**42**:302-4.

72 Thorpe JE, Steinberg D, Bernstein IL, Murlas CG. Bronchial reactivity increases soon after the immediate response in dual-responding asthmatic subjects. *Chest* 1987;**91**:21-5.

73 Twentyman OP, Holgate ST. The temporal development of increased bronchial responsiveness following allergen challenge and its relationship to the late asthmatic reaction. *Am Rev Respir Dis* 1988;**137**:135.

74 Chan-Yeung M, Lam S. Occupational asthma. *Am Rev Respir Dis* 1986;**133**:686-703.

75 Fabbri LM, Chiesura-Corona P, Dal Vecchio L *et al.* Prednisone inhibits late asthmatic reactions and the associated increase in airway responsiveness induced by toluene-diisocyanate in sensitized subjects. *Am Rev Respir Dis* 1985;**132**:1010-14.

76 Mapp CE, Corona PC, de Marzo N, Fabbri L. Persistent asthma due to isocyanates. *Am Rev Respir Dis* 1988;**137**:1326-9.

77 Mapp CE, Glacowo GR, Omini C, Broseghini C, Fabbri LM. Late, but not early asthmatic reactions induced by toluene-diisocyanate are associated with increased airway responsiveness to methacholine. *Eur J Respir Dis* 1986;**69**:276-84.

78 Mapp CE, Polato R, Maestrelli P, Hendrick DJ, Fabbri LM. Time course of the increase in airway responsiveness associated with late asthmatic reactions to toluene diisocyanate in sensitized subjects. *J Allergy Clin Immunol* 1985;**75**:568-72.

79 Boschetto P, Zocca E, Milani GF *et al.* Bronchoalveolar neutrophilia during late, but not early, asthmatic reactions induced by toluene diisocyanate (TDI). *J Allergy Clin Immunol* 1986;**77**:496A.

80 Fabbri LM, Boschetto P, Zocca E *et al.* Bronchoalveolar neutrophilia during late asthmatic reactions induced by toluene diisocyanate. *Am Rev Respir Dis* 1987;**136**:36-42.

81 Durham SR, Graneek BJ, Hawkins R, Newman Taylor AJ. The temporal relationship between increases in airway responsiveness to histamine and late asthmatic responses induced by occupational agents. *J Allergy Clin Immunol* 1987;**79**:398-406.

82 Mapp CE, Boschetto P, Dal Vecchio L *et al.* Protective effect of antiasthma drugs on late asthmatic reactions and increased airway responsiveness induced by toluene diisocyanate in sensitized subjects. *Am Rev Respir Dis* 1987;**136**:1403-7.

83 Boschetto P, Fabbri LM, Zocca E *et al.* Prednisone inhibits late asthmatic reactions and airway inflammation induced by toluene diisocyanate in sensitised subjects. *J Allergy Clin Immunol* 1987;**80**:261-7.

84 Lam S, Tan F, Chan H, Chan-Yeung M. Relationship between types of asthmatic reaction, nonspecific bronchial reactivity and specific IgE antibodies in patients with red cedar asthma. *J Allergy Clin Immunol* 1983;**72**:134-9.

85 Lam S, LeRiche J, Phillips D, Chan-Yeung M. Cellular and protein changes in bronchial lavage fluid after late asthmatic reaction in patients with red cedar asthma. *J Allergy Clin Immunol* 1987;**80**:44-50.

86 Seltzer J, Bigby BG, Stulbarg M *et al.* O$_3$-induced change in bronchial reactivity to methacholine and airway inflammation in humans. *J Appl Physiol* 1986;**60**:1321–6.

87 Kehrl HR, Vincent LM, Kowalsky RJ *et al.* Ozone exposure increases respiratory epithelial permeability in humans. *Am Rev Respir Dis* 1987;**135**:1124–8.

88 Holtzman MJ, Fabbri LM, O'Byrne PM *et al.* Importance of airway inflammation for hyperresponsiveness induced by ozone. *Am Rev Respir Dis* 1983;**127**:686–90.

89 Fabbri LM, Aizawa H, Alpert SE. Airway hyperresponsiveness and changes in cell counts in bronchoalveolar lavage after ozone exposure in dogs. *Am Rev Respir Dis* 1984;**129**:288–91.

90 Holtzman MJ, Fabbri LM, Skoogh BE *et al.* Time course of airway hyperresponsiveness induced by ozone in dogs. *J Appl Physiol* 1983;**55**:1232–6.

91 Evans TW, Brokaw JJ, Chung KF, Nadel JA, McDonald DM. Ozone-induced bronchial hyperresponsiveness in the rat is not accompanied by neutrophil influx or increased vascular permeability in the trachea. *Am Rev Respir Dis* 1988;**138**:140–4.

92 O'Byrne PM, Walters EH, Gold BD *et al.* Neutrophil depletion inhibits airway hyperresponsiveness induced by ozone exposure. *Am Rev Respir Dis* 1984;**130**:214–9.

93 Thompson JE, Scypinski LA, Gordon T, Sheppard D. Hydroxyurea inhibits airway hyperresponsiveness in guinea pigs by a granulocyte independent mechanism. *Am Rev Respir Dis* 1986;**134**:1213–8.

94 Murlas C, Roum JH. Bronchial hyperreactivity occurs in steroid-treated guinea pigs depleted of leukocytes by cyclophosphamide. *J Appl Physiol* 1985;**58**:1630–7.

95 Becket WS, Freed AN, Turner C, Menkes HA. Prolonged increased responsiveness of canine peripheral airways after exposure to ozone. *J Appl Physiol* 1988;**64**:605–10.

96 O'Byrne PM, Walters EH, Aizawa H, Fabbri LM, Holtzman MJ, Nadel JA. Indomethacin inhibits the airway hyperresponsiveness but not the neutrophil influx induced by ozone in dogs. *Am Rev Respir Dis* 1984;**130**:220–4.

97 Aizawa HA, Chung KF, Leikauf GD *et al.* Significance of thromboxane generation in ozone-induced airway hyperresponsiveness in dogs. *J Appl Physiol* 1985;**59**:1918–23.

98 Hulbert WM, Mclean T, Hogg JC. The effect of acute airway inflammation on bronchial reactivity in guinea pigs. *Am Rev Respir Dis* 1985;**132**:7–11.

99 Murlas CG, Roum JH. Sequence of pathologic changes in the airway mucosa of guinea pigs during ozone-induced bronchial hyperreactivity. *Am Rev Respir Dis* 1985;**131**:314–20.

100 Nadel JA. Role of inflammation in asthma. *Chest* 1985;**87**:171S.

101 Irvin CG, Baltopoulos G, Honour J, Seccombe JF, Henson PM. Lipid mediators released by activated human neutrophils which increase airways reactivity. *Am Rev Respir Dis* 1986;**133**:A175.

102 Holgate ST. Contribution of inflammatory mediators to the immediate asthmatic reaction. *Am Rev Respir Dis* 1987;**135**:S57–62.

103 Minor TE, Dick EC, Baker JW, Ouellette JJ, Cohen M, Reed CE. Rhinovirus and influenza type A infections as precipitants of asthma. *Am Rev Respir Dis* 1976;**113**:149–53.

104 Sherter LB, Polnitsky CA. The relationship of viral infections to subsequent asthma. *Clin Chest Med* 1981;**2**:67–78.

105 Halperin SA, Eggleston PA, Beasley P, Suratt P, Hendley JO, Gröschel DHM, Gwaltney JM Jr. Exacerbations of asthma in adults during experimental rhinovirus infection. *Am Rev Respir Dis* 1985;**132**:976–80.

106 Jenkins CR, Breslin ABX. Upper respiratory tract infections and airway reactivity in normal asthmatic subjects. *Am Rev Respir Dis* 1984;**130**:878–83.

107 Busse WW, Swenson CA, Borden EC, Treuhaft MW, Dick EC. Effect of influenza A virus on leukocyte histamine release. *J Allergy Clin Immunol* 1983;**71**:382–8.

108 O'Bryne PM. Allergen-induced airway hyperresponsiveness. *J Allergy Clin Immunol* 1988;**81**:119–27.

109 Boulet L-P, Cartier A, Thomson NC, Roberts RS, Dolovich J, Hargreave FE. Asthma and increases in nonallergic bronchial responsiveness from season pollen exposure. *J Allergy Clin Immunol* 1983;**71**:399–406.

110 Barbato A, Pisetta F, Ragusa A, Marcer G, Zacchello F. Modification of bronchial hyperreactivity during pollen season in children allergic to grass. *Ann Allergy* 1987;**58**:121–4.

111 Chan-Yeung M, Lam S, Koener S. Clinical features and natural history of occupational asthma due to western red cedar (Thuja plicata). *Am J Med* 1982;**72**:411–15.

112 Lam S, Wong R, Chan-Yeung M. Nonspecific bronchial reactivity in occupational asthma. *J Allergy Clin Immunol* 1979;**63**:28–34.

113 Sheppard D. Mechanisms of acute increases in airway responsiveness caused by environmental chemicals. *J Allergy Clin Immunol* 1988;**81**:128–32.

114 Holtzman MJ, Cunningham JH, Sheller JR, Irsigler GB, Nadel JA, Boushey HA. Effect of ozone on bronchial reactivity in atopic and nonatopic subjects. *Am Rev Respir Dis* 1979;**120**:1059–67.

115 Koenig JQ, Covert DS, Marshall SG, Van Belle G, Pierson WE. The effects of ozone and nitrogen dioxide on pulmonary function in healthy and in asthmatic adolescents. *Am Rev Respir Dis* 1987;**136**:1152–7.

116 Dimeo MJ, Glenn MG, Holtzman MJ, Sheller JR, Nadel JA, Boushey HA. Threshold concentration of ozone causing an increase in bronchial reactivity in humans and adaptation with repeated exposures. *Am Rev Respir Dis* 1981;**124**:245–8.

117 Islam MS, Vastag E, Ulmer WT. Sulphur-dioxide induced bronchial hyper-reactivity against acetylcholine. *Int Arch Arbeitsmed* 1972;**29**:221–32.

118 Härkönen H, Nordman H, Korhonen O, Winblad I. Long-term effects of exposure to sulfur dioxide. Lung function four years after a pyrite dust explosion. *Am Rev Respir Dis* 1983;**128**:890–3.

119 Wright WJ, Salome CM, Woolcock AJ. Review; SO$_2$ and asthma (in preparation).

120 Bauer MA, Utell MJ, Morrow PE, Speers DM, Gibb FR. Inhalation of 0.30 ppm nitrogen dioxide potentiates exercise-induced bronchospasm in asthmatics. *Am Rev Respir Dis* 1986;**134**:1203–8.

121 Orehek J, Massari JP, Cayrard P, Crimaud C, Charpin J. Effect of short-term, low level nitrogen dioxide exposure on bronchial sensitivity of asthmatic patients. *J Clin Invest* 1976;**57**:301–7.

122 Black JL, Schoeffel RE, Sundrum R, Berend N, Anderson SD. Increased responsiveness to methacholine and histamine after challenge with ultra-sonically nebulised water in asthmatic subjects. *Thorax* 1985;**40**:427–32.

123 Balmes JR, Frime JM, Christian D, Grodon T, Sheppard D. Acidity potentiates bronchoconstriction induced by hypoosmolar aerosols. *Am Rev Respir Dis* 1988;**138**:35–9.

124 Murray AB, Morrison BJ. The effect of cigarette smoke from the mother on bronchial responsiveness and severity of symptoms in children with asthma. *J Allergy Clin Immunol* 1986;**77**:575–81.

125 Knight A, Breslin ABX. Passive cigarette smoking and patients with asthma. *Med J Aust* 1985;**142**:194–5.

126 Wiedemann HP, Mahler DA, Loke J, Virgulto JA, Snyder P, Matthay RA. Acute effects of passive smoking on lung function and airway reactivity in asthmatic subjects. *Chest* 1986;**89**:180–5.

127 Martinez FD, Antognomi G, Macri F, Bonci E, Midulla F, de Castro G, Ronchetti R. Parental smoking enhances bronchial responsiveness in nine-year old children. *Am Rev Respir Dis* 1988;**138**:518–23.

128 Stevens WJ, Vermeire PA, van Schill LA. Bronchial hyperreactivity in rhinitis. *Eur J Respir Dis* 1983;64(Suppl. 128):72–80.

129 Braman SS, Barrows AA, DeCotiis BA, Settipane GA, Corrao WM. Airway hyperresponsiveness in allergic rhinitis. A risk factor for asthma. *Chest* 1987;91:671–4.

130 Henriksen JM, Wenzel A. Effect of an intranasally administered corticosteroid (budesonide) on nasal obstruction, mouth breathing and asthma. *Am Rev Respir Dis* 1984;130:1014–18.

131 Woolcock AJ, Salome CM, Wright W, Zhang YG, Tam WK, Nguyen-Dang TH. Benzylkonium chloride inhalation in asthmatic subjects (in preparation).

132 Cuss FM, Dixon CMS, Barnes PJ. Effects of inhaled platelet activating factor on pulmonary function and bronchial responsiveness in man. *Lancet* 1986;ii:189–92.

133 Chung KF, Barnes PJ. Effects of platelet activating factor on airway calibre, airway responsiveness and circulating cells in asthmatic subjects. *Thorax* 1989;44:108–15.

134 Wilson NM, Dixon C, Silverman M. Increased bronchial responsiveness caused by ingestion of ice. *Eur J Respir Dis* 1985;66:25–30.

135 Wilson N, Vickers H, Taylor G, Silverman M. Objective test for food sensitivity in asthmatic children; increased bronchial reactivity after 'cola' drinks. *Br Med J* 1982;284:1226–8.

136 Haripersad D, Wilson N, Dixon C, Silverman M. Oral tartrazine challenge in childhood asthma; effect on bronchial reactivity. *Clin Allergy* 1984;14:81–5.

137 Salome CM, Cheung NW, Lee A, McDougall A, Woolcock AJ. Mechanisms of action of inhaled propranolol (unpublished observations).

138 Kraan J, Köeter GH, Van der Mark ThW, Sluiter HJ, De Vries K. Changes in bronchial hyperreactivity induced by 4 weeks of treatment with anti-asthmatic drugs in patients with allergic asthma: A comparison between budesonide and terbutaline. *J Allergy Clin Immunol* 1985;76:628–36.

139 Kerrebijn KF, van Essen-Zandvliet EEM, Neijens HJ. Effect of long-term treatment with glucocorticosteroids and beta-agonists on bronchial responsiveness in asthmatic children. *J Allergy Clin Immunol* 1987;79:653–9.

140 Vathenen AS, Knox AJ, Higgins BG, Britton JR, Tattersfield AE. Rebound increase in bronchial responsiveness after treatment with inhaled terbutaline. *Lancet* 1988;i:554–8.

141 du Toit JI, Salome CM, Woolcock AJ. Inhaled corticosteroids reduce the severity of bronchial responsiveness in asthma, but oral theophylline does not. *Am Rev Respir Dis* 1987;136:1174–8.

142 Suzuki S, Chonan T, Sasaki H, Takishima T. Bronchial hyperresponsiveness to methacholine after exercise in asthmatics. *Ann Allergy* 1985;54:136–41.

143 Magnussen H, Reuss G, Jorres R. Airway response to methacholine during exercise induced refractoriness in asthma. *Thorax* 1986;41:667–70.

144 Schoeffel RE, Anderson SD, Gillam I, Lindsay DA. Multiple exercise and histamine challenge in asthmatic patients. *Thorax* 1980;35:164–70.

145 Poppius H, Stenius B. Changes in arterial oxygen saturation in patients with hyperreactive airways during a histamine inhalation test. *Scand J Respir Dis* 1977;58:1–4.

146 Salome CM, Schoeffel RE, Woolcock AJ. Effect of aerosol and oral fenoterol on histamine and methacholine challenge in asthmatic subjects. *Thorax* 1981;36:580–4.

147 Hanley SP, Garrett H, Britton JR, Hatfield J, Tattersfield AE. Differential effects of salbutamol and ipratropium bromide on airway calibre and reactivity to histamine in asthma. *Am Rev Respir Dis* 1986;4(Suppl. 133):A177.

148 Casterline GL, Evans R, Ward GW. The effect of atropine and albuterol aerosols on the human bronchial response to histamine. *J Allergy Clin Immunol* 1976;58:607–13.

149 Cockcroft DW, Rillian DN, Mellon JJA, Hargreave RE. Protective effect of drugs on histamine-induced asthma. *Thorax* 1977;32:429–37.

150 Casterline CL, Evans R. Further studies on the mechanism of human histamine-induced asthma. *J Allergy Clin Immunol* 1977;**59**:420–4.

151 Löwhagen O. Drug influence on bronchial responsiveness. In: Nadel JA, Pauwels R, Snashell PD eds. *Bronchial hyperresponsiveness, normal and abnormal control, assessment and therapy.* Oxford: Blackwell Scientific Publications 1988;385–408.

152 Kraan J, Koëter GH, Van der Mark ThW, Boorsma M, Kukler J, Sluiter HJ, De Vries K. Dosage and time effects of inhaled budesonide on bronchial hyperreactivity. *Am Rev Respir Dis* 1988;**137**:44–8.

153 Jenkins CR, Woolcock AJ. Effect of prednisone and beclomethasone dipropionate on airway responsiveness in asthma: a comparative study. *Thorax* 1988;**43**:378–84.

154 Löwhagen O, Rak S. Modification of bronchial hyperreactivity after treatment with sodium cromoglycate during pollen season. *J Allergy Clin Immunol* 1985;**75**:460–7.

155 Dorward AJ, Roberts JA, Thomson NC. Effect of nedocromil sodium on histamine airway responsiveness in grass-pollen sensitive asthmatics during the pollen season. *Clin Allergy* 1986;**16**:309–15.

156 Platts-Mills TAE, Heymann PW, Chapman MD, Mitchell EB. Bronchial hyperreactivity and allergen exposure. *Pro Respir Res* 1985;**19**:276–84.

157 Platts-Mills TAE, Tovey ER, Mitchell EB, Moszoro H, Nock P, Wilkins SR. Reduction of bronchial hyperreactivity during prolonged allergen avoidance. *Lancet* 1982;**ii**:675–7.

158 Ewer TC, Stewart DE. Improvement in bronchial hyperresponsiveness in patients with moderate asthma after treatment with a hypnotic technique: a randomised controlled trial. *Br Med J* 1986;**293**:1129–32.

159 Peat JK, Woolcock AJ, Cullen K. Rate of decline of lung function in subjects with asthma. *Eur J Respir Dis* 1987;**70**:171–9.

160 Kelly WJW, Hudson I, Raven J, Phelan PD, Pain MCF, Olinsky A. Childhood asthma and adult lung function. *Am Rev Respir Dis* 1988;**138**:26–30.

161 Gerritsen J, Koëter GH, Van Aalderen WMC, Knol K. The outcome of childhood asthma in early adult life. *Am Rev Respir Dis* 1987;**135** (Suppl.):A311.

162 Bleecker ER. Airway reactivity and asthma; significance and treatment. *J Allergy Clin Immunol* 1985;**75**:21–4.

163 Burrows B, Earle KH. Course and prognosis of chronic obstructive lung disease. *N Engl J Med* 1986;**280**:397–404.

164 Traver GA, Cline MG, Burrows B. Predictors of mortality in chronic obstructive pulmonary disease 15 year follow-up study. *Am Rev Respir Dis* 1979;**119**:895–902.

165 Postma DS, Burema J, Gimeno F *et al.* Prognosis in severe chronic obstructive pulmonary disease. *Am Rev Respir Dis* 1979;**119**:357–67.

166 Postma DS, Gimeno F, Van der Weele LTH, Sluiter HJ. Assessment of ventilatory variables in survival prediction of patients with chronic airflow obstruction: the importance of reversibility. *Eur J Respir Dis* 1985;**67**:360–8.

167 Postma DS, De Vries K, Koëter GH, Sluiter HJ. Independent influence of reversibility of airflow obstruction and non-specific hyperreactivity on the long term course of lung function in chronic airflow obstruction. *Am Rev Respir Dis* 1986;**134**:276–80.

168 Anthonisen NR, Wright EC, Hodgkin JE and the IPPB trial group. Prognosis in chronic obstructive pulmonary disease. *Am Rev Respir Dis* 1986;**133**:14–20.

169 Barter LE, Campbell AH. Relationship of constitutional factors and cigarette smoking to decrease in 1-second forced expiratory volume. *Am Rev Respir Dis* 1976;**133**:305–14.

170 Kanner RE, Renzetti AO, Klauber MR, Smith CB, Golden CA. Variables associated with changes in spirometry in patients with obstructive lung disease. *Am J Med* 1979;**67**:44–450.

171 *Early intervention for chronic obstruction pulmonary diseases.* Request for proposal CEP-NHLBI-84-1, National Institutes of Health, National Heart, Lung and Blood Institute, Bethesda, MD, 1983.

172 Mitchell EA. International trends in hospital admission rates for asthma. *Arch Dis Child* 1985;**68**:376–7.

173 Buist AS, Sears MR, Reid LM, Boushey HA, Spector SL, Sheffer AL. Asthma mortality: trends and determinants. *Am Rev Respir Dis* 1987;**136**:1037–9.

174 Burney PGJ. Asthma mortality in England and Wales: evidence for a further increase, 1974–84. *Lancet* 1986;ii:323–6.

175 Inman WHW, Adelstein AM. Rise and fall of asthma mortality in England and Wales in relation to use of pressurised aerosols. *Lancet* 1969;ii:279–85.

176 Fraser PM, Speizer FE, Waters SDM, Doll R, Mann NM. The circumstances preceding death from asthma in young people in 1968 to 1969. *Br J Dis Chest* 1971;**65**:71–84.

177 Stolley PD, Schinnar R. Association between asthma mortality and isoproterenol aerosols: a review. *Preventive Med* 1978;7:519–38.

178 Stolley PD. Asthma mortality. Why the United States was spared an epidemic of deaths due to asthma. *Am Rev Respir Dis* 1972;**105**:883–90.

179 Collins JM, McDevitt DG, Shanks RG, Swanton JG. The cardiotoxicity of isoprenaline during hypoxia. *Br J Pharmacol* 1969;**36**:35–45.

180 Taylor GJ, Harris WS. Cardiac toxicity of aerosol propellants. *JAMA* 1970;**214**:81–5.

181 Gandevia B. Pressurized sympathomimetic aerosols and their lack of relationship to asthma mortality in Australia. *Med J Aust* 1973;1:273–7.

182 Esdaile JM, Feinstein AR, Horwitz RI. A reappraisal of the United Kingdom epidemic of fatal asthma. Can general mortality data implicate a therapeutic agent? *Arch Intern Med* 1987;**147**:543–9.

183 Jackson RT, Beaglehold R, Rea HH, Sutherland DC. Mortality from asthma: a new epidemic in New Zealand. *Br Med J* 1982;**285**:771–4.

184 Sears MR, Rea HH, Beaglehole R *et al.* Asthma mortality in New Zealand: a two year national study. *NZ Med J* 1985;**98**:271–5.

185 Sears MR, Rea HH, de Boer G *et al.* Accuracy of certification of deaths due to asthma. A national study. *Am J Epidemiol* 1986;**124**:1004–11.

186 Sears MR. Why are deaths from asthma increasing? *Eur J Respir Dis* 1986;**69**(Suppl. 147):175–81.

187 Rea HH, Sears MR, Beaglehole R *et al.* Lessons from the national asthma mortality study; circumstances surrounding death. *NZ Med J* 1987;**100**:10–3.

188 Rothwell RPG, Rea HH, Sears MR *et al.* Lessons from the national asthma mortality study: deaths in hospital. *NZ Med J* 1987;**100**:199–202.

189 Sears MR, Rea HH, Fenwick J *et al.* 75 deaths in asthmatics prescribed home nebulisers. *Br Med J* 1987;**294**:477–80.

190 Sears MR, Rea HH, Rothwell RPG *et al.* Asthma mortality; comparison between New Zealand and England. *Br Med J* 1986;**293**:1342–5.

191 Sears MR, Rea HH, Beaglehole R. Asthma mortality: a review of recent experience in New Zealand. *J Allergy Clin Immunol* 1987;**80**:319–25.

192 Wilson JD, Sutherland DC, Thomas AC. Has the change to beta-agonists combined with oral theophylline increased cases of fatal asthma? *Lancet* 1981;i:1235–7.

193 Keating G, Mitchell EA, Jackson R, Beaglehole R, Rea H. Trends in sales of drugs for asthma in New Zealand, Australia and the United Kingdom, 1975–81. *Br Med J* 1984;**289**:348–51.

194 Paterson JW, Woolcock AJ, Shenfield GM. Bronchodilator drugs. *Am Rev Respir Dis* 1979;**120**:1149–88.

195 Prior JG, Cochrane GM, Raper SM, Ali C, Volans GN. Self-poisoning with oral salbutamol. *Br Med J* 1981;**282**:1932.

196 Haalboom JRE, Deenstra M, Struyvenberg A. Hypokalaemia induced by inhalation of fenoterol. *Lancet* 1985;i:1125–7.

197 Whyte KF, Reid C, Whitesmith R, Addis GJ, Reid JL. Theophylline increases salbutamol induced hypokalaemia and tachycardia. *Thorax* 1987;**42**:730.

198 Eidelman DH, Sami MH, McGregor M, Cosio MG. Combination of theophylline and salbutamol for arrhythmias in severe COPD. *Chest* 1987;**91**:808–12.

199 Hurwitz M, Howatt W, Crowley D, Ericson W. Effect of theophylline, beta adrenergic drugs, and hypoxia on cardiac rhythm and rate in acute childhood asthma. *J Allergy Clin Immunol* 1986;**77**:145.

200 Greenberg A, Piraino BH, Kroboth PD, Weiss J. Severe theophylline toxicity. Role of conservative measures, antiarrhythmic agents, and charcoal hemoperfusion. *Am J Med* 1984;**76**:854–60.

201 Beasley CRW, Rafferty P, Holgate ST. Bronchoconstrictor properties of preservatives in ipratropium bromide (Atrovent) nebuliser solution. *Br Med J* 1987;**294**:1197–8.

202 Harvey JE, Tattersfield AE. Airway response to salbutamol: effect of regular salbutamol inhalations in normal, atopic, and asthmatic patients. *Thorax* 1982;**37**:280–7.

203 Conolly ME, Tashkin DP, Hui KKP, Littner MR, Wolfe RN. Selective subsensitization of beta-adrenergic receptors in central airways of asthmatics and normal subjects during long-term therapy with inhaled salbutamol. *J Allergy Clin Immunol* 1982;**70**:423–31.

204 Svedmyr NLV, Larsson SA, Thiringer GK. Development of 'resistance' in beta-adrenegic receptors of asthmatic patients. *Chest* 1976;**69**:479–83.

205 Rossing TH, Fanta CH, McFadden ER. Effect of outpatient treatment of asthma with beta agonists on the response to sympathomimetics in an emergency room. *Am J Med* 1983;**75**:781–4.

206 Holgate ST, Baldwin CJ, Tattersfield AE. Beta-adrenergic resistance in normal human airways. *Lancet* 1977;**ii**:375–7.

207 Van Metre TE. Adverse effects of inhalation of excessive amounts of nebulized isoproterenol in status asthmaticus. *J Allergy* 1969;**43**:101–13.

208 Postma DS, Koëter G. Influence of inhaled terbutaline on bronchial responsiveness. *Lancet* 1988;**i**:1282.

209 Ormerod LP, Stableforth DE. Asthma mortality in Birmingham 1975–7: 53 deaths. *Br Med J* 1980;**280**:687–90.

210 MacDonald JB, Seaton A, Williams DA. Asthma deaths in Cardiff 1963–74: 90 deaths outside hospital. *Br Med J* 1976;**1**:1493–5.

211 Cochrane GM, Clark TJH. A survey of asthma mortality in patients between ages 35 and 64 in the Greater London hospitals in 1971. *Thorax* 1975;**30**:300–5.

212 Carswell F. Thirty deaths from asthma. *Arch Dis Child* 1985;**60**:25–8.

213 British Thoracic Association. Death from asthma in two regions of England. *Br Med J* 1982;**285**:1251–5.

214 Johnson AJ, Nunn AJ, Somner AR, Stableforth DE, Stewart CJ. Circumstances of death from asthma. *Br Med J* 1984;**288**:1870–2.

215 Sutherland DC, Beaglehole R, Fenwick J, Jackson RT, Mullins P, Rea HH. Death from asthma in Auckland: circumstances and validation of causes. *NZ Med J* 1984;**97**:845–8.

216 Rea HH, Scragg R, Jackson R, Beaglehole R, Fenwick J, Sutherland DC. A case-control study of deaths from asthma. *Thorax* 1986;**41**:833–9.

217 Sinclair BL, Clark DWJ, Sears MR. Use of anti-asthma drugs in New Zealand. *Thorax* 1987;**42**:670–5.

218 Harris JB, Weinberger MM, Nassif E, Smith G, Milavetz G, Stillerman A. Early intervention with short courses of prednisone to prevent progression of asthma in ambulatory patients incompletely responsive to bronchodilators. *J Pediatr* 1987;**110**:627–33.

219 Littenberg B, Gluck EH. A controlled trial of methylprednisolone in the emergency treatment of acute asthma. *N Engl J Med* 1986;**314**:150–2.

2: Pathology

L. M. Reid, G. J. Gleich, J. Hogg, J. Kleinerman &
L. A. Laitinen

In the light of relatively new clinically important information, it
must be remembered that there are several basic but, as yet,
unanswered questions on asthma. Factors causing an attack are
well known, but why some people, and not others, respond to a
given trigger is less clear. In some, genetic makeup is a determinant, but is it in all? While the differences in response between
asthmatic and non-asthmatic subjects are becoming more
clearly differentiated, the basic or inherited reason for the differences is not. Are the bronchial muscle or nerves abnormal in
asthmatics? At present it would appear not, therefore, where does
the difference lie?

The present discussion of the pathological features of asthma
serves two broad purposes:

1 *To identify subgroups of asthma and chronic bronchitis*, with the
aim of characterising them for separate study, so that our
hypotheses of pathogenesis and methods of treatment can be
precisely tested.

2 *To determine the role of inflammation in* (i) the asthmatic diathesis; (ii) triggering of an attack; (iii) amplification of the disease;
and (iv) the pathophysiology of signs and symptoms, between and
during attacks, and when the disease is fatal.

The first objective implies that there are subsets within the
disease categories. Thus, the role of inflammation whether in the
clinical or experimental setting, must be analysed separately for
the various subsets of asthma.

Certain premises form the basis of the discussion: that (i) there
are genetic cases in which the diathesis is inherited; (ii) in other
cases the cause is environmental; and (iii) there are probably
patients with a genetic predisposition, but for whom an environmental trigger can be identified. These simplified questions, however, represent a key issue: does category (ii) really exist clinically,
or is there always an unidentified genetic component? This means
that the nature of the inflammatory component and the patterns
of response need to be compared in cases that seem to represent
the extremes expressed by (i) and (ii).

Asthma, emphysema, and chronic bronchitis can each cause
airway obstruction. Because a patient may have more than one of
these conditions, it is important to recognise what is peculiar or
essential to each.[1] While it is necessary to recognise that the

various disease groups have identifiable subsets, it is also necessary to take into account the heterogeneity of inflammation. Rubor, calor, dolor, tumour, and mucus secretion still represent 'the black box' of inflammation. Various cellular and mediator cascades are capable of producing it, and so patterns or subsets of inflammation also need to be identified.

Investigations into asthma should follow a logical direction from the test tube or animal in the laboratory to the spontaneously occurring disease in man. Results obtained from human tissue are critical and central to our studies, but should be interpreted with care. The presence of a particular cell type does not mean that it is responsible for an attack: similarly, because a cell is capable of discharging active agents, it cannot be assumed that it does, or, that these agents have a key role in disease (i.e. essential to the development or evolution of an attack). Whereas one type of inflammation is perhaps relevant to the onset of an attack, the amplification of injury is likely to be based on different patterns. The information recently obtained from examining the patient's lung is an important consideration. This information can be from samples taken either from the large airways, by various biopsy techniques, or from less well defined sites using bronchoalveloar lavage (BAL).

PATHOLOGICAL FINDINGS IN ASTHMA USING BIOPSY TISSUE FROM LARGE AIRWAYS

Changes in the epithelial and inflammatory cells in the bronchial mucosa in asthma

Differences between early or mild cases of asthma and those that, clinically, were either late or severe, have been described. Laitinen *et al.* reported bronchial epithelial destruction, mucosal oedema, and an inflammatory cell population in specimens from the airways of asthmatic patients, all of whom showed increased bronchial reactivity.[2] In a more recent study, bronchial biopsy specimens were examined from 10 patients with mild to severe asthma ranging in duration from three months to 12 years. At the time of biopsy the patients were clinically stable as possible. No patient had had a viral infection for at least two months. This is important as such infections cause the same shedding of the bronchial mucosal epithelium as occurs in asthmatics.[3] Antigen challenge had not been performed for several months because this causes a marked increase in eosinophils in BAL fluid during the late reaction.[4] Long-term smokers (for 15 to 50 years), including some with symptoms compatible with chronic bronchitis, and patients with the hyperventilation syndrome, were used as controls.

Morphological studies of the mucosa in these biopsy specimens were made using a novel electron microscope method developed by Laitinen which uses slot grids without bars to prepare electron micrographs of a large area of tissue.[5] This method allowed the number of mast cells, neutrophils, and eosinophils within the airway epithelium to be determined.[6]

Light microscopy and low power transmission electron microscopy show that there is a striking difference in the bronchial mucosal structure of asthmatics, long-term smokers and controls. In the control specimens the airway mucosa had a firm appearance; the epithelium looked 'tight', and the ciliated and goblet cells were firmly attached to each other by tight junctions adjacent to the airway lumen. At the base they rested on the basement membrane along with basal cells (Table 2.1). Even in the long-term smokers, the epithelium was as firm as that in the

Table 2.1 Number of neutrophils, eosinophils, and mast cells in bronchial biopsy specimens from asthmatic patients, long term smokers, and controls*

Degree of severity	Duration (months)	Length of BM (µm)	Total number of cells			Number of cells per 500 µm of BM		
			N	M	E	N	M	E
Asthmatics								
A mild	12	816	0	5	3	0	3.1	1.8
B mild	24	1161	9	5	1	3.9	2.2	0.4
I mild	3	840	2	3	0	1.2	1.8	0
L mild	8	1071	3	2	0	1.4	0.9	0
C moderate	12	658	0	5	0	0	3.8	0
D moderate	60	1045	12	1	1	5.7	0.5	0.5
E moderate	3	1209	3	7	0	1.2	2.9	0
K mild	4	684	0	1	0	0	0.7	0
F severe	36	575	58	2	0	50	1.7	0
G severe	144	1284	61	2	0	24	0.8	0
Mean	30.3	934.3	14.8	3.3	0.5	8.74	1.84†	0.3
Long term smokers								
BR1		1217	0	0	0	0	0	0
BR2		956	2	0	0	1	0	0
BR3		677	2	0	0	1.5	0	0
BR4		1253	1	1	0	0.4	0.4	0
BR5		1218	1	3	0	0.4	1.2	0
Mean		1064.2	1.2	0.8	0	0.72	0.8†	0
Controls								
CO1		442	0	0	0	0	0	0
CO2		1816	0	2	0	0	0.6	0
Mean		1129	0	1	0	0	0.3†	0

*The numbers represent the mean of three specimens from three airway levels. BM, basement membrane; N, neutrophil; M, mast cell; E, eosinophil.
†Difference significant ($P < 0.05$).

controls. In most specimens the epithelium had a normal structure with ciliated, goblet, and basal cells. Occasionally, structural
changes like metaplasia could be seen. The numbers of other cells
in the epithelium and lamina propria were few compared with
those in the asthmatics (Table 2.1).

Electron microscopic examination confirmed findings from the
light microscope. In the controls the ciliated, goblet, and basal
cells formed the bulk of the airway epithelial cells. Intraepithelial
nerves containing vesicles, neurotubules and mitochondria were
also observed. At the base of the epithelium, neuroendocrine
(APUD-like; amine precursor uptake and decarboxylation) cells
containing many dense-cored small vesicles were found against
the basement membrane. Other cells in the airway epithelium
were rare.

In only a single case were mast cells (and then only two) seen
within the airway epithelium of controls. These two mast cells
contained well preserved, fully packed scroll-type substructures
in their granules. Other cells in the epithelium and lamina propria
were rare. Eosinophils and neutrophils were only occasionally
seen. The tissue around the mast cells, eosinophils, and neutrophils was intact, showing that tissue adjacent to these inflammatory cells is not always destroyed.

Within the airway epithelium of long-term smokers (Table 2.1),
in contrast to asthmatics, only small numbers of mast cells,
eosinophils, and neutrophils were present. The only cells regularly
seen in the epithelium of long-term smokers were lymphocytes.
Mast cells were seen in the lamina propria, but they had well
preserved granules.

Asthmatic patients—stable phase

In the asthmatics, the histological picture was very different, and
it was impossible to find a totally normal area of the bronchial
epithelium. These findings were in agreement with those from an
earlier study.[2] Typically, different types of change occurred in the
same specimen. Areas where only basal cells were resting on the
basment membrane were often seen. In most cases the specimen
showed epithelium, but this usually had a 'fragile' appearance. In
less damaged areas, homogeneous material, probably oedematous
fluid, had accumulated in widened intercellular spaces and at the
base of the epithelium. In extreme cases, this material seemed to
separate the columnar epithelial cells from the basement membrane and the basal cells. This effect of cells being 'pushed' away
from the basement membrane was often seen adjacent to foci of
epithelial destruction, where either only the basal cells were
present or the basement membrane was bare. Even when separated from basement membrane, the columnar epithelial cells were

often normal in appearance and still attached to each other at their luminal surface. Thus, the cells which were separated from the basement membrane did not necessarily show prominent intracellular damage to their organelles. The fragile look of the epithelium in the asthmatics arises partly from the changes within the cells. The ciliated cells, especially, seem to be swollen, vacuolised and often show loss of cilia. The basement membrane was usually, but not always, thickened, and the epithelium and lamina propria were crowded by various inflammatory cells.

The asthmatics showed great individual variation in the number of intraepithelial mast cells, eosinophils, and neutrophils. There were also some common features. All showed some degree of epithelial damage, with mast cells in the epithelium which in each case were degranulated, usually to a pronounced degree. The cell cytoplasm contained mainly empty granules and so the cell could be identified only by the presence of a few typical scroll granules (Figure 2.1). Ultrastructurally, degranulation was associated with replacement of the scroll structures by a small amount of dense homogeneous material left within an empty granule. Intermediate forms of the granules were common. The degranulation process had affected all granules, not only those close to the cell surface. Even the mild asthmatics, with less than a one year history of asthma, had highly degranulated mast cells within the epithelium. Cells with only empty granules were also observed, but, because they lacked features for mast cell identification, were not included in the mast cell counts. In the lamina propria in specimens both from asthmatic patients and control subjects, mast cells were found close to nerve fibres.

Eosinophils, identified by their crystalloid granules (Figure 2.2), were found in only three patients with moderate asthma, and they did not show features of degranulation.

Neutrophils, recognised by their azurophilic granules and their multinuclear pattern (Figure 2.2), were observed in high numbers only in severe asthmatics who had had the disease for several years. When present, neutrophils were located throughout the epithelium and close to the lumen between the tight junctions. If present within the epithelium, they were also seen in the lamina propria and blood vessels (Figure 2.3).

Other cells, such as macrophages, lymphocytes, and plasma cells were frequently observed in the lamina propria of asthmatics, including large numbers of transitional forms of lymphocyte to plasma cells.

During an asthma attack

There is little information on the morphology of the airways during worsening of symptoms, or during an attack. Bronchial

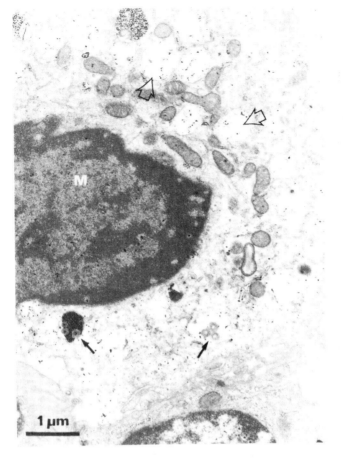

Fig. 2.1 Transmission electronmicrograph from the airway mucosa of a patient with clinically moderate asthma. The mast cell located in the airway epithelium shows highly degranulated granules. Several empty granules (open arrows) and some scroll type substructures (thin black arrows) by which the mast cell can be identified can be seen. M, mast cell; magnification × 26 000. (Reproduced with permission from Laitinen LA, Laitinen A. Review of the mechanisms involved in asthma. In: Howell JB ed. *Management of asthma.* Pennine Press 1987:12–16.)

biopsy specimens were taken from one asthmatic patient in this study during both a stable phase of the disease and an asthma attack. Compared with the stable state, there was a 100-fold increase in the number of eosinophils in the bronchial mucosa during the spontaneous asthma attack (Laitinen LA, Laitinen A, Haahtela T, unpublished observations).

These studies of early, mild, stable asthmatics emphasise that the asthma diathesis is associated with presence and activation of inflammatory cells within the epithelium of large airways—not just within the lamina propria. Injury to the airway epithelial layer is a continuous, active process, even when the patient has mild, seemingly inactive, disease. Correlation of these ultramicroscopic findings with other data indicates that activation of mast

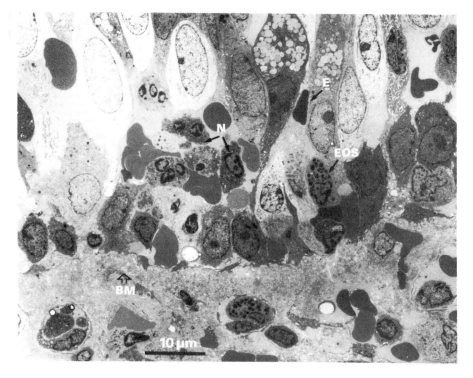

Fig. 2.2 Transmission electronmicrograph showing the basal part of the airway epithelium in a patient with clinically severe asthma, who has had the disease for several years. The intercellular spaces between the basal and columnar epithelial cells are widened and filled with homogeneous material, probably representing oedematous fluid. In the epithelium are many inflammatory cells, such as neutrophils and eosinophils. The lamina propria and the blood vessels beneath the epithelium are also filled with inflammatory cells. EOS, eosinophil; N, neutrophil; E, erythrocyte; BM, basement membrane; magnification × 3300.

cells might represent the diathesis, and that symptoms are associated with the presence of eosinophils in these large airways. In asthma of a longer duration or greater severity, eosinophils may be largely replaced by neutrophils. At all stages eosinophils seem to be present more peripherally in lung tissue. The various cell types identified and the pathological features described have implications for the pathogenesis of the asthma diathesis, the trigger of an attack, and for continuation or amplification of the disease.

The role of inflammatory cells in the pathogenesis of asthma

Mast cells

Mast cells are widely distributed in the body and are part of its defence against harmful agents. Within the airways they are

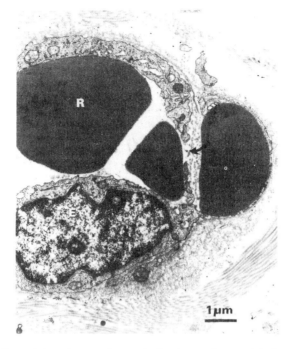

Fig. 2.3 Transmission electronmicrograph showing a microvessel in the airway mucosa beneath the epithelium in a moderate asthmatic. The vessel contains several red blood cells (R). One red blood cell in the lumen of the vessel is seen close to a gap (arrow) in the wall endothelium. E, endothelial cell; magnification × 20 000.

normally found in the connective tissue of the lamina propria. Release of their special cytoplasmic granules initiates the inflammatory response to certain stimuli. The granules contain several mediators that, experimentally, are chemotactic for inflammatory cells. The morphological state of mast cell granules reflects the cells' activity. Further study is needed on the location of mast cells in relation to several tissue structures, such as nerves, blood vessels, smooth muscle, epithelium and other inflammatory cells.

The critical feature in asthmatic patients is the presence, density, and degranulation of mast cells within epithelium. Preliminary results show that in the lamina propria the number of mast cells is similar in asthmatics and controls. It is mast cells within the epithelium that are greatly increased in asthmatics compared with either the long-term smokers or the controls. In asthmatics, the cell is highly degranulated and associated with epithelial injury. This is found even in mild asthmatics who have had the disease for less than a year. It cannot yet be decided which comes first—the tissue damage or the mast cells—but the mast cells represent one way in which inflammation can develop. The biopsy findings in early and mild cases point to the clinical importance of this cell type. The ability of activated mast cells to provoke allergic inflammation has been studied extensively in the skin.[7-9] In the nasal mucosa, mast cells are associated with development of allergic, but not infectious, inflammation.[10]

Mast cells may also have a role in the perpetuation of asthma or in its amplification, and mast cell mediators chemotactic for neutrophils[11-13] and for eosinophils have been described.[14]

Examination of BAL fluid has added to our understanding of the inflammatory events in asthmatic airways. Wardlaw *et al.*[15] found that in patients with mild, atopic asthma the percentage of mast cells showed a five to sixfold increase over control values. Even patients with mild asthma and short duration of the disease have highly degranulated mast cells in the epithelium.

Eosinophils

Although eosinophil infiltration is reported to be characteristic of asthmatic airways in necropsy specimens,[16] in only a few of the stable asthmatic patients in our series were they present within the airway epithelium. Eosinophils were seen in patients with mild to moderate asthma, but curiously enough, not in those with severe disease. The influx of eosinophils into the airway mucosa seems to be associated with a worsening of symptoms. Inhalation of an allergen results in a pronounced increase in eosinophils in BAL fluid during the late reaction.[4] This is in agreement with Laitinen's findings that eosinophils are present in large numbers in the bronchial mucosa during acute asthma attacks.

Several lavage studies have shown that eosinophils occur in the BAL fluid of all patients with asthma.[17-19] Increased numbers of eosinophils have been found in asthmatics with clinical evidence of active disease.[15] The amount of major basic protein (MBP) was measured in the latter study, and the authors suggested that it was a more specific indicator of increased eosinophil activity than the eosinophil count. During relatively inactive stages of the disease, MBP is present at the lung periphery, but is not typically found in central airways. During an acute attack, it increases noticeably and is then seen even in large airways. The presence and activity of eosinophils seems to be a marker of an asthma attack. The amount of MBP of eosinophils is raised and provides an indicator of the number and activity of the eosinophils; the products of eosinophils injure tissue. Eosinophils release a variety of mediators, including leukotriene C4, platelet activating factor (PAF), and also basic proteins such as MBP and eosinophilic cationic protein, which are toxic to airway epithelium. The findings of recent studies have associated eosinophils and, especially, eosinophil MBP with epithelial damage in asthma.[20]

In three out of the 10 asthmatics no neutrophils were found in the epithelium, but if the patients had had severe asthma for a long time, high numbers of neutrophils were present. It therefore seems that chronic asthma with impaired lung function is associated with the epithelial neutrophil influx.

The presence of a few neutrophils in the epithelium is probably normal, because even healthy subjects may have neutrophils in their lavage fluid.[21] The numbers of neutrophils and eosinophils are increased during the late asthmatic response to allergen challenge tests, thought to mimic spontaneous asthma.[22,23]

The clinical importance of neutrophils is unclear. These cells have been studied experimentally with somewhat conflicting results, perhaps reflecting differences between species. They have been associated with bronchial hyperresponsiveness (BHR).[24] Holzman and his colleagues claimed that these cells were active participants in epithelial damage, based on the results of administering ozone to dogs,[25] which caused BHR with a concomitant increase in neutrophils. Murlas and Roum,[26] however, described similar epithelial changes in guinea-pigs after two hours of exposure to ozone. They showed that this hyperreactivity was not dependent on inflammatory cell infiltration.[27] This is similar to the results of Hulbert *et al.* who showed BHR, but no neutrophil infiltration, in guinea-pigs half an hour after exposure to cigarette smoke.[28]

Secondary effects of epithelial injury

In recent years, an epithelial derived factor that inhibits bronchial smooth muscle contraction has been described.[29] Afferent nerve endings are numerous in bronchial epithelium, and injury to either the epithelium, or stimulation of the nerve could influence the behaviour of axon reflexes.[30] It has been shown that transient hyperresponsiveness occurs in otherwise healthy subjects during respiratory viral infections,[31,32] or in dogs after exposure to ozone,[33] and it was suggested that this reflex relied on an ecosanoid product from the epithelial cells. Prostaglandin or thromboxane newly released from activated neutrophils can act directly on airway smooth muscle or nerves to increase responsiveness.[34]

Epithelial injury can thus directly increase hyperreactivity of bronchial smooth muscle. This is an important clinical response, and because it occurs, albeit temporarily, in people who are not asthmatics, it would be well to understand it. Control of the response by an antagonist would improve treatment of airway infection and might also help to establish whether such injury contributes to, or is directly responsible for, the asthma diathesis. Is this one way in which acquired asthma develops? Is it the same pathogenesis as for the inherited diathesis? Is there a common functional disturbance between the 'soggy epithelium' described in chronic asthmatics and the acute injury of the experimental model?

Neural effect

Surface epithelium, as well as all airway coats and their included structures, are well supplied with nerves (Figure 2.4).[5] It is unlikely that there is a neural role in the development of the diathesis, because direct studies of nerve fibres, and of bronchial smooth muscle, have not indicated any abnormality. Neural effects have been provoked experimentally. Inflammatory mediators affecting blood vessel walls lead to congestion and oedema of the airway wall.[35-37] Oedema and increased susceptibility to BHR after infection have been reported. Oedema of the wall causes a narrowing of the lumen which has a greater effect in small, compared to large, airways.[38]

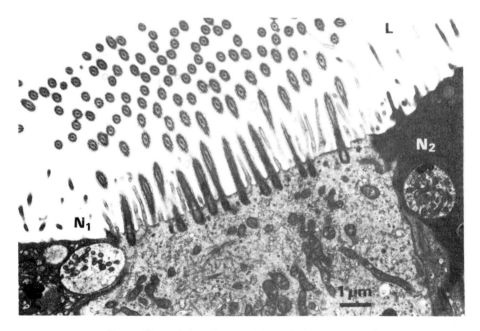

Fig. 2.4 Transmission electronmicrograph showing normal airway epithelium from a normal control subject. Two nerve profiles are located between ciliated and goblet cells close to the airway lumen. The nerve profiles contain many mitochondria, neurotubules, and vesicles. L, lumen; N_1 and N_2, nerve profiles; magnification × 13 000. (Reproduced with permission from Laitinen LA, Heino M, Laitinen A, Kava T, Haahtela T. Damage of the airway epithelium and bronchial reactivity in patients with asthma. *Am Rev Respir Dis* 1985;131:599–606.)

The neural role is speculative. It may, again, be a mechanism of amplification. A neural reflex is unlikely to be important in the development of the diathesis, as studies of bronchial smooth muscle behaviour suggest that the fibres are normal. A role for neural pathways in the characteristics of an attack, be it oedema or bronchial constriction, however, *is* likely.

Healing of bronchial epithelial damage

The understanding and control of asthma requires knowledge not only of amplification, but also of resolution, of the inflammatory process involved. What are the interactions, the stimuli, that convert 'protection' to disease, maintaining or amplifying inflammation after the cause is removed?

The mechanisms behind the destruction, turnover, and repair of bronchial epithelium are not known, but, at other sites, it seems that fibronectin and related substances have an important role in the healing of epithelial ulcers. Fibronectin is the term for a group of structurally and immunologically related high molecular weight glycoproteins that are present in plasma and extracellular matrix. It is important in cell–cell and cell–matrix interactions. *In vitro*, its secretion mediates adhesion of cultured cells to non-biological material.[39] *In vivo*, fibronectin seems to help migration and adhesion of cells on biological surfaces.[40,41] After tissue injury fibronectin can be identified at the site.[42–45]

In the cornea, fibronectin is rapidly deposited, together with fibrin, at the basement membrane, where it is thought to serve as a natural glue anchoring the epithelial cells.[46,47] These are temporary components of the extracellular matrix during healing of the wound, and fibronectin has been used therapeutically to enhance corneal resurfacing.[48,49] It is, however, susceptible to even mild proteolytic activity.

The presence of fibronectin in the bronchial mucosa of eight non-smoking asthmatic patients and two control subjects was investigated by light and electron microscopy using a fluorescence antibody (Laitinen A *et al.*, unpublished observations). In asthmatic patients the basement membrane was thickened, with fibronectin located superficially. In the basement membrane beneath healthy epithelium (whether in control subjects or mild asthmatics) no reaction was identified; but at the bottom of an ulcer, or in epithelium adjacent to such an ulcer, there was fluorescence at the basement membrane. Where epithelial loss was complete, sometimes no immunoreaction was identified. The presence of fibronectin in ulcerated epithelium in these asthmatics suggests that in the airway epithelium also this compound may have a role in wound healing.

FATAL CASES OF ASTHMA

Pathological findings in asthma in a forensic population

Deaths due to allergic bronchial asthma are uncommon among hospital admissions. However, a recent review of a coroner's necropsies indicated that deaths due to asthma were more common than generally expected.[50-52] In a recent study, Kleinerman and Adelson[50] analysed the histological findings in the lungs of the cases recorded as bronchial asthma. Using standardised semiquantitative methods, they were able to verify the presence of acceptable histological criteria for the diagnosis of allergic bronchial asthma, and evaluated the severity and extent of these asthmatic lesions. They also determined the presence of evidence for other disease in the lungs of the subjects dying from asthma, and compared their findings with those from appropriately matched control groups from the same coroner's population.

The available histological slides and the necropsy protocols of 39 deaths from the files of the coroner's office of Cuyahoga County, (coded according to the International Classification of Disease as Code 112, Asthma) comprised the index cases. These necropsies were performed between January 1979 and April 1986. A similar number of control cases matched for age, sex, and race were selected from deaths occurring during the same period. The eight histopathological criteria listed below were selected for analysis.

1 Infiltration of bronchial and bronchiolar walls by eosinophils (BE).

2 Bronchial and bronchiolar smooth muscle hypertrophy (SMH).

3 Bronchial epithelial desquamation (ED).

4 Bronchial and bronchiolar mucus plugs (MP).

5 Bronchial epithelial goblet cell metaplasia (GCM).

6 Bronchial and bronchiolar basement membrane thickening (BMT).

7 Infiltration of lung parenchyma by eosinophils or eosinophilic pneumonia.

8 Chronic respiratory bronchiolitis (CRB).

The lesion caused by CRB is composed of clusters of large alveolar macrophages, containing brown granular material, in the alveolar spaces opening from a respiratory bronchiolus. The respiratory bronchiolar wall may be thickened, contain a small number of chronic inflammatory cells and have an abnormal epithelial surface. This lesion has been observed in young cigarette smokers and has been regarded as a precursor of centriacinar emphysema.

For every index and control case, five slides, each holding one section of lung and bronchus, were evaluated. Grading of each of the above criteria was performed semiquantitatively on a scale of o to $+4$, with o as no evidence of the lesion and $+4$ as the most intense lesion observed. In all slides in every case, each criterion was graded and severity of the lesions in the large bronchi, membranous bronchi, and respiratory bronchioli evaluated. The total intensity for each airway size was then divided by the number of airways of that type to obtain the mean value of intensity for that section. Thus, a mean value for intensity of bronchial eosinophilia in large bronchi, in membranous bronchi and in respiratory bronchioli was determined for each slide. The case mean was then calculated for each parameter, and for the three bronchial groups, by summing the intensity mean for all five slides and dividing by five. Finally, a grand mean for each parameter and bronchial or bronchiolar size was calculated by summing the mean values for each case and dividing the total number of asthmatic cases by 39. A similar semiquantitative analysis was performed on the control slides.

The grand means of all 39 asthma and 39 control groups were subjected to statistical analysis by two non-parametric methods,[53] the Wilcoxon Rank sum test and the Mann–Whitney U test, using the NPAR test of the SPSS/PC program.* The results were obtained in terms of a two-tailed t test. A P value equal to, or less than, 0.05 was regarded as significant.

A total of 197 large cartilaginous bronchi, 375 membranous or non-cartilaginous bronchi and 583 respiratory bronchioli were studied in the 39 index cases. A similar number of airways was studied in the control group.

Little or no clinical data are available with which to correlate these pathological findings. All patients died suddenly either at home or in a public place without benefit of medical attention. The ages of the asthmatics ranged from seven to 60; 24 patients were black, 15 were white, the male to female ratio was one to 1.7, and five of the 39 patients were children.

Analysis identified the criteria that were most useful for the diagnosis of asthma. Infiltration of bronchial walls by eosinophils, bronchial and bronchiolar muscle hypertrophy, and basement membrane thickening were found significantly more often in asthmatics than in controls. These are considered to be classic histopathological findings in patients with allergic bronchial asthma.[54,55] Neither epithelial desquamation nor goblet cell metaplasia were found more often in the asthmatics than in controls. Airway plugging with mucus was found more often in respiratory bronchioli of asthmatics than in the cartilaginous bronchi, but it was only in the non-cartilaginous airways and

---

*SPSS/PC+ V2.0 *Base Manual, Nonparametic Tests; Procedure NPAR Tests.* Chapter 16, B-177–197, Norusis/SPSS.

the bronchioli that mucus plugs were found more often in asthmatics than in controls. The possibility that resuscitative manoeuvres or tissue handling had shifted this mucus cannot be excluded.

In 27 of the 39 cases of asthma, a striking eosinophilic infiltration was found in the alveolar spaces in the vicinity of airways. This was found in the lung adjacent to non-cartilaginous airways. This is different from the diffuse or chronic eosinophilic pneumonia that is distributed more widely through lung tissue. This 'splinting' of airway wall by periairway consolidation might change the physical properties of the airways sufficiently to contribute to airway obstruction.[56]

The CRB associated with cigarette smoking was found as often in asthmatics as in controls. It suggests that there was a similar number of patients smoking in both groups and that the habit of cigarette smoking is not a factor in provoking or increasing fatal asthmatic episodes.

These findings are consistent with the results reported in the biopsy study. Eosinophils tend to inhabit the periphery except during an acute attack when central airways are also affected. The alveolar component is detected in the BAL fluid even when not present in large airway tissue. Epithelial desquamation is not a distinguishing feature of these cases. Neither cigarette smoking nor obstruction by retained mucus differentiates these asthmatics from the control cases. These deaths, then, are different from those in 'the classic' cases of death from asthma—that is, cases of status asthmaticus which are typical of a hospital population.

In spite of the impression given by published findings, the pathological findings in patients who die from asthma vary widely. Three recognisable patterns point to differences in the pathophysiological basis of an attack of asthma, and therefore of death, and perhaps to the clinical subset of asthma.[57,58]

Endobronchial mucus plugging—suffocation

Death occurs from suffocation because of blockage of the airways by mucus.[57,58] This type of death is typically described as status asthmaticus.[54,59] It occurs in patients who die in hospital after some days of treatment for asthma, and the findings are virtually identical with those already published. The airways are plugged with a secretion that is highly viscid and extremely difficult to remove except by cutting. Microscopically, the luminal mucus is often seen to be continuous with the intracellular mucus.

Sudden death from asthma with empty airways

At the other extreme is the known asthmatic who dies suddenly in an acute attack and whose airways are empty of mucus.[57,58] Even if some evidence of allergy is present—eosinophils in tissue or thickened airway basement membrane—no mechanical reason for the obstruction is found. Therefore, if the patient had clinical airways obstruction before death then this may represent sudden marked bronchial constriction. This may be caused by an over-whelming dose of antigen, or, drug treatment that, while adequate for a hospital regimen, may not be adequate for the home environment. This is exemplified by a patient who, in hospital, was in an excellent condition, but once returned home, was *in extremis* within a couple of hours and died in the ambulance while returning to hospital. At necropsy this patient had empty or dry airways.

Cardiac arrhythmia could cause sudden death with or without major airway symptoms.[60] Thus empty airways could also be found if the cause of death is cardiac or the result of drug sensitivity. Myocardial contraction bands have been described in which a pattern of necrosis is seen which is different from that of myocardial infarction.[61] Myocardial contraction band necrosis is characterised by transverse bands that are densely eosinophilic and alternate with lighter staining granular cytoplasm. It occurs in association with intracranial trauma, with severe emotional states, after administration of large amounts of adrenergic agents and, from reperfusion after coronary block. It is possible that myocardial contraction band necrosis may cause cardiac arryth-mia, or, alternatively, increase the susceptibility of the heart to certain drugs.

The clinical picture is important in interpreting the importance of empty airways. In status asthmaticus cardiac arrhythmia could be the actual cause of death although, if airway mucus is abundant, the cardiac lesion may well be missed. To determine whether heart failure is the cause, microscopic examination of the heart is essential and so should be performed in all fatal cases of asthma.

Unexpected death in asthma with mild mucus plugging

Between deaths due to mucus plugging of the airways and those associated with empty airways is the mild degree of mucus accumulation. Perhaps the patient was not 'at their best', but certainly the clinical features were not severe enough to prepare family or medical attendants for rapid deterioration and death. Understanding the death of these patients often depends on anecdotal evidence. One particular patient played football in the afternoon, wheezed a little in the evening, took some medicine, but died within an hour or two, having clearly had airways obstruction (CAO) as the major symptom in the hours before death. In such a case there may be definite, even if not severe, mucus plugging as evidence of mechanical obstruction. The findings suggest that a couple of hours before death, when the patient seemed asymptomatic, the clinical condition was not optimal. Either the treatment regimen was inadequate or, within the previous hours to days, something had changed to render a suitable regimen inappropriate. An acute infection or an overwhelming dose of allergen would suffice.

Even in some patients admitted to hospital, death occurs quite quickly and rather unexpectedly. A known asthmatic may have increasing respiratory problems, but not enough to unduly concern either the patient, the family, or the physician, and can die 'unexpectedly' in hospital. Such a patient is probably better represented in the forensic population reported above than in hospital reports, but such cases are increasingly being seen in hospital. In this setting it is sometimes difficult to convince the pathologist and then the physician, that a cause of death is provided by findings in the lung, so conditioned are we to the typically reported picture of status asthmaticus. This apparent contradiction leads to analysis of the pathophysiology of an attack of asthma and of death in the patient with asthma.

PATHOPHYSIOLOGY OF THE SIGNS AND SYMPTOMS OF ASTHMA

The symptoms of wheezing and sputum production are related to the following pathological findings: CAO, mucus secretion, and turgesence of airway walls, from congestion or oedema. Cough reflects irritation/stimulation of nerve receptors.

Mechanisms contributing to the pathophysiology of airway narrowing in asthma

Bronchial constriction is often equated to airway narrowing, but as mentioned elsewhere, the responsiveness of the muscle cell *in vitro* seems to be no greater than normal. And so the hypothesis that exaggerated smooth muscle shortening is the only important change is untenable because several studies have failed to show a correlation between *in vivo* airway responsiveness and *in vitro* smooth muscle sensitivity.[62-64] These studies indicate that the BHR which characterises asthma is a property of intact airways, and that abnormal behaviour of airway smooth muscle is only one factor contributing to this abnormal response. An alternative hypothesis—that the thickening of airway walls associated with the chronic inflammatory process gives rise to exaggerated changes in airway calibre when the smooth muscle shortens normally—has been put forward by several authors.[65,66] An analysis of this hypothesis showed that small changes in airway

wall thickness which have little effect on baseline airways resistance, can considerably increase airway responsiveness to inhaled
agonists.[67]

In a series of studies, Hogg and his co-workers have tested
this hypothesis. They showed that the internal perimeter and wall
area of airways remain constant at different lung volumes and
with different degrees of airway smooth muscle shortening.[68,69]
Recently, they used this information to measure airways of
different size, reconstruct their relaxed dimensions, and calculate
the degree of muscle shortening required to occlude the airway
lumen.[70] These findings are reviewed here with reference to the
relative importance of wall thickness and smooth muscle shortening to BHR in asthma. The data suggest that the inflammatory
process is important in asthma, and that both the exudate and the
proliferation of interstitial connective tissue in the repair process
thicken the submucosa.

The 'control' studies of airway contraction and wall thickness
were performed on lung tissue obtained from lobes resected
because of a solitary peripheral lung carcinoma.[69] The resected
specimens were inflated with Krebs' solution, bisected in the
sagittal plane, and each half was placed in Krebs' solution
containing either supersaturated theophylline or carbachol
10^{-3} M for 30 minutes at room temperature. The Krebs'
solution was then replaced with 2.5% buffered glutaraldehyde
and the specimens were left in this fixative for 24 hours. After
fixation, blocks of tissue containing large and small airways were
taken from the apposing cut surfaces of the specimens to observe
the effect of relaxation and contraction on airways from a similar
region of the same lung.

Histological studies were also made on lung specimens obtained
at necropsy from 18 patients with asthma.[70] These patients
ranged in age from nine to 71 years (34 ± 23; mean $\pm$ SD) and
had a diagnosis of asthma which was based on a history of
recurrent wheeze and shortness of breath. Seventeen of these
patients were classified as having severe asthma (steroid dependent, frequent hospital admissions, and/or one or more admissions requiring ventilatory assistance), and one patient as 'mild'
(occasional use of bronchodilators). Asthma was the cause of
death in 11 cases and death was sudden and unexplained
(probably from asthma) in four others. The causes of death in the
remaining three patients were carbon monoxide poisoning, pulmonary embolus, and anaphylaxis after administration of radio-
opaque contrast material. Airways from 23 patients who

CHAPTER 2
Pathology

53

had died suddenly without evidence of chronic or acute lung disease at necropsy served as controls.

The airway dimensions measured (Figure 2.5) included the internal perimeter (Pi) and internal area (Ai) defined by the luminal surface of the epithelium, and the external perimeter (Pe) and external area (Ae) defined by the outer border of the smooth muscle. Where the smooth muscle was discontinuous, the external perimeter was interpolated between the ends of the adjacent portions of muscle. In cartilaginous bronchi where the muscle is present only in portions of the airway perimeter, the interpolation was made in the border between the dense and loose connective tissue underlying the cartilage. Wall area (WA) was calculated by

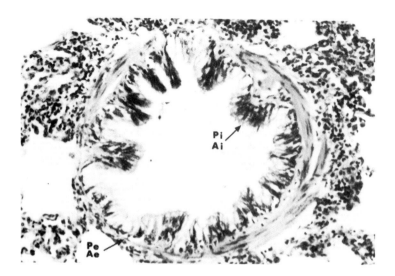

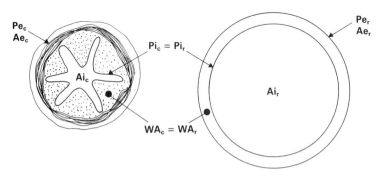

Fig. 2.5 Data showing a photomicrograph and schematic drawing of a membranous bronchiole illustrating measurements which were made. Pi, internal perimeter; Ai, internal area; Pe, external perimeter; Ae, external area; WA, wall area; c, contracted; r, relaxed. Because $Pi_c = Pi_r$ and $WA_c = WA_r$ the 'relaxed' airway dimensions can be calculated using the measured dimensions of the contracted airway. (Reproduced with permission from James AL, Pare PD, Hogg JC. Mechanisms of airway narrowing in asthma. *Am Rev Respir Dis* (in press).)

subtracting internal area from external area (WA = Ae − Ai). In the studies of asthmatic lungs,[70] WA was normalised for each airway by expressing it as a portion of its own 'relaxed/dilated' external area. The degree of muscle shortening present in the observed airway was calculated as the change in muscle length from the relaxed airway dimension to that measured in the tissue specimen and the degree of muscle shortening required to produce airway closure was calculated as the change from the relaxed dimension to the muscle length when the lumen area is reduced to zero.

The effect of airway wall thickening on airway responsiveness was estimated by calculating the increase in airway resistance which would occur with varying degrees of smooth muscle shortening, where airways resistance was calculated using the equation from Moreno *et al.*[67]

Study of resected lungs

The data showed that treatment of the resected lungs with carbachol 10^{-3} M produced contraction of both large and small airways and caused the luminal area to decrease and the mucosal surface to fold (Figure 2.5). It also showed that when the square root of WA was plotted against Pi (Figure 2.6) there was a linear relationship.

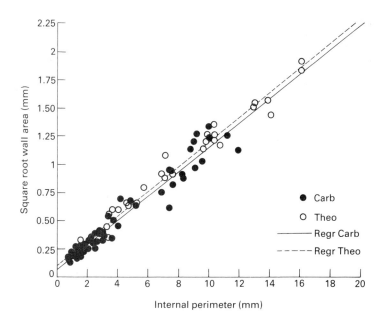

Fig. 2.6 Linear relationship between the square root of wall area and the internal perimeter of airways when they are either contracted with carbacholamine or relaxed with theophylline. (Reproduced with permission from James AL, Hogg JC, Dunn LA, Pare PD. The use of internal perimeter to compare airway size and calculate smooth muscle shortening. *Am Rev Respir Dis* 1988;**138**:136–9.)

The absolute wall areas of airways from asthmatic patients were greater than those of non-asthmatic patients. In the membranous bronchioli measuring less than 2 mm in internal perimeter, mean ($\pm$ SD) airway wall area was 0.065 ± 0.049 mm^2 in the asthmatic patient and 0.044 ± 0.017 mm^2 in the non-asthmatic patients. For membranous airways greater than 2 mm internal perimeter and both groups of cartilaginous airways, wall areas were 0.444 ± 0.379 mm^2, 1.852 ± 0.139 mm^2 and 4.486 ± 3.209 mm^2 for asthmatic patients, and 0.176 ± 0.079 mm^2, 0.458 ± 0.324 mm^2, and 1.728 ± 1.221 mm^2 for non-asthmatic patients, respectively ($P < 0.05$ for all four groups). In the asthmatic, compared to control, patients, the WA relative to the relaxed external area was greater in both the membranous and cartilaginous airways ($P < 0.001$) (Figure 2.7).

The areas of epithelium, submucosa and muscle were greater in the airways of asthmatic patients except for the area of muscle in membranous bronchioli less than 2 mm Pi (Table 2.2). The sections of airways of the asthmatic patients were infiltrated with inflammatory cells and there was thickening of the basement membrane, mucous gland and goblet cell prominence and partial occlusion of the lumen with mucus and cellular debris. There was

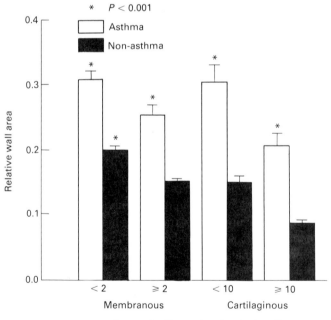

Fig. 2.7 Relative wall areas of the different size groups of airways of non-asthmatic and asthmatic subjects (mean $\pm$ SE). (Reproduced with permission from James AL, Pare PD, Hogg JC. Mechanisms of airway narrowing in asthma. *Am Rev Respir Dis* (in press).)

Table 2.2 Area (mm²) of epithelium, submucosa and muscle in the airway walls of non-asthmatic and asthmatic subjects

	Membranous airway (internal perimeter)		Cartilaginous airway (internal perimeter)	
	< 2 mm	> 2 mm	< 10 mm	> 10 mm
Epithelium				
Asthma	0.030 ± 0.022**	0.156 ± 0.084**	0.46 ± 0.22**	0.88 ± 0.30*
Non-asthma	0.018 ± 0.006	0.069 ± 0.037	0.18 ± 0.09	0.56 ± 0.29
Submucosa				
Asthma	0.020 ± 0.020**	0.135 ± 0.134*	0.73 ± 0.45**	1.35 ± 0.87**
Non-asthma	0.010 ± 0.004	0.049 ± 0.037	0.20 ± 0.18	0.71 ± 0.54
Muscle				
Asthma	0.015 ± 0.012	0.152 ± 0.177*	0.67 ± 0.45**	1.57 ± 0.87**
Non-asthma	0.014 ± 0.007	0.051 ± 0.031	0.14 ± 0.09	0.46 ± 0.39

*$P < 0.05$.
**$P < 0.01$ compared to non-asthmatic group.
Values are mean ± SD.

also pronounced folding of the epithelium in some airways with a prominent circular layer of muscle.

The calculated muscle shortening required to cause airway closure was less ($P < 0.001$) in the asthmatic patients than in the non-asthmatic patients.[70] Figure 2.8 shows that smooth muscle shortening of 40% results in about a 15-fold increase in resistance of the 'airway' of the non-asthmatic subjects; the same degree

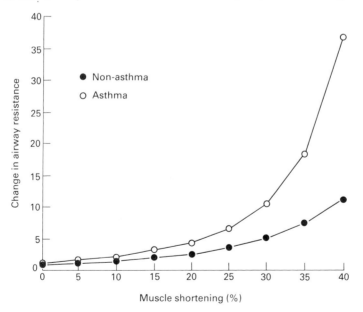

Fig. 2.8 Changes in resistance of cartilaginous airways (Pi < 10 mm) calculated using the mean dimensions measured in non-asthmatic and asthmatic subjects. (Reproduced with permission from James AL, Pare PD, Hogg JC. Mechanisms of airway narrowing in asthma. *Am Rev Respir Dis* (in press).)

of muscle shortening caused about a 290-fold increase in resistance (data point off scale) in the 'airway' of the asthmatic subjects. The increases in resistance with 40% smooth muscle shortening for the 'airways' of asthmatic subjects were 256-, 72-, and 37-fold for membranous airways of < 2 mm, membranous airways of > 2 mm, and cartilaginous bronchi of > 10 mm Pi, respectively. Corresponding values for the airways of non-asthmatic subjects showed 20-, 13-, and nine-fold increases in the resistance of these airways.

An important feature of asthma is the rapid reversibility of airway obstruction with drugs that relax smooth muscle. Although this bronchodilatation is usually attributed to a reversal of excessive smooth muscle contraction, this need not be the case. Smooth muscle shortening within the normal range acting in tandem with a thickened airway wall, would have the same effect on airway calibre as excessive muscle shortening with a normal wall. In both cases, reversing the muscle contraction would increase airway calibre and rapidly lower resistance. Because increased wall thickness has been a feature of several studies of asthmatic assays,[71] and there is little or no evidence for abnormal smooth muscle function in hyperresponsive airways[62–64], it seems prudent to consider that the major problem in the asthmatic airways may be the wall thickening associated with the chronic inflammatory process. These and other studies show that this thickening is due to cellular infiltration, deposition of connective tissue, hypertrophy of smooth muscle, goblet cell metaplasia of the epithelium, and an inflammatory exudate containing mucus in the airway lumen.[71–82] These findings strongly suggest that the treatment of asthma should focus on drugs that will reverse the inflammatory changes responsible for the thickening of the airway wall and the exudate into the lumen, as well as on those that relax airway smooth muscle.

Markers of disease

It is important to identify the markers of the asthma diathesis and of an asthma attack. Mast cells within the epithelium of large airways, and eosinophils in the peripheral small ones, seem to indicate the presence of the asthma diathesis. Their great increase in number and activity point to a prominent role for eosinophils during an attack. In considering the asthma diathesis, it seems that eosinophils are capable of inducing BHR, but whether this is transient or long-term is a critical question still to be answered. Here we are mainly concerned with considering their role in an attack, and their response to an allergen or to other laboratory stimuli.

Since the early part of this century, it has been known that

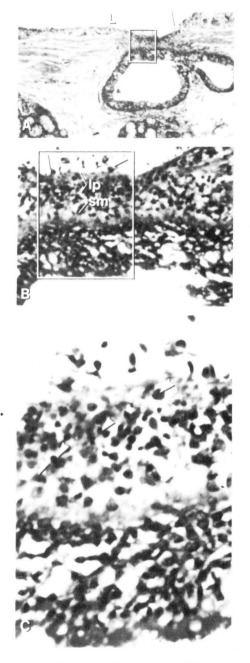

Fig. 2.9 Sputum samples from patients with asthma. (A) elongated ciliated cells (arrowhead) desquamated from bronchial epithelium. When cells are viewed in a wet preparation, the cilia are often extremely motile, propelling themselves in a circular path. (Papanicolaou stain; original magnification × 300.) (B) Creola body, a compact cluster of epithelial cells shed from the bronchial epithelium. (Papanicolaou stain.) (C) Charcot–Leyden crystals (arrowheads) and eosinophils identified by their large refractile granules and bilobed nuclei. (Original magnification × 400.) (Reproduced with permission from Frigas E, Gleich GJ. The eosinophil and the pathophysiology of asthma. *J Allergy Clin Immunol* 1986;77:527.)

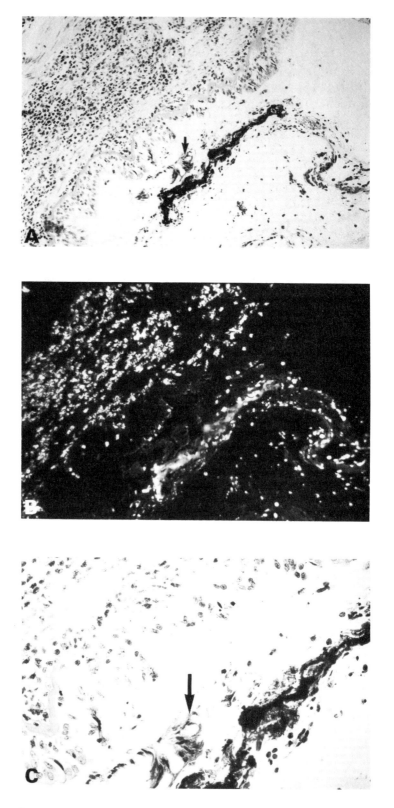

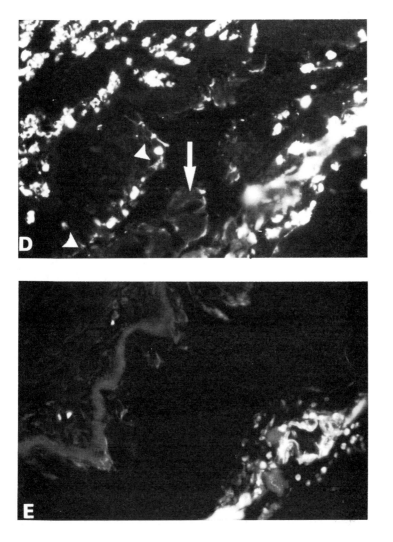

Fig. 2.10 Photomicrographs showing localisation of MBP in lung epithelium of a patient dying of asthma. (A) Haematoxylin and eosin-stained epithelium with striking submucosal eosinophil infiltration and a cluster of desquamated epithelial cells in the bronchial lumen (arrow) next to a 'stringy' deposit of a black-appearing substance, presumably soot. (Original magnification × 160.) (B) Section stained by MBP by immunofluorescence showing bright staining of eosinophils in the submucosa. There is also MBP staining of the epithelial cells on their luminal surfaces. (Original magnification × 160.) (C) Higher power view of A illustrating areas of mainly intact epithelium (left) and desquamated epithelium (top centre). Note the thickened basement membrane zone and the cluster of desquamated epithelial cells (arrow). (Original magnification × 400.) (D) Higher power view of B showing MBP deposition on the desquamated epithelial cells (arrow). Note deposition of MBP on the luminal surfaces and outlining the more superficial epithelial cells (arrowheads). (Original magnification × 400.) (E) A control section stained with normal rabbit IgG. There is rather bright, non-specific staining of the soot noted in (A) and weaker staining of the basement membrane zone. (Reproduced with permission from Gleich GJ, Flavahan NA, Fujisawa T, Vanhoutte PM. The eosinophil as a mediator of damage to respiratory epithelium; a model for bronchial hyperreactivity. *J Allergy Clin Immunol* 1988;81:776.)

bronchial asthma is sometimes associated with eosinophilia of the blood and lung,[83] and in the 1970s it was reported that peripheral blood eosinophilia was inversely correlated with the severity of asthma, as measured by FEV_1 (Figure 2.9).[84] These associations stimulated study of a toxic protein released from the eosinophil granule—namely, MBP—as a result of respiratory epithelial damage.[85-87] The epithelial damage and desquamation caused by MBP are remarkably similar to the pathological changes in asthma,[88] and so sputum MBP concentrations of patients with various inflammatory diseases, including asthma, were measured (Figure 2.10).[87] Sputum MBP concentrations in patients with asthma had a geometric mean of 8 µg/ml and ranged as high as 93 µg/ml; *in vitro* MBP concentrations as low as 10 µg/ml caused damage to tracheal rings.[86] Treatment of patients with asthma brings about an improvement in measurements of airflow with a concomitant drop in the sputum MBP concentration.[87] Immunofluorescence staining of specimens from patients dying from asthma showed that MBP is deposited at sites of damage to bronchial epithelium, in mucus plugs and in amorphous deposits beneath the epithelium.[20] Such evidence for eosinophils as mediators of damage in asthma has been reviewed elsewhere in more detail.[89-92]

EOSINOPHIL GRANULE PROTEINS AND DAMAGE TO RESPIRATORY EPITHELIUM

Eosinophil granule proteins

There are four principal basic proteins in the eosinophil granule: MBP, eosinophil-derived neurotoxin (EDN), eosinophil cationic protein (ECP),[92] and eosinophil peroxidase (EPO).

MBP has a molecular weight of about 14 000 and is very basic with an isoelectric point of almost 11.[93] It contains 17 arginines —accounting for its basic properties—and nine half-cysteines. At least four reactive sulphydryl groups are present and this could explain its noticeable propensity to aggregate with itself and with other proteins. The functions of MBP, especially its toxicity to parasites and mammalian cells and its stimulation of histamine release from basophils and mast cells, have been reviewed elsewhere.[92]

EDN and ECP have been partially sequenced to about residue 62.[94,95] In their sequence analysis EDN and ECP display remarkable homology—37 of the first 55 residues are identical (67% homology, including the four cysteine residues). Surprisingly, both EDN and ECP sequences show pronounced homology to ribonuclease from various species.[94] Subsequent study shows what both ECP and EDN possess ribonuclease activity as judged by spectrophotometric analysis of acid soluble nucleotides formed from yeast RNA.[96,97] Finally, EPO has been partially sequenced and its light chain distinguished from MBP.[98] EPO in combination with H_2O_2 and halide kills a variety of micro-organisms.[92] To date, the preferred halide seems to be iodide *in vitro*, but recent studies indicate that EPO preferentially uses the bromide that is present in physiological fluids.[99]

Effects of eosinophil granule proteins on respiratory epithelium—species comparison

The cationic MBP damages both guinea-pig and human respiratory epithelium,[85-87] as well as human and rat pneumocytes.[100] Because eosinophils possess several cationic proteins, their effects were tested on guinea-pig epithelium and compared with the cytotoxic effects of MBP.[101] Comparison of native MBP (with reactive sulphydryl groups) and alkylated MBP (whose sulphydryl groups are not reactive) indicates that native MBP produces the same effects as the mildly reduced and alkylated MBP. The same changes—namely, exfoliation of respiratory epithelial cells, bleb formation in epithelial cells, and partial or complete ciliostasis—were produced by both forms of MBP. A test of the effect of ECP showed that concentrations lower than 100 µg/ml caused no visible changes in the tracheal rings, while 100 µ/ml (5.4×10^{-6} M) caused exfoliation of cells; this was less pronounced than that caused by either form of MBP. Surprisingly, EDN, which is strikingly similar to ECP in amino acid sequence and in possessing ribonuclease activity, did not alter the rings even at concentrations up to 200 µg/ml (1.1×10^{-5} M).

Analysis of the effects of the EPO + H_2O_2 + halide system on guinea-pig tracheal epithelium indicated that EPO in the presence of H_2O_2, and chloride (0.11 M) or iodide (10^{-4} M), causes exfoliation, bleb formation, and ciliostasis. These effects were reduced or lost by deletion of EPO itself (as by heating of EPO, by deletion of glucose oxidase, and by addition of catalase). These findings agree with those of Agosti *et al.* who previously showed that the EPO + glucose oxidate + glucose + halide system is toxic to pneumocytes.[102] While 10 U/ml of EPO by itself caused only slight bleb formation, addition of 50 U/ml EPO, caused partial ciliostatis and bleb formation, suggesting that EPO itself might be toxic. Increasing concentrations of EPO caused dose-related damage to the epithelium, but there is about a 30-fold reduction in the toxic potency of EPO when it acts alone compared with its effect in the presence of H_2O_2 and halide. These results indicate that MBP, ECP, and EPO are each toxic to respiratory epithelium or pneumocytes.

Mechanisms for MBP injury of respiratory epithelium

Early studies showed that MBP abolishes ciliary activity of respiratory mucosa.[85–87] This effect was restudied by analysing the rate of ciliary beat using rabbit tracheal rings.[103] Application of native human MBP at 100 µg/ml (7×10^{-6} M) reduces the rate of ciliary beat in the rings but more strikingly reduces the zones of ciliary activity. Studies on isolated axonemes indicated that the effect of MBP is to inhibit the adenosine triphosphatase (ATPase) activity necessary for the ciliary function.

The effect of MBP on the electrical properties of respiratory epithelium has been studied using tracheal membranes of dogs mounted in Ussing chambers.[23] Addition of MBP (5×10^{-6} M) to the mucosal side of the membrane produced an increase in short circuit current and net chloride secretion. In contrast, exposure of the submucosal surface to MBP (5×10^{-6} M), did not alter short circuit current. The effect of MBP on the tracheal epithelium was evidently not cytotoxic because lactic dehydrogenase was not detected in the solution bathing the mucosal epithelium after exposure to MBP. In patients with acute asthma, MBP could contribute to a change in airway secretions and ciliary function by stimulating the airway epithelial chloride and water secretion.

Asthma and bronchial eosinophilia

If eosinophils damage tissues in asthma, their presence and activity should correlate with markers of the severity of asthma such as BHR. Three studies have shown a correlation between peripheral blood eosinophilia and BHR,[104–106] but a more direct manner of assessment is with eosinophils and their products in bronchial secretions. Striking bronchial eosinophilia was found in patients with extrinsic asthma and idiosyncratic reactions to aspirin; indeed, in fluids from these patients, only eosinophils were increased.[18] Subsequently, BAL has been performed in asthmatics in whom allergen challenge induced late phase reactions, and in patients with chronic symptomatic asthma without such provocation.

Late phase asthmatic reactions

The late phase reaction after allergen challenge has been reviewed by O'Byrne *et al.*[107] During the time of the late phase reaction eosinophils are increased in the BAL fluid; this was associated with an increased ECP:albumin ratio in the fluid, suggesting that eosinophils degranulate during the late reaction.[22] (An increase in numbers of neutrophils in BAL fluid was not found in this study.)

Secondly, of 12 atopic patients studied 'out of season' after bronchoprovocation with allergen, the results were compared with those in five normal subjects.[108] Within four hours of allergen exposure, the number of neutrophils significantly increased in BAL fluid. The number of eosinophils was significantly increased at both four and 24 hours. Transmission electron photomicrographs showed that in the cells from the asthmatic patients there was degranulation of mast cells and loss of core material from eosinophils. Similar changes were observed in the patients with allergic asthma during spontaneous environmental exposures. It seems that eosinophils and neutrophils infiltrate the bronchi after bronchoprovocation,[108] and it is the eosinophils that remain.

Thirdly, the cellular changes of BAL fluid after the late asthmatic reaction include, as well as an increase in eosinophils, an increase in the sloughed bronchial epithelial cells, and in degenerated cells—mainly epithelial cells and macrophages. Increased vascular permeability was shown by an increase in albumin in the BAL fluid. A significant increase in neutrophils was not found until 48 hours after bronchial challenge.[109]

Finally, in the late asthmatic reactions induced by toluene diisocyanate (TDI), the numbers of neutrophils are increased in the BAL fluid at two and eight hours after challenge, whereas eosinophils are increased only at eight hours. This is an important difference in the pattern of cell accumulation in this chemically induced reaction from that induced by allergen.

Spontaneous asthma

Since the first report of the findings in the BAL fluid of patients with asthma and idiosyncratic reactions to aspirin,[18] several additional studies have been conducted. Firstly, a study of ten patients with extrinsic asthma and 14 controls showed that numbers of mast cells and eosinophils were significantly increased in the BAL fluid.[110] Secondly, 10 'stable' asthmatics with airway hyperresponsiveness and 10 non-asthmatic subjects were investigated by studying their BAL fluid.[111] 'Metachromatic cells' and eosinophils were significantly increased in both the BAL fluid and the bronchial washings of asthmatics compared with non-asthmatics. In the asthmatics there was close correlation between the increased number of mast cells and increased BHR, and to a lesser extent, with the eosinophils in BAL fluid. Measurement of the MBP in lavage and blood did not differentiate between asthmatics and non-asthmatics. This study concluded that there is evidence of cellular inflammation in the airways of stable asthmatics which involves both metachromatic cells and eosinophils, but not the MBP.

Thirdly, BAL was performed on 17 mild atopic asthmatics (nine of whom were symptomatic, and eight asymptomatic), and 14 non-asthmatic controls (including six patients with hay fever and eight non-atopic subjects).[15] A significant increase in the percentage of mast cells in both groups of asthmatics was observed, although the counts were no different than those previously reported in a number of other respiratory diseases such as sarcoidosis and fibrosing alveolitis.[112] Patients with asthma with BHR showed significant increases in spontaneous histamine release from luminal mast cells. Significant increases in the eosinophil count and in the concentration of MBP in the BAL fluids were also found in the symptomatic asthmatics. The amounts of MBP recovered and the percentage of eosinophils in the fluid, were positively correlated. These changes were even more striking when asthmatics with BHR were compared with subjects with normoreactive airways. There was also a significant increase in the percentage of epithelial cells in the hyperreactive asthmatics. Inverse correlations between airway hyperreactivity (PC_{20} < 4 mg/ml) and the percentage of eosinophils, epithelial cells and the quantity of MBP in the BAL fluid, were observed. This study supports the hypothesis that BHR may be secondary to epithelial cell damage mediated through eosinophil-derived products. Thus, studies of spontaneous asthma have shown increases in both mast cells and eosinophils in the BAL fluids and have shown that BHR is inversely related to the numbers of mast cells, eosinophils, and epithelial cells.

Finally, in a continuing study of BAL fluid from patients with asthma, Godard *et al.* have reported that there were significant increases in the number of alveolar macrophages, lymphocytes, neutrophils, and eosinophils.[113] This contrasts with the findings of their earlier report[18] that the number of eosinophils alone were increased in patients with bronchial asthma and sensitivity to aspirin. This suggests that a variety of inflammatory cells are increased in number. It becomes important, therefore, to establish the timing of the accumulation of the cells and also any degranulation.

Late phase reactions in experimental animals

The rabbit model of the late asthmatic response has been extensively investigated by Larsen *et al.*[114] Rabbits immunised neonatally to *Alternaria tenuis* develop only IgE antibodies but they show both early and late phase asthmatic reactions. Both of these reactions can be passively transferred by serum rich in IgE antibodies. The presence of antigen specific IgG antibodies was not associated with the development of the late reactions: it even seemed to blunt an increase in pulmonary resistance during the late reaction.

The importance of polymorphonuclear leucocytes has been shown in this model, with experiments showing that neutropenia induced by administration of nitrogen mustard prevents the late asthmatic reaction. At the time of exposure to ragweed, transfusion with granulocytes (mainly neutrophils and some eosinophils) to granulocytopenic rabbits immunised to ragweed, restored the ability of these animals to develop a late asthmatic reaction. These studies suggest that cells of the granulocyte series, and especially neutrophils, are important in the late asthmatic reaction. On the other hand, study of the granulocytes infiltrating the bronchioli of control and immunised rabbits has shown that during the early response (30 minutes after antigen challenge) most granulocytes in the airway are neutrophils, but during the late response (six hours) 20–40% of the granulocytes are eosinophils in both control and immunised rabbits. Forty-eight hours after antigen exposure, eosinophils comprised more than 80% of the granulocytes in the animals with late asthmatic responses, but less than half of the granulocytes in the control rabbits. Thus the relative contribution of neutrophils and eosinophils in rabbits is still to be established.

The late asthmatic reaction has also been studied in guinea-pigs. Of guinea-pigs immunised with *Ascaris suum* extract, about 40% showed dual asthmatic reactions after challenge, the late reaction occurring three to six hours after the immediate one.[115] This suggests that there is a genetic factor in guinea-pigs which determines the presence of the double reaction. Analysis of BAL fluid of the guinea-pigs with late asthmatic reactions showed that neutrophils were increased in number, suggesting that it is these cells which are critical for expression of the late reaction. Examination of the lungs, however, showed that there was also eosinophil infiltration of the walls which was more prominent than in guinea-pigs with only the immediate reaction. Furthermore, no significant difference was found in the neutrophil infiltration within the airway walls between guinea-pigs with dual or with only an immediate reaction. This, therefore, points to an important role for eosinophils even in the late reaction. It also indicates that analysis of the inflammatory cells should be conducted not only by BAL, but also by biopsy of lung tissue.

Hutson *et al.* found two late phase asthmatic responses when guinea-pigs were immunised with ovalbumin by nebulisation —one at 17 hours and the other at 72 hours.[116] Study of BAL fluid showed a sevenfold increase in neutrophils at six hours and a 17-fold increase at 17 hours, after which the numbers of neutrophils returned to baseline. The eosinophilia in the BAL fluid developed gradually and until 17 hours was not significantly different in animals challenged with saline compared to those challenged with ovalbumin. By 72 hours, however, eosinophils constituted about half of the cells in BAL fluid. Histological examination showed progressive eosinophil infiltration of the respiratory tract, and electron microscopic examination at 17 hours showed loss of the eosinophil granule crystalline core substance—namely, MBP[117] and goblet cell mucus discharge.

During the late phase reaction in guinea-pigs, eosinophils were increased in number in BAL fluid by 18 hours after antigen challenge and remained significantly increased for seven days; at 17 hours the eosinophils accounted for 37% of the BAL leucocytes, at 54 hours for 30%, and at seven days for 31%.[118] Histologically, eight minutes after challenge peribronchial and peribronchiolar vessels showed a pronounced margination of eosinophils and neutrophils. By 30 minutes the eosinophils had migrated into the peribronchial and peribronchiolar connective tissue while the neutrophils had not left the blood vessels. By six and 18 hours, eosinophil infiltration around the peribronchial and peribronchiolar smooth muscle was intense; neutrophils and mononuclear cells were not prominent. By 18 hours, eosinophils had reached the lumen of the respiratory passages and they continued to infiltrate the smooth muscle and epithelium for up to seven days. These findings nicely corroborate those noted above,[115,116] and the authors concluded that eosinophils probably have a role in the late phase response.

Finally, elimination of circulating neutrophils by antisera to neutrophils in guinea-pigs did not inhibit the late reactions.[119] Their results suggest that although neutrophils infiltrate the lung during the peak of the late asthmatic reaction, their presence is not critical for the expression of the late asthmatic reaction. Thus the studies of late reactions in guinea-pigs[115,116,118,119] are in overall agreement in showing a major and clinically important role for eosinophils—at least in this species.

THE CREOLA BODY

Creola bodies and Charcot–Leyden crystals are found in the sputum of patients with asthma (Figure 2.9).[83,88,120–126] The Creola body was first called an epithelialzellballen by von Hoesslin in 1921,[127] and then rediscovered and renamed by Naylor in the 1960s.[128] In 1957, Naylor examined the sputum of a 44 year old patient admitted to the University of Michigan Medical School whose first name was Creola; she was wheezing and had pulmonary infiltrates on the chest radiograph. At first, carcinoma was diagnosed because of the hundreds of non-ciliated fragments of bronchial epithelium in the sputum, but at the bronchoscopy no abnormalities were found. Subsequently, sputum specimens, still reported as containing carcinoma cells, showed fewer clusters of cells, some ciliated, suggesting that the condition was benign and indicating that these cells were derived from surface bronchial epithelium rather than from solid glandular structures in the bronchial wall. Furthermore, the infiltrates, presumed to be neoplastic, were disappearing. The patient stopped wheezing and left hospital, somewhat perplexed by all the excitement her illness had generated. Naylor pursued the importance of the Creola bodies, the term he applied to the clusters of bronchial epithelial cells, and discovered that they were associated with bronchial asthma and were more common during an attack.[129]

The way a Creola body is formed remains obscure. The possibility that the eosinophil granule MBP is implicated was suggested by the finding that MBP causes desquamation of tracheal epithelial cells[85-87] and, subsequently, Creola bodies have been shown to be coated with MBP (Figure 2.10).[130] Attempts to determine whether expectorated Creola bodies in the sputum of patients with asthma are coated with MBP have been frustrated by the bright staining of the sputum itself. In other words, asthmatic sputum containing Creola bodies also contains sufficiently high concentrations of MBP to give bright immunoflurorescence staining for MBP, thus making it difficult to determine if the MBP is in the Creola bodies or simply coating it. Obviously, further study of the mechanism(s) of Creola body formation (and those of respiratory epithelial desquamation) are needed.

MECHANISM FOR INDUCTION OF BHR IN ASTHMA

The information summarised above indicates that damage to, and desquamation of, bronchial epithelial cells are regular features of asthma. Dysfunction, or loss, of respiratory epithelial cells can contribute to BHR in several ways.[131,132] Changing osmolarity of the surface mucosa,[132] or exposing underlying sensory nerves,[131] could stimulate a reflex to bronchoconstriction. Epithelial cells may also release a relaxing factor(s), causing relaxation of the underlying smooth muscle. Loss of epithelium leads to changed reactivity in canine bronchi; sensitivity of the smooth muscle to acetycholine, 5-hydroxytryptamine, and histamine increase and the relaxant effect of isoproterenol is reduced.[29] Preliminary support for the existence of diffusible epithelial-derived relaxing factor(s) was obtained in various bioassay studies.[29,133-140] By interfering with release of this relaxing factor, damage to the respiratory epithelial cells could cause hyperreactivity of bronchial smooth muscle.

To determine whether MBP might mediate increased respiratory smooth muscle reactivity, its effect on the contractility of rings of guinea-pig trachea was analysed. When muscle strips denuded of epithelium were incubated with histamine, with or without MBP, no effect was seen on muscle contractility. In contrast, the tension generated by graded doses of acetylcholine in rings of guinea-pig trachea incubated with MBP depended on whether the epithelium was intact (Figure 2.11). In the absence of epithelium MBP did not alter the effect of the drug. MBP, therefore, could inhibit release of the epithelial-derived relaxing factor or could stimulate generation of constrictor factors.[134]

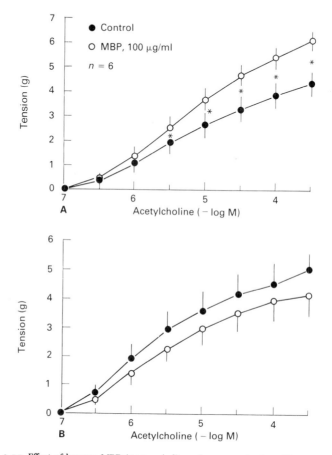

Fig. 2.11 Effect of human MBP (100 µg/ml) on the concentration-effect curve to acetylcholine in rings of guinea-pig trachea with (A) and without (B) epithelium. Data are presented as means ± SE for number of observations shown. Asterisk indicates effect of MBP is significant $P < 0.05$. In rings of trachea with epithelium the effect of human MBP is consistent with an upward shift in the concentration-effect curve, increasing the maximal response evoked by acetylcholine but not significantly affecting the ED_{50} value. The ED_{50} value represents the concentration of the agonist producing 50% of the maximal response to that agonist. In denuded rings, MBP was without effect and no change was observed in the maximal response or in the ED_{50} values. (Reproduced with permission from Flavahan NA, Slifman NR, Gleich GJ, Vanhoutte PM. Human eosinophil major basic protein causes hyperreactivity of respiratory smooth muscle. Role of the epithelium. *Am Rev Respir Dis* 1988;138:685.)

Support for the latter hypothesis comes from observations by Brofman and his associates who analysed the effect of removing epithelial cells and injecting MBP intraepithelially into underlying canine tracheal smooth muscle *in vivo*.[141] Here a dual *in situ* tracheal preparation was used that allowed adjacent areas of the epithelium to be compared. Evidence in dogs showed that intra-epithelial injection of MBP increases the response of the airway to intra-arterial administration of acetylcholine; no change was found in the tension of the control segment after intraepithelial injection of vehicle alone. Injection of MBP directly into the subepithelial muscle did not alter its contraction. After epithelial excision, no significant differences in contractile response to acetylcholine or to the relaxation response were observed.[141] These results suggest that MBP promotes secretion, by the epithelium, of a factor that enhances muscarinic reactivity. The results of these two studies are consistent with the conclusion that MBP alters respiratory smooth muscle contractility through an effect on the epithelium, possibly by the production of a constricting factor.

Experimental studies

Respiratory smooth muscle hyperreactivity has also been investigated in animal models. The administration of endotoxin produces an increase in neutrophils and monocytes in BAL fluid between four and 24 hours.[142] After 24 hours the numbers of eosinophils and lymphocytes are also increased. Histologically, at both times neutrophils are found in the trachea. There was no difference in the maximum response or in the slope of dose–response curves for carbachol or histamine between the smooth muscle of control animals and that of those exposed to endotoxin. The responsiveness to histamine was slightly decreased. *In vivo*, an increase in bronchial resistance induced by histamine was significantly reduced by about 35% in the exposed group. These authors concluded that the influx of inflammatory cells stimulated by endotoxin injury induces hyporeactivity of the guinea-pig respiratory tract.[142] Finally, it has been reported that induction of an increase of eosinophils in BAL fluid in Cynomolgus monkeys (*Macaca fascicularis*) is associated with an increase in airway reactivity to inhaled methacholine.[143]

Further studies are needed to determine: (i) the mechanisms responsible for eosinophil infiltration into tissues and eosinophil activation; (ii) the mechanism(s) of respiratory epithelial desquamation and Creola body formation; (iii) the ability of eosinophil granule proteins to alter respiratory smooth muscle reactivity *in vitro*; and to isolate (iv) the putative epithelial-derived relaxing and contracting factors.

MUCUS IN NORMAL AIRWAYS, HYPERSECRETORY
DISEASES AND ASTHMA

Although many patients with asthma have more goblet cells than is normal, this is not always the case, and persistent mucus hypersecretion is by no means present in all patients. In the necropsy study of forensic deaths, Kleinerman found no increase in the number of goblet cells in patients with asthma.[50] Whereas mucus hypersecretion is the diagnostic hallmark of the patient with chronic bronchitis, in typical extrinsic asthma it is rare, and sputum production is often only a feature of the end of an attack. In attempting to identify subsets of asthma it is important to emphasise that mucus hypersecretion is *not* a consistent feature of asthma.[1,144,145]

It has recently been shown that in normal airways, bronchial mucus does not include typical glycoprotein; in fact, the glyco-conjugate is a proteoglycan.[146-150] This has been shown in normal human and canine aspirates, and confirmed by following a canine model of bronchitis.[147,151] In aspirates from normal dogs before exposure to SO_2, no typical glycoprotein is identified. On exposure to the irritant, a typical epithelial glycoprotein can be identified before there is any clear increase in the amount of secretion. This, therefore seems to be a qualitative marker of irritation before the signs of hypersecretion are apparent.[152-154] It has also been shown that, whereas in normal dogs the lipids are mainly neutral, under irritation other lipids, notably glycolipids, appear quite quickly. This is also before hypersecretion develops.

Recently, we analysed the mucus removed from the airways of a patient dying in status asthmaticus. The material was extremely viscid and needed to be cut from the large airways.[58] No typical epithelial glycoprotein was identified in the secretion. This, there-fore, poses the question as to what stimulates the secretion and why this is retained in patients with asthma.

Studies of the mucus secreted by patients with quadriplegia offer another paradox. In patients with high cervical injury, excessive mucus production often develops quickly. In about 25% of patients this is clinically so serious that it necessitates tracheos-tomy. If the mucus hypersecretion does not prove fatal, such patients typically show spontaneous recovery within a couple of months. This suggests that the hypersecretion is a functional disturbance not based on mucous gland hypertrophy. For this reason, we expected the secretion to resemble the high volume low macromolecular yield mucus of a patient with pituitous catarrh or bronchitis serosa. On the contrary, we found that it has all the features of chronic bronchitis. This suggests that the secretion of typical epithelial glycoprotein and lipids can be maintained from structurally normal airways, and that their excessive production, even over some months, is reversible. Some patients with asthma may have an intermittent hypersecretion of mucus of the kind typical of chronic bronchitis.

Many different agents have been shown to increase the volume of secretion, amongst them neuromimetic agents and mediators of inflammation. Selective secretion by certain cells also adds to the complexity of the mucus secretion story.[150,152] Secretion by surface cells is different from that by glands. In studying the acute effect of agonists, it emerged that some agents that are powerful releasers of mucus into culture medium produce this effect by emptying the gland duct, not the cells.[154]

REFERENCES

1 Reid L. Chronic obstructive pulmonary diseases. In: Fishman AP ed. *Pulmonary diseases and disorders*. Volume 2. New York: McGraw-Hill, 1988:1247–72.
2 Laitinen LA, Heino M, Laitinen A, Kava T, Haahtela T. Damage of the airway epithelium and bronchial reactivity in patients with asthma. *Am Rev Respir Dis* 1985;**131**:599–606.
3 Hers JFPH. Disturbances of the ciliated epithelium due to influenza virus. *Am Rev Respir Dis* 1966;**93**:162–71.
4 Frigas E, Gleich GJ. The eosinophil and the pathology of asthma. *J Allergy Clin Immunol* 1986;**77**:527–37.
5 Laitinen A. Ultrastructural organization of intraepithelial nerves in the human airway tract. *Thorax* 1985;**40**:488–92.
6 Laitinen LA, Laitinen A. Mucosal inflammation and bronchial hyperreactivity. *Eur Respir J* 1988;**5**:488–9.
7 Oertel HL, Kaliner MA. The biological activity of mast cell granules. III. Purification of inflammatory factors of anaphylaxis (IF-A) responsible for causing late-phase reactions. *J Immunol* 1981;**112**:1398–402.
8 Solley GO, Gleich GJ, Jordan Scroeter AL. Late phase of the immediate wheal and flare skin reaction: its dependence on IgE antibodies. *J Clin Invest* 1976;**58**:408–20.
9 Tannenbaum S, Oertel H, Hederson WR, Kaliner M. The biologic activity of mast cell granules. I. Elicitation of inflammatory responses in rat skin. *J Immunol* 1980;**125**:325–35.
10 Meleb J, Pipkorn U. Mast cells on the surface of the mucous membrane—a general feature in inflammatory reactions in the nose? *Rhinology* 1985;**23**:187.
11 Goetzl EJ, Phillips MJ, Gold WM. Stimulus specificity of the generation of leukotrienes by dog mastocytoma cells. *J Exp Med* 1983;**158**:731–7.
12 Nagy L, Lee TH, Kay AB. Neutrophil chemotactic activity in antigen-induced asthmatic reactions. *N Engl J Med* 1982;**306**:497–501.
13 Phillips MJ, Calonico L, Gold WM. Morphological and pharmacological characterization of dog mastocytoma cells. *Am Rev Respir Dis* 1982;**125**:63A.
14 Goetzel EJ, Austen KF. Purification and synthesis of eosinophilotactic tetrapeptides of human lung tissue: identification as eosinophil chemotactic factor of anaphylaxis. *Proc Natl Acad Sci USA* 1985;**72**:4123–7.
15 Wardlaw AJ, Dunnette S, Gleich GJ, Collins JV, Kay AB. Eosinophils and mast cells in bronchoalveolar lavage in subjects with mild asthma. *Am Rev Respir Dis* 1988;**137**:62–9.

16 Dunnill MA. The morphology of the airways in bronchial asthma. Park Ridge III. *Am Coll Chest Physicians Bull* 1975:213–321.

17 Flint KC, Leung KBP, Hudspith BN, Brostoff J, Pearce FL, Johnson N McI. Bronchoalveolar mast cells in extrinsic asthma: a mechanism for the initiation of antigen specific bronchoconstriction. *Br Med J* 1985;**291**:923.

18 Godard P, Chaintreuil J, Damon M *et al.* Functional assessment of alveolar macrophages: comparison of cells from asthmatics and normal subjects. *J Allergy Clin Immunol* 1982;**70**:88–94.

19 Tomioka M, Ida S, Shindoh Y, Ishihara T, Takishima T. Mast cells in bronchoalveolar lumen of patients with bronchial asthma. *Am Rev Respir Dis* 1984;**129**:1000–5.

20 Filley WC, Holley KE, Kephart GM, Gleich GJ. Identification by immunofluorescence of eosinophil granule major basic protein in lung tissues of patients with bronchial asthma. *Lancet* 1982;**ii**:11–15.

21 Crystal RG, Reynolds HY, Kalica AR. Bronchoalveolar lavage. The report of an international congress. *Chest* 1986;**90**:122–8.

22 De Monchy JGR, Kauffman HF, Venge P *et al.* Bronchoalveolar eosinophilia during allergen-induced late asthmatic reactions. *Am Rev Respir Dis* 1985;**131**:373–6.

23 Fabbri LM, Boschetto P, Zocca E *et al.* Bronchoalveolar neutrophilia during late asthmatic reactions induced by toluene di-isocyanate. *Am Rev Respir Dis* 1987;**136**:36–42.

24 Boushey HA, Holtzman MJ. Experimental airway inflammation and hyperreactivity. *Am Rev Respir Dis* 1985;**3**:312–3.

25 Holtzman MJ, Fabbri LM, O'Byrne PM *et al.* Importance of airway inflammation for hyperresponsiveness induced by ozone. *Am Rev Respir Dis* 1983;**127**:686–90.

26 Murlas C, Roum JH. Sequence of pathological change in the airway mucosa of guinea-pigs during ozone induced bronchial hyperreactivity. *Am Rev Respir Dis* 1985;**131**:314–20.

27 Murlas C, Roum JH. Bronchial hyperreactivity occurs in steroid treated guinea-pigs depleted of leukocytes by cyclophosphamide. *J Appl Physiol* 1985;**58**:1630–7.

28 Hulbert WM, McLean T, Hogg JC. The effect of acute airway inflammation on bronchial reactivity in guinea-pigs. *Am Rev Respir Dis* 1985;**132**:7–11.

29 Flavahan NA, Aarhus LL, Rimele TJ, Vanhoutte PM. Respiratory epithelium inhibits bronchial smooth muscle tone. *J Appl Physiol* 1985;**58**:834–8.

30 Barnes PJ. Asthma as an axon reflex. *Lancet* 1986;**i**:242–4.

31 Empey DW, Laitinen LA, Jacobs L, Gold WM, Nadel JA. Mechanism of bronchial hyperreactivity in normal subjects after upper respiratory tract infections. *Am Rev Respir Dis* 1976;**113**:131–9.

32 Laitinen LA, Elkin RB, Empey DW, Mills J, Gold WM, Nadel JA. Changes in bronchial reactivity after administration of live attenuated influenza virus. *Am Rev Respir Dis* 1976;**113**:194.

33 Lee L-Y, Bleecker ER, Nadel JA. Effect of ozone on bronchometer response to inhaled histamine aerosol in dog. *J Appl Physiol* 1977;**43**:626–31.

34 Nadel J. Inflammation and asthma. *J Allergy Clin Immunol* 1984;**73**:651–3.

35 Laitinen LA, Laitinen A, Widdicombe JG. Effects of inflammatory and other mediators on airway vascular beds. *Am Rev Respir Dis* 1987;**135**(Suppl. 6):S67–S70.

36 Laitinen LA, Laitinen A, Widdicombe JG. Dose-related affects of pharmacological mediators on tracheal vascular resistance in dogs. *Br J Pharmacol* 1987;**92**:703–9.

37 Laitinen LA, Laitinen A, Salonen RO, Widdicombe JG. Vascular actions of airway neuropeptides. *Am Rev Respir Dis* 1987;**136**:S59–S64.

38 Laitinen LA, Robinson NP, Laitinen A, Widdicombe JG. Relationship between mucosal thickness and vascular resistance in dogs. *J Appl Physiol* 1986;**61**:2186–93.

74

39 Yamada KM, Olden K. Fibronectin-adhesive glycoproteins of cell surface and blood. *Nature* 1987;**275**:179–84.

40 Hedman K, Vaheri A, Wartiovaara J. External fibronectin of cultured human fibroplasts is predominately a matrix protein. *J Cell Biol* 1978;**76**:748–60.

41 Pearlstein E. Plasma membrane glycoprotein which mediates adhesion of fibroplasts to collagen. *Nature* 1976;**262**:497–500.

42 Clark RAF, Dvorak HF, Colvin RB. Fibronectin in delayed-type hypersensitivity skin reactions. *J Immunol* 1981;**126**:787–93.

43 Grinnel F, Billingham RE, Burgess L. Distribution of fibronectin during wound healing *in vivo*. *J Invest Dermatol* 1981;**76**:181–9.

44 Saksela O, Alitalo K, Kiistala U, Vaheri A. Basal lamina components in experimentally induced skin blisters. *J Invest Dermatol* 1981;**77**:283–6.

45 Vaheri A, Salonen E-M, Vartio T, Hedman K, Stenman S. Fibronectin and tissue injury. In; Wolf N ed. *Biology and pathology of the vessel wall*. Eastbourne: Praeger 1983;161.

46 Zuckerman KS, Wicha MS. Extracellular matrix production by the adherent cells of long-term murine bone marrow cultures. *Blood* 1983;**61**:540–7.

47 Tervo T, Sulonen J, Valtonen S, Vannas A, Virtanen I. Distribution of fibronectin in human and rabbit corneas. *Exp Eye Res* 1986;**42**:399–406.

48 Nishida T, Ohashi Y, Awata T, Suda T, Manabe R. Fibronectin; a new therapy for corneal topic ulcer. *Arch Ophthalmol* 1983;**101**:1046–8.

49 Salonen E-M, Tervo T, Törmä E, Tarkkanen A, Vaheri A. Plasmin in tear fluid of patients with corneal ulcers; basis for new therapy. *Acta Ophthalmol* 1987;**65**:3–12.

50 Kleinerman J, Adelson L. A study of asthma deaths in a coroner's population. *J Allergy Clin Immunol* 1987;**80**:406–9.

51 Copeland AR. Asthmatic deaths in the medical examiners population. *Forensic Sci Int* 1986;**31**:7–12.

52 Preston HV, Bowen DAL. Asthma deaths; a review. *Med Sci Law* 1987;**27**:89–99.

53 Wilcoxon F. Individual comparisons by ranking methods. *Biometrics Bull* 1945;**1**:80–3.

54 Cardell BS, Pearson RSB. Deaths in asthmatics. *Thorax* 1959;**14**:341–52.

55 Dunnill MS. The pathology of asthma with special reference to changes in the bronchial mucosa. *J Clin Pathol* 1960;**13**:27–33.

56 Roche WR, Beasley R, Williams JH, Holgate ST. Subepithelial fibrosis in the bronchi of asthmatics. *Lancet* 1989;**i**:520–4.

57 Reid LM. Workshop on pathology; summary of workshop manuscripts and discussion with recommendations from the panel. *J Allergy Clin Immunol* 1987;**80**(Suppl.):403–6.

58 Reid LM. The presence or absence of bronchial mucus in fatal asthma. *J Allergy Clin Immunol* 1987;**80**(Suppl.):415–6.

59 Bhaskar KR, O'Sullivan DD, Coles SJ, Kozakewich H, Vawter GF, Reid LM. Characterization of airway mucus from a fatal case of *status asthmaticus*. *Pediatr Pulmon* 1988;**5**:176–82.

60 Schoen FJ, Cardiac pathology in asthma. *J Allergy Clin Immunol* 1987;**80**(Suppl.):419–22.

61 Drislane FW, Samuels MA, Kozakewich H, Schoen FJ, Strunk RC. Myocardial contraction band lesions in patients with fatal asthma; possible neurocardiologic mechanisms. *Am Rev Respir Dis* 1987;**135**:498–501.

62 Armour CL, Lazar NM, Schellenberg RR *et al.* A comparison of *in vivo* and *in vitro* human airway reactivity to histamine. *Am Rev Respir Dis* 1984;**129**:907–10.

63 Cerrina J, Ladurie ML, Labat C, Raffestin B, Bayol A, Brink C. Comparison of human bronchial muscle responses to histamine *in vivo* with histamine and isoproteronol *in vitro*. *Am Rev Respir Dis* 1986;**134**:51–61.

64 Vincenc KS, Black JL, Yan K, Armour CL, Donnelly PD, Woolcock AJ. A comparison of *in vivo* and *in vitro* responses to histamine in human airway. *Am Rev Respir Dis* 1983;**128**:875–9.

65 Benson MK. Bronchial hyperreactivity. *Br J Dis Chest* 1975;**69**:227–39.

66 Freedman BJ. The functional geometry of the bronchi. *Bull Physiopathol Respir* 1972;**8**:545–51.

67 Moreno RH, Hogg JC, Pare PD. Mechanisms of airway narrowing. *Am Rev Respir Dis* 1986;**133**:1171–80.

68 James AL, Pare PD, Moreno RH, Hogg JC. Quantitative measurement of smooth muscle shortening in the isolated pig trachea. *J Appl Physiol* 1987;**63**:1360–5.

69 James AL, Hogg JC, Dunn LA, Pare PD. The use of internal perimeter to compare airway size and calculate smooth muscle shortening. *Am Rev Respir Dis* 1988;**138**:136–9.

70 James AL, Pare PD, Hogg JC. Mechanisms of airway narrowing in asthma. *Am Rev Respir Dis* (in press).

71 Unger L. Pathology of bronchial asthma. *Southern Med J* 1945;**38**:513–22.

72 Bullen SS. Correlation of clinical and autopsy findings in 176 cases of asthma. *J Allergy* 1952;**23**:193–203.

73 Messer J, Peters GA, Bennet WA. Cause of death and pathological findings in 304 cases of bronchial asthma. *Dis Chest* 1960;**38**:616–24.

74 Dunnill MS. The pathology of asthma with special reference to changes in the bronchial mucosa. *J Clin Pathol* 1960;**13**:27–33.

75 Richards W, Patrick JR. Death from asthma in children. *Am J Dis Child* 1965;**110**:4–21.

76 Houston JC, De Vavasquez S, Trounce JR. A clinical and pathological study of fatal cases of status asthmaticus. *Thorax* 1953;**8**:207–13.

77 Dunnill MS, Massarella GR, Anderson JA. A comparison of the quantitative anatomy of the bronchi in normal subjects, in status asthmaticus, in chronic bronchitis and in emphysema. *Thorax* 1969;**24**:176–9.

78 Heard BE, Hossain S. Hyperplasia of bronchial muscle in asthma. *J Pathol* 1971;**110**:319–31.

79 Cutz E, Levison H, Cooper DM. Ultrastructure of airways in children with asthma. *Histopathology* 1978;**2**:407–21.

80 Takizawa T, Thurlbeck WM. Muscle and mucous gland size in the major bronchi of patients with chronic bronchitis, asthma and asthmatic bronchitis. *Am Rev Respir Dis* 1971;**104**:331–6.

81 Salvato G. Some histologic changes in chronic bronchitis and asthma. *Thorax* 1968;**23**:168–72.

82 Huber HL, Koessler KK. The pathology of bronchial asthma. *Arch Intern Med* 1922;**30**:689–760.

83 Ellis AG. The pathological anatomy of bronchial asthma. *Am J Med Sci* 1908;**136**:407–29.

84 Horn BR, Robin ED, Theodore JA, Van Kessel A. Total eosinophil counts in the management of bronchial asthma. *N Engl J Med* 1975;**292**:1152–5.

85 Gleich GJ, Frigas E, Loegering DA, Wassom DL, Steinmuller D. Cytotoxic properties of eosinophil major basic protein. *J Immunol* 1979;**123**:2925–7.

86 Frigas E, Loegering DA, Gleich GJ. Cytotoxic effects of the guinea pig eosinophil major basic protein on tracheal epithelium. *Lab Invest* 1980;**42**:35–43.

87 Frigas E, Loegering DA, Solley GO, Farrow GM, Gleich GJ. Elevated levels of eosinophil granule major basic protein in the sputum of patients with bronchial asthma. *Mayo Clin Proc* 1981;**56**:345–53.

88 Dunnill MS. The pathology of asthma with special reference to changes in the bronchial mucosa. *J Clin Pathol* 1960;**13**:27–33.

89 Frigas E, Gleich GJ. The eosinophil and the pathophysiology of asthma. *J Allergy Clin Immunol* 1986;**77**:527–37.

90 Wardlaw AJ, Kay AB. The role of the eosinophil in the pathogenesis of asthma. *Allergy* 1987;**42**:321–35.

91 Venge P, Hakansson L, Peterson CGB. Eosinophil activation in allergic disease. *Int Arch Allergy Appl Immun* 1987;**82**:333–7.

92 Gleich GJ, Adolphson CR. The eosinophilic leukocyte; structure and function. *Adv Immunol* 1986;**39**:177–253.

93 Wasmoen TL, Bell MP, Loegering DA, Gleich GJ, Prendergast FG, McKean DJ. Biochemical and amino acid sequence analysis of human eosinophil granule major basic protein. *J Biol Chem* 1988;**236**:12559–63.

94 Gleich GJ, Loegering DA, Bell MP, Checkel JL, Ackerman SJ, McKean DJ. Biochemical and functional similarities between human eosinophil-derived neurotoxin and eosinophil cationic protein; homology with ribonuclease. *Proc Natl Acad Sci USA* 1986;**83**:3146–50.

95 Olsson I, Persson A-M, Winqvist I. Biochemical properties of the eosinophil cationic protein (ECP) and studies of its biosynthesis *in vitro* in marrow cells from patients with an eosinophila. *Blood* 1986;**67**:498–503.

96 Slifman NR, Loegering DA, McKean DJ, Gleich GJ. Ribonuclease activity associated with human eosinophil-derived neurotoxin and eosinophil cationic protein. *J Immunol* 1986;**137**:2913–17.

97 Gullberg U, Widegren B, Arnason U, Egesten A, Olsson I. The cytotoxic eosinophil cationic protein has RNase activity. *Biochem Biophys Res Commun* 1986;**139**:1239–42.

98 Weller PF, Ackerman SJ, Smith JA. Eosinophil granule cationic proteins; major basic protein is distinct from the smaller subunit of eosinophil peroxidase. *J Leukocyte Biol* 1988;**43**:1–40.

99 Weiss SJ, Test ST, Eckmann CM, Roos D, Regiani S. Brominating oxidants generated by human eosinophils. *Science* 1986;**234**:200–3.

100 Ayars GH, Altman LC, Gleich GJ, Loegering DA, Baker EB. Eosinophil – and eosinophil granule – mediated pneumocyte injury. *J Allergy Clin Immunol* 1985;**76**:595–604.

101 Motojima S, Frigas E, Loegering DA, Gleich GJ. Toxicity of eosinophil cationic proteins for guinea pig tracheal epithelium *in vitro*. *Am Rev Respir Dis* (in press).

102 Agosti JM, Altman LC, Ayars GH, Loegering DA, Gleich GJ, Klebanoff SJ. The injurious effects of eosinophil peroxidase, hydrogen peroxide and halides on pneumocytes *in vitro*. *J Allergy Clin Immunol* 1987;**79**:496–504.

103 Hastie AT, Loegering DA, Gleich GJ, Kueppers F. The effect of purified human eosinophil major basic protein on mammalian ciliary activity. *Am Rev Respir Dis* 1987;**135**:848–53.

104 Durham SR, Kay AB. Eosinophils, bronchial hyperreactivity and late-phase asthmatic reactions. *Clin Allergy* 1985;**40**:411–8.

105 Iijima M, Adachi M, Kobayashi H, Takahashi T. Relationship between airway hyperreactivity and various atopic factors in bronchial asthma (English abstract). *Arerugi* 1985;**34**:226–33.

106 Taylor KJ, Luksza AR. Peripheral blood eosinophil counts and bronchial responsiveness. *Thorax* 1987;**42**:452–6.

107 O'Byrne PM, Dolovich J, Hargreave FE. Late asthmatic responses. *Am Rev Respir Dis* 1987;**136**:740–51.

108 Metzger WJ, Zavala D, Richerson HB *et al*. Local allergen challenge and bronchoalveolar lavage of allergic asthmatic lungs. *Am Rev Respir Dis* 1987;**135**:433–40.

109 Lam S, Le Riche J, Phillips D, Chan-Yeung M. Cellular and protein changes in bronchial lavage fluid after late asthmatic reaction in patients with red cedar asthma. *J Allergy Clin Immunol* 1987;**80**:44–50.

110 Flint KC, Leung KBP, Hudspith BN, Brostoff J, Pearce FL, Johnson NM. Bronchoalveolar mast cells in extrinsic asthma; a mechanism for the initiation of antigen specific bronchoconstriction. *Br J Med* 1985;**291**:923–6.

111 Kirby JG, Hargreave FE, Gleich GJ, O'Byrne PM. Bronchoalveolar cell profiles of asthmatic and nonasthmatic subjects. *Am Rev Respir Dis* 1987;**136**:379–83.

112 Wardlaw AJ, Cromwell O, Celestino D *et al*. Morphological and secretory

properties of bronchoalveolar lavage mast cells in respiratory diseases. *Clin Allergy* 1986;**16**:163–73.

113 Godard P, Bousquet J, Lebel B, Michel FB. Bronchoalveolar lavage in the asthmatic. *Bull Eur Physiopathol Respir* 1987;**23**:73–85.

114 Larsen GL, Wilson MC, Clark RAF, Behrens BL. The inflammatory reaction in the airways in an animal model of the late asthmatic response. *Fed Proc* 1987;**46**:105–12.

115 Iijima H, Ishii M, Yamauchi K *et al*. Bronchoalveolar lavage and histologic characterization of late asthmatic response in guinea pigs. *Am Rev Respir Dis* 1987;**136**:922–9.

116 Hutson PA, Church MK, Clay TP, Miller P, Holgate ST. Early and late-phase bronchoconstriction after allergen challenge of nonanesthetized guinea pigs. I. The association of disordered airway physiology to leukocyte infiltration. *Am Rev Respir Dis* 1988;**137**:548–57.

117 Lewis DM, Lewis JC, Loegering DA, Gleich GJ. Localization of the guinea-pig eosinophil major basic protein to the core of the granule. *J Cell Biol* 1978;**77**:702–13.

118 Dunn CJ, Elliot GA, Oostveen JA, Richards IM. Development of a prolonged eosinophil-rich inflammatory leukocyte infiltration in the guinea-pig asthmatic response to ovalbumin inhalation. *Am Rev Respir Dis* 1988;**137**:541–7.

119 Church MK, Hutson PA, Sanjar S, Holgate ST. Neutrophils do not participate in the development of the late asthmatic reaction in guinea-pigs. *J Allergy Clin Immunol* 1988;**81**:234.

120 Huber HL, Koessler KK. The pathology of bronchial asthma. *Arch Intern Med* 1922;**30**:689–760.

121 Cardell BS, Pearson RSB. Death in asthmatics. *Thorax* 1959;**14**:341–52.

122 Houston JC, De Navasquez S, Trounce JR. A clinical and pathological study of fatal cases of status asthmaticus. *Thorax* 1953;**8**:207–13.

123 Glynn AA, Michaels L. Bronchial biopsy in chronic bronchitis and asthma. *Thorax* 1960;**15**:142–53.

124 Gough J. Post-mortem differences in 'asthma' and in chronic bronchitis. *Acta Allergol* 1961;**16**:391–9.

125 Carabelli AA. Cytologic patterns in bronchopulmonary disease. *Am Rev Tuberculosis* 1958;**77**:22–31.

126 Leyden Z, Konigsberg E, Zur Kenntniss des bronchial asthma. *Arch Pathol Anat Physiol* 1872;**54**:324–52.

127 Von Hoesslin H. *Das sputum*. Berlin: Springer 1921.

128 Naylor B. The shedding of the mucosa of the bronchial tree in asthma. *Thorax* 1962;**17**:69–72.

129 Naylor B. Creola bodies; their discovery and significance. *Cytotechnologist Bull* 1985;**22**:33–4.

130 Gleich GJ, Flavahan NA, Fujisawa T, Vanhoutte PM. The eosinophil as a mediator of damage to respiratory epithelium; a model for bronchial hyper-reactivity. *J Allergy Clin Immunol* 1988;**81**:776–81.

131 Nadel JA. Bronchial reactivity. *Adv Intern Med* 1983;**28**:207–23.

132 Hogg JC, Eggleston PA. Is asthma an epithelial disease? *Am Rev Respir Dis* 1984;**129**:207–8.

133 Flavahan NA, Slifman NR, Gleich GJ, Vanhoutte PM. Human eosinophil major basic protein causes hyperreactivity of respiratory smooth muscle. Role of the epithelium. *Am Rev Respir Dis* 1988;**138**:685–8.

134 Flavahan NA, Vanhoutte PM. The respiratory epithelium releases a smooth muscle relaxing factor. *Chest* 1985;**87**(Suppl.):189s.

135 Vanhoutte PM, Flavahan NA. Modulation of cholinergic neurotransmission in the airways. In: Kaliner M, Barnes P eds. *Neural regulation of the airways*. New York: Marcel Dekker 1987:203–16.

136 Ilhan M, Sahil I. Tracheal epithelium releases a vascular smooth muscle relaxing factor; demonstration by bioassay. *Eur J Pharmacol* 1986;**131**:293–6.

137 Hay DWP, Muccitelli RM, Hostemeyer DL, Wilson KA, Raeburn D. Demonstration of the release of an epithelium-derived inhibitory factor from a novel preparation of guinea pig trachea. *Eur J Pharmacol* 1987;**136**:247–50.

138 Vanhoutte PM. Airway epithelium and bronchial reactivity. *Can J Physiol Pharmacol* 1987;**65**:448–50.

139 Reaburn D, Hay DWP, Robinson VA, Farmer SG, Fleming WW, Fedan JS. The effect of verapamil is reduced in isolated airway smooth muscle preparations lacking the epithelium. *Life Sci* 1986;**38**:809–16.

140 Barnes PJ, Cuss FM, Palmer JB. The effect of airway epithelium on smooth muscle contractility in bovine trachea. *Br J Pharmacol* 1985;**86**:685–91.

141 Brofman JD, White SR, Blake JS, Munoz NM, Gleich GJ, Leff AR. Augmentation of tracheal smooth muscle contraction by major basic protein of eosinophils *in vivo*. *J Appl Physiol* (in press).

142 Folkerts G, Henricks PAJ, Slootweg PJ, Nijkamp FP. Endotoxin-induced inflammation and injury of the guinea pig respiratory airways cause bronchial hyporeactivity. *Am Rev Respir Dis* 1988;**137**:1441–8.

143 Gundel RH, Gerritsen ME, Wagner CD. Increase in airway eosinophils is associated with increase in airway reactivity in monkeys (abstract). *Am Rev Respir Dis* 1988;**137**:281.

144 Reid L. The pathology of obstructive and inflammatory airway diseases. Inflammation; its clinical relevance in airway diseases. *Eur J Respir Dis* 1986;**69**(Suppl.):26–37.

145 Lopez-Vidrerio MT, Reid LM. Bronchial mucus in asthma. In; Weiss EB, Segal MS, Stein M eds. *Bronchial asthma mechanisms and therapeutics*, 2nd edition. Boston: Little & Brown 1985:218–35.

146 Bhaskar KR, O'Sullivan DD, Seltzer J, Rossing T, Drazen J, Reid L. Density gradient study of bronchial mucus aspirates from healthy volunteers (smokers and nonsmokers) and from patients with tracheostomy. *Exp Lung Res* 1985;**9**:289–308.

147 Bhaskar KR, Drazen J, O'Sullivan DD, Scanlon P, Reid L. Transition from normal to hypersecretory bronchial mucus in a canine model of bronchitis; changes in yield and composition. *Exp Lung Res* 1988;**14**:101–20.

148 O'Sullivan DD, Bhaskar KR, Opaskar-Hincman H, Reid LM. Proteoglycans in airway secretions. Respiratory tract secretions. *Eur J Respir Dis* 1987;**71**(Suppl):274–5.

149 Koshino T, Bhaskar KR, Reid LM *et al.* Increased expression of an epitope recognized by a monoclonal antibody to human airway epithelial glycoprotein during exposure to SO_2 gas in dogs (in press).

150 Kim KC, Hincman HO, Bhaskar KR. Secretions from primary hamster tracheal epithelial cells in culture; mucins, proteoglycans and lipids. *Exp Lung Res* 1989;**15**:299–314.

151 Bhaskar KR, O'Sullivan DD, Opaskar-Hincman H, Reid L, Coles S. Density gradient analysis of secretions produced *in vitro* by human and canine airway mucosa; identification of lipids and proteoglycans in such secretions. *Exp Lung Res* 1986;**10**:401–22.

152 Reid LM, Bhaskar KR. Macromolecular and lipid constituents of bronchial epithelial mucus. In; Chantler E ed. *International symposium on mucus and related topics*. Society of Experimental Biology (in press).

153 Bhaskar KR, O'Sullivan DD, Opaskar-Hincman H, Reid LM. Lipids in airway secretions. Respiratory tract secretions. *Eur J Respir Dis* 1987;**71**(Suppl.):215–21.

154 Reid LM, O'Sullivan DD, Bhaskar KR. Pathophysiology of bronchial hypersecretion. Respiratory tract secretions. *Eur J Respir Dis* 1987;**71**(Suppl.):19–25.

3: Diagnostic Procedures

F. E. Hargreave, G. Marone & T. Platts-Mills

Current evidence suggests that asthma is a disease caused by a special type of inflammation in the airways of the lungs which can give rise to various clinical manifestations. Special characteristics of the inflammation are eosinophilia, increases in metachromatic cells (mast cells or basophils), shedding of epithelial cells and increased releasability of mediators. The clinical manifestations including cough, hypersecretion, variable airflow limitation, and airway hyperresponsiveness (BHR) all appear to be a consequence of the inflammation. BHR is a determinant of the severity of the variable airflow limitation. This chapter will deal with the diagnostic procedures required to identify airway inflammation, BHR (which in addition to other clinical characteristics needs to be correlated with this) and the causes of the inflammation.

DIAGNOSIS OF AIRWAY INFLAMMATION

The presence of airway inflammation can be recognised directly or inferred from indirect correlates. Direct investigative methods include histopathology of lung tissue removed at surgery or autopsy, or of bronchial biopsies[1-4] or brushings.[5] Additionally, providing there is no disease of the peripheral respiratory tissues, cytology of bronchoalveolar lavage (BAL),[6-16] bronchial washings,[13,15,16] and sputum[17] can be used. Indirect correlates of asthmatic airway inflammation include heightened airway responsiveness, increased bronchodilator requirements, sputum production, and increased blood eosinophil and basophil counts.

Direct examination of airway tissue or cells is required to improve our understanding of asthma and BHR, because it documents the characteristics of inflammation as well as its presence. Studies are needed to compare the histopathology and cytology from the different methods, as well as to correlate these with other clinical characteristics. To date, only limited studies have been performed.

The use of sputum to study the pathogenesis of airway disease is advantageous because it is a non-invasive technique. Recently, Gibson and co-workers[17] described a method in which both total and differential cell counts were reproducible between sputum samples from the same specimen and between specimens from two consecutive days. To obtain a representative sample, the method requires adequate sample collection, the microscopic selection of the portion of the sputum for analysis, and the examination of more than one portion of the specimen. Initial observations using this method suggest that inflammation associated with an exacerbation of asthma is characterised by eosinophilia and an increase in metachromatic cells. Both types of cells were few or absent in the sputum of cigarette smokers with chronic bronchitis which was not complicated by acute infection, airflow limitation, or methacholine BHR. No differences were observed in the numbers of other cell types. These observations are in keeping with those from BAL and bronchial washings[15,16] of mild stable asthmatics, with the exception that these have smaller increases in cell counts and have also identified the excess shedding of bronchial epithelial cells.[16]

Comparisons have been made between the direct examination for airway inflammation and indirect correlates. Studies of asthmatic responses induced by allergen or chemical sensitisers suggest that the cellular phase of inflammation is especially associated with late asthmatic responses and the prolonged heightening of histamine or methacholine airway responsiveness.[8,12] Other features of exacerbations, which would be expected to be associated with inflammation, are increased bronchodilator requirements, sputum production and an increase in peripheral blood eosinophil and basophil counts.[18,19]

DIAGNOSIS OF AIRWAY HYPERRESPONSIVENESS

BHR can be measured by a variety of stimuli which act through different specific mechanisms.[20] Thus, categorisation of airway responsiveness into specific and non-specific is confusing. The term 'specific' was introduced to refer to the responsiveness induced by allergens and chemical sensitisers which affected only those people hypersensitive to them. 'Non-specific' was used to describe the variety of nonallergic or nonsensitising stimuli which affected the majority of people with variable airflow limitation. However, the relative airway responsiveness to these different 'non-specific' stimuli can differ between individuals. The terms 'specific' and 'non-specific' should therefore be discontinued and substituted by the agent being used to measure responsiveness, e.g. methacholine airway responsiveness.[21,22]

The most common method of measuring airway responsiveness has been by inhalation with histamine or methacholine (or other cholinergic agonists), or by exercise tests. More recently, however, other stimuli have been used. The type of stimulus to be used requires discussion, and the interpretation of results necessitates careful regulation of the tests and the correlation of results with clinical and histopathological features.

Which stimulus?

The most effective stimulus to identify airway inflammation of the type which occurs in asthma is not known. Histamine and methacholine (or other cholinergic agonists like acetylcholine or carbachol) have been most extensively used to measure airway responsiveness.[23-26] Other stimuli have included exercise,[23,25] isocapnic hyperventilation of ambient or cold dry air,[23,25] or inhalation of distilled water,[27] hypertonic saline,[28] leukotrienes (LT) D_4 and C_4,[29] prostaglandins (PG) F_{2a} and D_2,[30,31] neurokinin A,[32] adenosine,[33] adenosine monophosphate (AMP),[34] propranolol,[35] bradykinin,[36] and methoxamine.[37]

The various stimuli act through different specific mechanisms which are complex and incompletely understood. A simple classification has been to divide them into those which are thought to act chiefly through a direct effect on smooth muscle, e.g. methacholine, and those which are considered to exert their effects indirectly via nerves or the release of a number of chemical mediators, e.g. exercise.[20] The way in which they stimulate airway constriction and the extent to which different components are involved will vary between stimuli. Some may act chiefly on airway smooth muscle, while others may involve capillary permeability or secretions. Furthermore, some stimuli may have effects which will minimise the response; for example, exercise is considered to stimulate the release of bronchodilator catecholamines from the adrenal,[38] and high doses of histamine can stimulate H_2 receptors to release the dilator prostaglandin E_2.[39] There is clearly a need to learn more about the mechanisms through which the different stimuli act.

Airway responsiveness to inhaled histamine correlates very closely with that to inhaled methacholine.[24,26] Responsiveness to inhaled histamine is an important determinant of the response to inhaled allergen which involves the release of a variety of chemical mediators. It is, therefore, not surprising that initial correlations were found between responsiveness to histamine or methacholine and responsiveness to exercise, hyperventilation, PGF_{2a}, LTC_4 and LTD_4.[24,26,29,30] However, the correlations were not as close as those between histamine and methacholine, and some studies were unable to show any. Subsequently, no correlation was found between airway responsiveness to histamine or methacholine and water or hypertonic saline,[27,28] propranolol,[35] and adenosine,[33] or AMP.[34] There have been few studies comparing responsiveness between stimuli other than histamine or cholinergic agonists. Responsiveness to exercise is similar to that to distilled water, presumably because the mechanisms involved are similar.[40] Further studies are needed in the same subjects to investigate correlations between responsiveness to a variety of stimuli in addition to histamine or methacholine.

CHAPTER 3
Diagnostic
Procedures

The clinical relevance of airway responsiveness has chiefly been examined using inhaled histamine or methacholine.[24,26] This has usefully demonstrated that; asthma can be transient or persistent, airway inflammation can increase airway responsiveness, the degree of BHR is closely related to the degree of variable airflow limitation, and the degree of responsiveness is an important determinant of the response to certain stimuli such as allergens, exercise, and hyperventilation. However, these measurements have also documented discrepancies between responsiveness and clinical characteristics which suggest that BHR to histamine or methacholine is not the most specific indicator of airway inflammation of the asthmatic type. For example, responsiveness can be normal when variable airflow limitation (and presumed airway inflammation) is triggered by occupational chemical sensitisers or allergens.[41] It may also be normal when there is chronic cough and the production of sputum which has the same cell characteristics as asthma and responds similarly to treatment with corticosteroids.[42] However, it can be abnormal in smokers with chronic airflow limitation who are not considered to have asthma.[37,43–45] Such individuals, in contrast to asthmatics, do not respond to hyperventilation of cold dry air,[43] to methoxamine,[37] or to propranolol.[46] These observations with stimuli which are considered to act via release of chemical mediators, have indicated that they might be better at identifying asthmatic-type airway inflammation. Further studies are required to correlate objective evidence of inflammation with measurements of airway responsiveness to different stimuli to determine whether some are able to identify its presence more clearly than others.

Methods of inhalation challenge tests

The methods of inhalation challenge tests have been standardised so that results are reproducible and can be accurately interpreted and compared. Inhalation tests involve generation and inhalation of the aerosol, measurement of the response, construction of dose–response curves, and expression of the results. One method involves continuous generation and inhalation by tidal breathing for a defined time.[47] A second consists of generation of a puff of aerosol by a nebuliser attached to a dosimeter,[48,49] or by a hand operated nebuliser, during a specified number of inspired breaths.[50] The methods are well described, but it is common for laboratories to be imprecise and to ignore the factors which influence the dose that actually reaches the airways. These factors include nebuliser output for both methods, and speed of inhalation and duration of breathhold for the puff delivery methods. The response is usually expressed as a point on the deep linear part of the dose–response curve which indicates the position of the curve, e.g. the provocation concentration or dose to cause a fall in FEV_1 of 20%. In future, however, the presence of a maximal response plateau will also need consideration in the definition of normal responsiveness.[21,51-53]

DIAGNOSIS OF THE CAUSES OF INFLAMMATION

Causes of airway inflammation in asthma include allergic responses to inhaled allergens, reactions to certain chemical sensitisers usually encountered in occupations (e.g. isocyanates and plicatic acid), and viral infections. Altered releasability of inflammatory cells may be one of the factors responsible for the persistence of the inflammation.

Allergy sensitisation

Since the initial findings indicating an association between exposure to airborne allergens and asthma, all the evidence has related to immediate hypersensitivity. That is, only patients who have developed immediate hypersensitivity to house dust,[54] dust mites,[55] cat dander allergens,[56] or pollen,[57-59] are at risk of developing asthma on continued exposure. This section is, therefore, restricted to the identification of immediate skin sensitivity or serum IgE antibody. However, it is important to recognise that much of the inflammatory response to allergen exposure may involve other forms of immunity, i.e. T-cell or IgG antibody as well as IgE antibody.[60] At present, there are no practical methods of diagnosing this form of T-cell or IgG antibody sensitisation, therefore IgE antibody is used as the marker for sensitisation associated with asthma.

Skin tests for immediate hypersensitivity

Skin testing was first carried out by scratching the skin under an extract and watching for the development of a weal and flare response. In patients who are profoundly reactive, there is no difficulty in identifying a positive reaction.

However, in order to use the test for epidemiological studies and to compare results between centres, it is necessary to define conditions for the skin test, to grade the results, and to define a cut-off point. The major issues in skin testing are the technique, i.e. scratch, prick or intradermal, the safety and the standardisation of the extracts used.

Method: There are several different varieties of prick test in use. One, established by Pepys[61] and widely used, uses a 25 gauge needle to lift the skin through the extract. However, various special needles can be used, e.g. the Morrow Brown plastic disposable needle which gives a very consistent reaction and requires less skill, and the bifurcated needle which was originally developed for scarification. Many attempts have been made to produce a non-painful skin test technique, particularly for use in surveys of children. Using a lance to scrape the surface of the skin to remove epidermal layers can be successful, but has not been widely used. The multitest, a plastic disposable needle with multiple points, was developed for delayed hypersensitivity testing and has not yet been validated for use with immediate hyper-sensitivity.

The size of the weal graded as positive has been very variable. Commonly, skin tests are graded by their mean diameter relative to the negative control or a histamine control. While weals 2 mm greater than the negative control may sometimes be significant, there are problems using weal sizes this small. There are several ways of judging the reliability of a skin test response. Firstly, is it repeatable on that day? It has been clearly shown that different parts of the skin give different responses, so repeating responses at separate sites improves reliability. Secondly, how consistent are responses when repeated on a subsequent occasion? When studies of this kind were done, it has been clear that weals with a size of 3 mm diameter (or less) are often *not* reproduced six months later, while weal sizes of ≥ 5 mm diameter almost always (i.e. $\geq 95\%$) are. It seems likely that ≥ 4 mm mean diameter is a suitable cut-off for a positive response. The third criterion is to observe the way in which skin responses correlate with *in vitro* assays of IgE antibody. Here also, weal sizes less than 4 mm have been found to correlate poorly with IgE antibodies, while weals ≥ 5 mm have a better than 80% correlation with results for serum IgE antibody. In part, this is because the skin tests are more sensitive. In conclusion, prick test responses are best graded by mean weal size, and can be related to histamine or control. Weals of 5 mm are definitely positive, and those ≥ 8 mm $\pm$ pseudopods are strongly positive. Given the variability of the system, a more detailed gradation than this is inappropriate.

Intradermal skin testing is used for two completely different purposes; to increase sensitivity with allergens, such as the fungi, in clinical practice, and to increase precision in testing sensitivity to purified allergens. An intradermal test using 0.03 ml represents approximately 1000-fold more allergen than the prick test and it carries considerably more risk of anaphylaxis. When carried out as an end point dilution test, it is considered to be the most accurate assessment of skin sensitivity and is used for assessing skin sensitivity to purified allergens in genetic studies. To give an 8 mm weal,[59,62] results vary from concentrations of $\geq$ 10^{-2} µg/ml (i.e. negative) to 10^{-6} µg/ml. Intradermal testing with crude extracts may be useful in clinical practice, but has very few advantages in defining sensitivity because, unless the extract is defined very accurately, the dilution used becomes critical. The increased risk and pain of intradermal testing are strong arguments against its use for surveys.

Standardisation of extracts: In all skin testing, the nature of the extract used is critical, and for most extracts the present situation is unsatisfactory. For some allergens the source material used to make the extract is important. Simple examples include the use of cat washings rather than cat pelt, isolated mites or whole mite culture, different growth media for mites, different strains of fungi, and spores versus mycelial extracts. Each of these can affect not only the overall potency of extracts, but also the relative strength of individual allergenic proteins within an extract. However, the major problem with extracts is the establishment and recording of their potency or allergen content in units which maintain their meaning. In the past, allergen standardisation has often used skin testing to provide data in biological units or allergy units which are extremely difficult to reproduce and cannot be compared from one allergen to another. Similarly, *in vitro* tests using human allergic serum (i.e. radioallergosorbent (RAST) inhibition) give results in units which are difficult to reproduce in different laboratories or over a period of time. The most consistent techniques available have used measurements of marker proteins in an extract (usually one or more major allergens). Typical examples include *Amb a* I (antigen E) of ragweed, *Fel d* I (cat I) in cat extracts, *Lol p* I in rye grass extracts and Group I (*Der p* I and *Der f* I) allergens in dust mite extracts.[63] Over the last few years there has been a progressive improvement in techniques available for measuring allergens. These include radial immunodiffusion, radioimmunoassay, two-site monoclonal antibody radioimmunoassays and enzyme immunoassays.[60,64] There are several advantages of measuring specific antigens. Firstly, the reagents used can be defined allowing assays to be maintained constant and results to be related to national or international standards. Secondly, assay results can be given in absolute units, i.e. µg, which can be easily understood. Thirdly, results (in µg) of one allergen can be directly compared with those of others in the same extract or in extracts of different allergens. Fourthly, very similar assays can be used for measurements of environmental exposure.

Most commercially available pollen extracts or mite extracts marketed for prick tests contain between 10 and 70 µg of major allergen/ml. Some extracts, e.g. cat, are more difficult to maintain at this level, but the 'standardised' or acetone precipitated extracts commonly contain > 10 µg *Fel d* I/ml. For many other allergens, e.g. all the fungi, it has been very difficult to define a specific major allergen or a method of measuring allergen, so that it is not possible to make any firm statement about the level. Nonetheless, it seems reasonable to propose that prick test reagents should contain between 10 and 70 µg of major allergen/ml.

In vitro assays of IgE antibody

Soon after the discovery of IgE, it became possible to measure the specific IgE antibodies in serum using solid phase antigen and radiolabelled anti IgE; the RAST technique. Since that time, there have been many commercial modifications of the technique with different solid phases or different methods of identifying bound IgE, e.g. enzyme or fluorescent markers. However, none of the modifications have significantly altered the principle, and most have presented more problems than the original assay. Over the last few years it has been recognised that RAST results can be expressed in units which can be related to absolute quantities of IgE antibody. The quantity of the bound antibody is a direct function of the quantity of IgE present. Thus, it is possible to relate results to ng of IgE antibodies and to propose levels of specific IgE antibodies that should be regarded as significant. In general, values of 5 ng of IgE antibody are well above both the background and the fluctuations in background caused by anything except very high levels of total serum IgE (> 2000 iu/ml). Total serum IgE alone is not a useful test for the diagnosis of specific allergy, but it may be of value if considered in conjunction with specific tests. Firstly, total serum IgE is important in interpreting the results of solid phase *in vitro* assays (i.e. RAST). Secondly, a low total IgE is helpful in 'confirming' negative skin tests or RAST results, although it is important to remember that even very low levels such as 20 iu (1 iu = 2.4 ng IgE) do not exclude an important specific sensitivity. Thirdly, a very high total IgE, i.e. > 500 iu/ml may lead to further diagnostic tests or suggest the possibility of bronchopulmonary aspergillosis.

Using *in vitro* assays, the choice of extract is just as critical as with skin tests. Most commercially available assays give no indication as to what extract is being used. Indeed, some companies pride themselves on keeping the nature of the extracts secret. The quantity of relevant allergen in the solid phase will depend on several variables which include the efficacy of the linking procedure, the proportion of irrelevant (i.e. non-allergic) material in the extract, and the surface area of the solid phase.

Most assays have used either a matrix or a bead, e.g. sepharose or microcellulose, which have a very high surface area, or a cellulose disc which uses the same linking technique (usually cyanogen bromide activation).[65] More recently, several efforts have been made to use microwells directly as the solid phase. This has the disadvantage that the surface area is generally smaller making the quality of the extract even more important. At present, many of the techniques used to link proteins to plastic wells are secret or still in development. This makes it very difficult to evaluate their reliability in general use. However, the important conclusion is that with further modifications of the binding procedure and improvements of extract quality, it is highly likely that IgE antibody assays for inhalant allergens will become simpler and more rapid, and will be accepted as a reliable part of routine practice.

Conclusions on skin tests and in vitro assays of IgE activity

Allergen exposure is established as a major risk factor for symptomatic asthma among children over 5 years old and adults under 50 years old, and this risk is restricted to individuals who have developed immediate hypersensitivity. Thus, the diagnosis of specific immediate hypersensitivity is an essential part of evaluating most patients with asthma. It is certainly not possible to educate about allergen avoidance without being clear about specific sensitivity, and histories of allergen exposure are not sufficient. Diagnosis of immediate hypersensitivity can be made either by skin tests or *in vitro* assays. While there are no internationally accepted criteria for establishing sensitivity, standards can be proposed. Thus, a prick test weal response of 5 mm using an extract containing between 10 and 70 µg of major allergen/ml can be regarded as a definite positive. Similarly, the presence of 5 ng of IgE antibody/ml of serum is a definite positive result. A high level of 20 ng of IgE antibody is very broadly equivalent to a weal response > 7 mm. The primary concern is to establish definitely whether or not a patient is specifically sensitive. The relevance of quantitating higher degrees of sensitivity is not clear. Thus, although it is possible and desirable to grade skin tests or RAST results, it is unclear whether such grading changes the interpretation of the results. However, higher grades do increase the level of reliability of the result and, thus, increase the confidence with which they can be interpreted in relation to symptoms.

Allergen inhalation tests

Allergen inhalation tests are not required to confirm the clinical relevance of allergens in asthma.[26] Like skin tests and RAST, their effects will depend on the potency or allergen content of the extracts. Their effect is also determined by the degree of airway responsiveness to histamine (or methacholine) and, therefore, the dose required to cause an early asthmatic response can be predicted from skin sensitivity to the allergen extract and the degree of histamine airway responsiveness.[66] Allergen inhalation tests are, however, useful in research, and have been important in the recognition of the relationship between the cellular phase of inflammation in the airways and the heightening of airway responsiveness to histamine or methacholine.[8,10,12,19] The methods are described elsewhere.[25,26]

Measurement of allergen exposure

It is generally recognised that the frequency of sensitisation, i.e. IgE antibody protection, is related to the quantity of exposure to allergens. Thus, for many antigens the prevalence of sensitisation is much lower in areas where the allergen is at low levels or absent. Exposure to pollen outside can be estimated from pollen counts, and in some areas there is a direct relationship, not only between maximum pollen counts and sensitisation, but also between asthma exacerbations and seasonal peaks in airborne pollen.[57-59]. Until recently, it has been difficult to measure exposure to the most important indoor allergens and, therefore, impossible to define the levels of exposure that should be regarded as relevant to sensitisation or the development of BHR. Counting mites in house dust has provided a background understanding of the relationship between the exposure to mites and allergic disease.[55,67] The problem with identifying and counting mites is that it is time consuming, skilled, and difficult to standardise. The first assays of allergens in house dust used RAST inhibition; however, it is generally only possible to express the results in relative units and again the results are difficult to standardise because of the requirement for a serum pool.[65,68] Over the last 10 years, several major indoor allergens have been purified including; *Fel d* I, a salivary protein from the cat;[56,69] *Der p* I and *Der f* I, which are digestive enzymes of mites of the genus *Dermatophagoides*;[70,71] two major allergens from *Blatella germanica*, the German cockroach;[72,73] and *Mus d* I, a urinary protein from the rat or mouse. In each case, purification has allowed the development of specific assays that can be applied to house dust extracts.[69,70,72,73] More recently, assays have been developed using monoclonal antibodies.[64] The major advantage of assaying specific proteins is that the results can be expressed in absolute units (i.e. μg), which can be standardised relative to national or international standards. Consequently, it is possible to compare the levels of different indoor allergens. The monoclonal antibody two-site assays add further advantages because they are simpler and faster than most other assays, and the reagents used (i.e. ascites containing monoclonal antibodies) can be produced consistently in large quantities.[64] Assays of specific major allergens do not necessarily reflect the total potency of an allergen extract because other important allergens may be present in very different proportions. Examples of this are strikingly different ratios of Group I (*Der p* I and *Der f* I) and Group II (*Der p* II and *Der f* II) allergens in dust mite extracts, or of *Fel d* I and cat albumin in cat extracts.[56,74] However, in house dust these ratios are generally consistent and a single marker protein can be used to indicate the quantity of allergen in a house dust sample.

Patients actually inhale airborne allergen and, theoretically, exposure levels should be based on airborne measurements. However, because of major problems with airborne measurements, it is advisable to use floor dust as a marker of exposure for the present. Airborne levels of allergen are generally very low, i.e. $1-20$ ng/m^3 which means that either very sensitive assays are required or large volumes have to be sampled.[75–78] In addition, the particle size of airborne allergens may be critically important. For example, in one study airborne mite allergen *Der p* I was found to be $\geq 90\%$ large particles and the number of particles representing 20 ng was estimated at 100.[75,79] In another house studied for cat allergen, 60% of the allergen was on particles ≤ 2.5 μm and it was estimated that the 5 ng airborne/m^3 was carried on $> 10^6$ particles.[77,78,80] Thus, without measurements of particle size it may be difficult to evaluate airborne measurements. At present, several different techniques are in use and the results obtained have varied. Furthermore, while it is clear that disturbance can dramatically change airborne levels, it is not possible to define the degree of disturbance. The exact procedure used for collecting floor samples is easily described,[81] but because of variations in the efficacy of dust collection, it is best to express all results in μg/g of dust rather than as total μg or μg/surface area.[81]

The levels of mite allergen measured in floor samples have ranged from ≤ 0.01 to ≥ 100 μg/g of dust.[60,75,81] This range appears to apply to most of the allergens studied to date, i.e. mite, cat, cockroach, rat urine. While there seems little doubt that larger quantities will progressively increase the risk of disease, it is much easier to evaluate results or to recommend intervention if significance is defined at a particular level. Although values are necessarily provisional, there is enough data for mite allergens to recommend levels, and these were published as part of the report of an international workshop on the relationship between mites and asthma.[81] Two levels were proposed; one which was a risk for sensitisation (i.e. IgE antibody formation) and development of BHR, and a second higher level which was a risk for acute attacks of asthma among individuals allergic to mite (Table 3.1). At the

Table 3.1 Provisional standards for indoor levels of dust mites and dust mite allergens

1 Level that is a risk for the development of IgE antibody and persistent bronchial reactivity	2 µg Group I* mite allergen/g dust (≃ 100 mites or 0.6 mg guanine/g dust)
2 Level that represents a risk for acute asthma and a level at which most mite allergic patients will experience symptoms	10 µg Group I mite allergen/g dust (≃ 500 mites/g dust)

* Group I mite allergen is the sum of *Der p* I and *Der f* I from *D. pteronyssinus* and *D. farinae*, respectively (modified from reference 81).

workshop, it was generally agreed that 2 µg of *Der p* I is equivalent to 100 mites/g or 0.6 mg of guanine/g of dust.[75,81,82]

The justification for these proposed levels comes from several different studies, both on mite numbers and on mite allergen levels (Figure 3.1). The first suggestion that a given level of mites was significant came from Spieksma[55] who regarded 200 mites/g of dust as a level above which most mite allergen individuals would have symptoms. More recently, Korsgaard, on the basis of a formal epidemiological study in Denmark, concluded that ≥ 100 mites/g of dust was a sevenfold risk factor for the development of

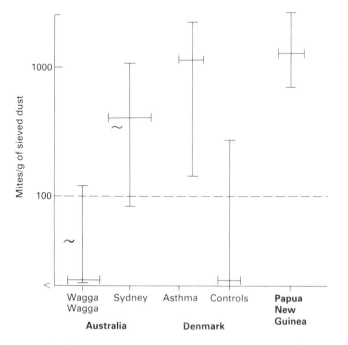

Fig. 3.1 Levels of dust mites in: houses from two towns in Australia:[84] houses of patients with asthma and controls from Aarhus in Denmark:[83] blankets being used by natives in Papua, New Guinea, who developed mite allergy and asthma.[85]

mite allergic asthma.[83] In Australia, Woolcock, Green and their co-workers[84] studied two communities with very different climates, a dry inland town where the house dust contained on average < 100 mites/g, and a coastal town where more than 90% of the samples contained > 100 mites/g. They found a strong association between positive skin tests to mites and BHR in children in the coastal town, but no such association in the inland town. In another striking study, the introduction of blankets to a native community in the South Fore region of Papua, New Guinea, represented the first site of mite growth in their houses.[85] This was followed by a dramatic increase in asthma and BHR from < 0.7% to 7%. The number of mites in dust from the blankets was ~ 1000/g and the individuals who developed asthma had all become allergic to mites, with both positive skin tests and IgE antibody.[86]

The studies that relate levels of mite allergen in dust to asthma are different but lead to the same conclusions (Figure 3.2). Houses of symptomatic mite allergic asthmatic individuals, both in the United States and Europe, have generally been found to contain dust with 10 μg *Der p* I/g of dust.[65,87,88] By contrast, 39/41 dust samples from houses in North California, where mite allergy was not an apparent risk factor for asthma, contained < 2 μg Group I

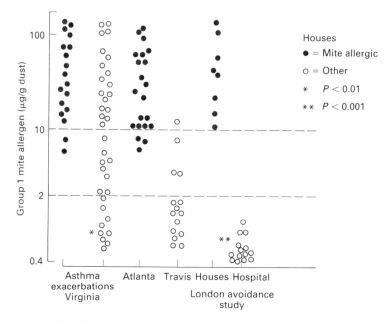

Fig. 3.2 Mite allergen levels in dust from houses of asthmatic patients in Virginia (mite allergic (●) compared to non-mite allergic (○)).[88] Mite allergen levels in dust from houses of mite allergic asthmatic children in Atlanta compared to levels from the houses of patients in Travis, North California, presenting with asthma during the pollen season.[87] Finally, the results from an avoidance study in London 1982 comparing levels in patients' houses with those in an 'allergen free' room.[89]

protein/g of dust.[57] When seven asthmatic patients were moved from houses with a mean level of $13 \, \mu g/g$ of dust to hospital rooms with $< 0.2 \, \mu g/g$ of dust, they all improved, and five had a progressive reduction in BHR.[89] As yet, it has not been shown that seasonal rises in mite allergen levels above a threshold can increase severity of symptoms. However, there have been reports of seasonal increases in asthma symptoms among mite allergic asthmatics in some areas, and the levels of mites and allergen in dust can increase dramatically during humid periods of the year.[55,67,88] Indeed, individual carpets can change from $< 1 \, \mu g$ to $50 \, \mu g$ Group I protein/g of dust.[88] Thus, while the data are obviously incomplete, it appears reasonable to propose the levels of mites and mite allergen exposure shown in Table 3.1. It is clearly premature to specify the quantitative or percent decrease in allergen exposure that would be necessary to produce an improvement in symptoms. However, it seems likely that a decrease of at least 10-fold in exposure would be necessary to produce a significant change in a controlled trial. The techniques necessary for decreasing the levels of mite or other allergens in houses are not well established. However, there is currently much interest in acaricides to mill mites and in air filtration and other techniques to reduce airborne cat allergen levels.

In conclusion, it is now possible to measure the levels of several different allergens in houses and the techniques are becoming progressively more simple. The levels that are relevant for mites are in the range $1-10 \, \mu g$ Group I protein/g dust, and it seems likely that levels for cockroach and cat proteins will be in a similar range although their distribution in the house is very different. In the next few years it should be possible to define the risk levels for many of the indoor allergens relevant to asthma. Ideally, one would define the risk associated with given levels of sensitivity and exposure. There is no level of exposure or sensitivity that guarantees the development of asthma, since some highly sensitive patients develop atopic dermatitis without wheezing or developing BHR. However, it now seems clear that increasing sensitivity and increasing exposure to either perennial or seasonal allergens, represents a progressively higher risk for the development of BHR and symptomatic asthma.

Sensitisation to chemical sensitisers

Chemicals encountered in the workplace are an important cause of sensitisation and asthma.[90] Allergic hypersensitivity to some chemicals, e.g. platinum salts, nickel, and acid anhydrides, can be identified by skin tests or RAST. However, with many chemicals e.g. isocyanates, plicatic acid, and colophony, there is no simple test. Sensitisation can be established in these people by controlled inhalation exposure tests in the laboratory, which are specialised and time consuming procedures.

An alternative approach to the objective confirmation of occupational asthma is to follow peak flow rates and methacholine airway responsiveness during periods both at work and away.[26,91] The problem is to distinguish occupational asthma caused by sensitisation to a chemical from non-occupational asthma where symptoms and variable airflow limitation may be worse at work because of the effects of triggers such as exercise, dust, and fumes acting on hyperresponsive airways. Occupational asthma is inferred if there are falls in peak flow rates and heightened airway responsiveness during periods at work, with improvement away from work. Non-occupational asthma, in contrast, causes an increase in peak flow rate variability at work without changes in airway responsiveness.

Releasability

In the 1960s it was a widely held belief that the quantitation and characterisation of the immunoglobulins involved in allergic responses would explain all their pathophysiological manifestations. However, once it became possible to measure and characterise human IgE and IgG antibodies against various allergens, it also became clear that these alone would not predict the extent of an allergic response.[92,93] Although IgE antibody responses to antigen are the classical means of distinguishing allergic from non-allergic individuals,[94] it is now generally agreed that these parameters alone cannot explain allergic rhinitis and asthma.

In the mid 1970s it began to be appreciated that alterations of effector cells (e.g. basophils and mast cells) might play a role in the pathogenesis of allergic disorders through the release of histamine, and other chemical mediators, secreted by these cells in response to immunological and non-immunological stimuli. In addition, it was demonstrated that a basophil that had 5000 IgE molecules on the membrane surface responded about as well to anti-IgE as one with 500 000. Similarly, Conroy, Adkinson and Lichtenstein,[95] studying the basophils from different patients, each with 100 000 IgE antibody molecules/cell, found that histamine release induced by the same concentration of anti-IgE could range from 10% to 95%. Thus, the response of these different cells was obviously influenced by something other than the antigen–antibody interaction.

The latter observation is the biochemical basis for the concept of releasability, defined *in vitro*. The term 'releasability' implies that biochemical events in basophils and mast cells, not only the surface density of the IgE molecules, determine the capacity of these cells to release mediators in response to activating stimuli.[96]

Additional evidence in support of the concept of releasability came from clinical observations. A study of patients allergic to insect venoms showed that subjects with identical levels of IgE anti-venom antibodies, the same amounts of IgG anti-venom antibodies and similar skin tests, had very different reactions when stung. For instance, one patient suffered severe anaphylaxis, whereas another was completely unaffected.[97] Similar observations have been made in individuals with positive skin tests to inhalant allergens. It is well known that patients with positive skin tests may suffer no symptoms during the appropriate season, whereas others with similar skin test results are clinically ill. In patients with food allergy, more than 50% of individuals with positive food skin tests will have no reaction on the ingestion of these foods, whereas the remaining 50% will respond.[98]

Taken together, these observations suggest that allergic individuals have both an altered IgE response to various allergens and an intrinsic alteration of the capacity of the effector cells to release chemical mediators in response to IgE, and possibly non-IgE-mediated, stimuli. Furthermore, studies of end organ responsiveness have identified other separate, but possibly related, abnormalities in these patients. For example, *in vivo* airway responsiveness to various chemical mediators is increased in most asthmatics[26] and the degree of this BHR is an important determinant of the airway constrictive response to allergic[66,99] and non-allergic stimuli, such as exercise and hyperventilation.[26,100] Although alterations of the IgE antibody response to antigen and BHR to various chemical mediators have been extensively studied in asthmatic and allergic individuals, the third category of abnormalities, basophil, and mast cell releasability, has received less attention.

Genetic and biochemical basis of releasability

Despite evidence to support the belief that basophil and mast cell releasability could be involved in the pathophysiology of allergic disorders, releasability was still not a tangible concept because it lacked a biochemical or genetic basis. The study of basophil and mast cell releasability was hampered by the lack of highly purified cells for appropriate biochemical studies. Therefore, attention focused on the possibility of providing a genetic basis for the concept of releasability.

To date, only one study, in monozygotic and dizygotic twins, has attempted to ascertain the influence of genetic and environmental factors on the releasability of basophils.[101] In this study, the release mechanisms of basophils were studied using three releasing agents; an IgE-specific stimulus (rabbit anti-IgE), the formylated tripepitide (formyl-L-methionyl-L-leucyl-L-phenylalan-

95

ine; the f-met peptide) which interacts with a specific cell surface receptor and is not cross-desensitised with anti-IgE,[102] and the Ca^{2+} ionophore, A23187, which causes release by allowing transmembrane Ca^{2+} influx and bypasses some of the early stages of the release process.[103] This study employed basophils obtained from 14 monozygotic and 13 dizygotic twins exposed to a range of concentrations of stimuli optimal for histamine release. The results indicated that both IgE-mediated releasability and basophil sensitivity to anti-IgE were influenced by genetic factors. The response to A23187 seemed to be mainly controlled by genetic factors, whereas the response to f-met peptide was only slightly influenced by these factors, if at all. The results of this study indicated that IgE-mediated releasability is determined by genetic factors, thus confirming the importance of this parameter in the control of mediator release from human inflammatory cells.

Several studies have demonstrated that the total serum IgE level and BHR are under genetic control.[104-106] Interestingly, no correlation was found between serum IgE levels and the maximal percentage of anti-IgE-induced histamine release in either monozygotic or dizygotic twins.[101] This suggests that IgE-mediated releasability, as well as BHR and serum IgE level (the hallmarks of the atopic state) are influenced by separate genetic factors, and this might account for the polymorphic genetic traits of allergic individuals.

Additional investigations are necessary to characterise further the genetic control of basophil releasability. Similar studies using different types of human mast cells, need to be made in order to evaluate whether this type of genetic control applies also to these cells. There may be differences because it is now well established that human basophils and mast cells are different from a biochemical, ultrastructural and pharmacological point of view.[107-109]

Altered releasability

Allergic rhinitis: Few studies have evaluated IgE- and non IgE-mediated releasability in detail in patients with allergic rhinitis. Basophils of patients with allergic rhinitis are more responsive to exposure to heavy water (D_2O) compared to normal individuals.[110] Indeed, basophils of patients with allergic rhinitis degranulate and release histamine in the apparent absence of a stimulus when cells are incubated *in vitro* using a buffer in which the water normally used has been substituted with 44% D_2O. The cells of approximately 32% of patients with allergic rhinitis released more histamine in D_2O-based buffer than controls. It was suggested that the release caused by D_2O was due to *in vivo* activation of basophils.[111] It is not known whether this enhanced state of basophil activation is due to exposure to suboptimal concentrations of an 'endogenous' releasing agent(s), or to qualitative alterations of IgE molecules on the membrane surface. It is of interest that a similar hyperresponsiveness to D_2O has been found in approximately 60% of patients with atopic dermatitis, another atopic disease.[112]

Releasability of basophils from patients with allergic rhinitis was also evaluated in a study in which spontaneous releasability of basophils from patients with allergic rhinitis was similar to that of controls. In contrast, the response to concanavalin A was significantly greater in patients with allergic rhinitis.[113] This observation calls for additional studies because, although there is evidence that concanavalin A interacts with human IgE, this molecule does not activate human lung mast cells.[114] In a recent study using basophils from patients with allergic rhinitis challenged with optimal concentrations of anti-IgE, f-met peptide and A23187, it was found that IgE-mediated releasability was slightly greater than that from control basophils.[115] No differences were detected when releasability induced by f-met peptide and A23187 were compared to controls.

Asthma: Few studies have evaluated releasability in patients with asthma. Initially, basophils from patients with steroid-dependent and non-steroid-dependent perennial asthma of unknown cause were compared to normal individuals.[116] It was found that release to anti-IgE, A23187, and mannitol, did not differ significantly between normal individuals and each group of asthmatics. Release to C5a and f-met peptide was the same in non-steroid-dependent asthmatics as in normal individuals, but was significantly lower in steroid-dependent asthmatics. These results were attributed to desensitisation caused by *in vivo* exposure to C5a and f-met peptide-like molecules. However, they may also represent effects of prolonged corticosteroid treatment on the response to C5a and f-met peptide. In fact, after basophils have been cultured with corticosteroids for 24 hours, they lose much of their capacity to release in response to anti-IgE.[117] Prolonged *in vivo* exposure to corticosteroids may also inhibit release to other stimuli.

In another study, IgE- and non-IgE-mediated releasability of basophils isolated from adult patients with allergic or non-allergic asthma, was compared to that of normal subjects.[118] In this study, the allergic asthmatics had at least one positive response to skin tests with common allergens, whereas the non-allergic patients had negative skin tests. Basophil histamine release to concanavalin A and anti-IgE was significantly greater in both allergic and non-allergic asthmatic patients compared to normal subjects. In contrast, basophil histamine release to Ca^{2+} ionophore A23187 was similar in leucocytes from normal subjects and asthmatic patients. In this study, the IgE-mediated releasability was also correlated with *in vivo* airway responsiveness. Interestingly, an inverse correlation was found between the basophil histamine release to anti-IgE and the provocative dose of inhaled histamine required to produce a 20% decrease in FEV_1. This observation suggests that the degree of enhanced IgE-mediated basophil releasability correlates with the degree of BHR to histamine in asthma.

Only two studies from the same group of investigators have examined in some detail the relationship between basophil releasability and BHR to histamine in children with asthma.[119,120] The release of histamine induced by the A23187[120] and by anti-IgE[119] from the basophils of asthmatic children was greater in asthmatics compared to age-matched healthy children. There was also a significant correlation between BHR to histamine and the histamine release *in vitro* to D_2O.[119]

It is obvious that there are significant differences in the results obtained by the few groups working in this area. It is possible that the differences reported so far are due to differences in the patients evaluated, their age, the types of asthma (extrinsic or intrinsic), degree of asthma, and the type of immunotherapy or drug therapy. Perhaps equally important is the lack of consistency in the nomenclature used to describe the different parameters evaluated in the study of basophil and mast cell releasability. However, it is clear that further studies are needed to probe the effects of the above factors in IgE- and non-IgE-mediated basophil and mast cell releasability in patients with asthma.

Marone *et al.* (unpublished observations) focused on the response to a single agent, D_2O, of basophils in 27 patients with extrinsic asthma and 20 patients with allergic rhinitis compared to 18 skin test negative controls (Figure 3.3). When 44% of the water in the isotonic buffer was replaced by D_2O, the vast majority (> 95%) of basophils from the non-atopic controls did not release histamine. In contrast, more than one-third of patients with allergic rhinitis, and approximately 50% of asthmatic patients were hyperresponsive to D_2O. These data indicate that D_2O responsiveness defines a subset of individuals with respiratory allergies whose basophils release more than 5% of their cellular histamine in response to 44% D_2O. Taken together, they confirm and extend previous observations that basophils of a percentage of asthmatics and, to a lesser extent, allergic rhinitis patients degranulate in the apparent absence of a stimulus.[112,121]

In another study, basophil releasability of 29 adult patients with extrinsic asthma and positive skin tests to *Dermatophagoides pteronyssinus* was compared with that of 31 skin test negative controls.[115] The response to a wide range of concentrations of anti-IgE (10^{-2} to 1 µg/ml) on the basophils of patients with

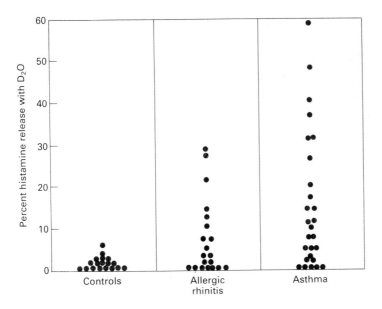

Fig. 3.3 Effect on leukocyte histamine release of using 44% heavy water (D_2O) in the isotonic buffer instead of water (H_2O). Peripheral blood leucocytes from 18 normal donors, 20 patients with allergic rhinitis and 27 patients with extrinsic asthma were incubated in the presence of 44% D_2O for 60 minutes at 37°C. The mean percent $\pm$ SD histamine in controls was 1.7 ± 0.4, in rhinitis was 7.3 ± 2.1 ($P < 0.01$ vs controls), and in asthmatics was 13.6 ± 2.8 ($P < 0.001$ vs controls).

asthma was significantly increased compared with controls. In addition, the maximum percent histamine release induced by anti-IgE in asthmatics was higher than in controls. Interestingly, there was an excellent linear correlation between the maximum percent histamine release caused by anti-IgE and the maximum percent histamine release induced by the purified allergen, *Der p* I, from basophils of the asthmatic patients. This correlation tends to support the notion that the increased IgE-mediated releasability of basophils from asthmatic patients is, to some extent, relevant to their allergic condition. In this study, the non-IgE-mediated basophil releasability was also examined. Similar to previous reports in adults,[114,118] but in contrast to those in children,[119,120] the basophil reactivity to the Ca^{2+} ionophore, A23187, was similar in asthmatics to controls. In contrast, however, the percent histamine release induced by all concentrations (10^{-8} to 10^{-5} M) of f-met peptide was significantly increased in the asthmatics.

These results were obtained with basophilic leucocytes, inflammatory cells involved in a wide group of allergic conditions.[108] In addition to basophils, however, it is likely that mast cells at the bronchoalveolar level are the first type of inflammatory cells involved, through the allergen-IgE interaction, in asthmatic subjects inhaling allergens. The cellular and immunological analysis of BAL is now widely used in the evaluation of patients with asthma and other pulmonary diseases. Data are rapidly accumulating in this area suggesting that histamine and other pro-inflammatory mediators are present in higher concentrations in BAL fluids obtained from asthmatics compared to normal subjects.

Previous BAL studies have demonstrated increased percentages of mast cells and eosinophils in subjects with asthma.[6,7,15,16] These cellular abnormalities have been inversely correlated with either baseline pulmonary function or BHR to histamine or methacholine.[7,15,16]

Mast cell- and eosinophil-derived mediators such as histamine, PGD_2, and peptide leukotrienes, presumably play a major role in the pathophysiology of asthma. Several groups have evaluated the concentrations of these mediators in BAL fluids from normal subjects and from asthmatic patients. Histamine levels in normal subjects have ranged from 11 to 300 pg/ml BAL fluid;[7,114,122–124] in asthmatics, while some studies have shown elevations of four to 10-fold.[114,123,125] others have shown no increase.[124,126] In addition to histamine, PGD_2 appears to be the predominant arachidonic acid metabolite found in asthmatics compared to normal subjects.

Mast cells are probably the source of both histamine and PGD_2 present in BAL fluids in asthmatic patients. Therefore, it has been appropriate to examine releasability of mast cells in the BAL fluid of patients with asthma. Casolaro et al.[114] have looked at IgE- and non-IgE-mediated releasability of BAL mast cells obtained from patients with asthma and from control subjects. BAL mast cells from both controls and asthmatics were unresponsive to f-met peptide and equally responsive to compound A23187. In contrast, the BAL mast cells of asthmatics, compared to controls, were sensitive to anti-IgE. In this study, the histamine content of BAL fluid from the asthmatics was approximately four times higher than that of controls. Therefore, it is possible that the increased releasability of BAL mast cells is, at least in part, responsible for the increased levels of inflammatory mediators found in asthmatic subjects, which is evidence of chronic inflammation in these patients.

In conclusion, the results of several studies suggest that altered basophil and mast cell releasability is one of the hallmarks of asthma. The results obtained so far are occasionally contradictory. Asthma is a heterogeneous condition; therefore a better characterisation of patients, type and degree of asthma, age of donors, and types of therapy, is necessary to establish the degree of altered releasability in these patients. However, the release of chemical mediators in response to standard stimuli (e.g. cellular releasability) is an important parameter that is just starting to be characterised. Releasability needs to be evaluated separately in basophils and mast cells from different tissues. It must also be defined with respect to each stimulus, since profound differences exist between IgE- and non-IgE-mediated releasability. In addition, it is important to note that releasability is influenced by genetic and environmental factors that have not yet been defined. Furthermore, IgE- and non-IgE-mediated releasability are influenced by an age-dependent factor that should be taken into account when designing future studies.

Despite all these problems, the evaluation of basophil and mast cell releasability could already be useful in defining different types of allergic disorders.

REFERENCES

1 Laitenen LA. Epithelial damage. In; Malo JL, Hargreave F, Hogg J eds. *Glucocorticoids and mechanisms of asthma*. Excerpta Medica (in press).

2 Jeffrey PK, Nelson FC, Wardlaw A, Kay AB, Collins JV. Quantitative analysis of bronchial biopsies in asthma. *Am Rev Respir Dis* 1987;**135**:A316.

3 Lozewicz S, Gomez E, Ferguson H, Davies RJ. Inflammatory cells in the airways in mild asthma. *Br Med J* 1988;**297**:1515–6.

4 Beasley R, Roche RW, Roberts JA, Holgate ST. Cellular events in the bronchi in mild asthma and after bronchial provocation. *Am Rev Respir Dis* 1989 (in press).

5 Gibson P, Mattoli S, Dolovich J, Denburg J, Hargreave FE. Airway inflammation in asthma; characterization using sputum analysis and bronchial brushings. *J Allergy Clin Immunol* 1988;**81**(1):247.

6 Tomioka M, Ida S, Shindoh Y, Ishihara T, Takishima T. Mast cells in bronchoalveolar lumen of patients with bronchial asthma. *Am Rev Respir Dis* 1984;**129**:1000–5.

7 Flint KC, Leung KBP, Hudspith BN, Brostoff J, Pearce FL, Johnson NM. Bronchoalveolar mast cells in extrinsic asthma; a mechanism for the initiation of antigen specific bronchoconstriction. *Br Med J* 1985;**291**:923–6.

8 De Monche JGR, Kauffman HF, Venge P *et al*. Bronchoalveolar eosinophilia during allergen-induced late asthmatic reactions. *Am Rev Respir Dis* 1985;**131**:373–6.

9 Summary and recommendations of a workshop on the investigative use of fiberoptic bronchoscopy and bronchoalveolar lavage in asthmatics. *Am Rev Respir Dis* 1985;**132**:180–2.

10 Metzger WJ, Richerson HB, Worden K, Monick M, Hunninghake GW. Bronchoalveolar lavage of allergic asthmatic patients following allergen bronchoprovocation. *Chest* 1986;**89**:477–83.

11 Casale TB, Wood D, Richerson HB, Zehr B, Zavala D, Hunninghake GW. Direct evidence of a role for mast cells in the pathogenesis of antigen-induced bronchoconstriction. *J Clin Invest* 1987;**80**:1507–11.

12 Fabbri L, Boschetto P, Zocca E *et al*. Broncho-alveolar neutrophilia during late asthmatic reactions induced by toluene diisocyanate. *Am Rev Respir Dis* 1987;**136**:36–42.

13 Lam S, Leriche JC, Kijek K, Phillips D. Effect of bronchoalveolar lavage volume on cellular and protein recovery. *Chest* 1985;**88**:856–9.

14 Fick RB Jr, Richerson HB, Zavala DC, Hunninghake GW. Bronchoalveolar lavage in allergic asthmatics. *Am Rev Respir Dis* 1987;**135**:1204–9.

15 Kirby JG, Hargreave FE, Gleich GH, O'Byrne PM. Bronchoalveolar cell profiles of asthmatic and nonasthmatic subjects. *Am Rev Respir Dis* 1987;**136**:379–83.

16 Wardlaw AJ, Dunnette S, Gleich GJ, Collins JV, Kay AB. Eosinophils and mast cells in bronchoalveolar lavage in subjects with mild asthma. Relationship to bronchial hyperreactivity. *Am Rev Respir Dis* 1988;**137**:62–9.

17 Gibson PG, Girgis-Gabardo A, Morris MM *et al.* Cellular characteristics of sputum from patients with asthma and chronic bronchitis. *Thorax* (in press).

18 Cookson WOCM, Craddock CF, Benson MK, Durham SR. Falls in peripheral eosinophil counts parallel the late asthmatic response. *Am Rev Respir Dis* 1989;**139**:458–62.

19 Gibson PG, Manning PJ, Girgis-Gabardo A *et al.* Progenitors during the late asthmatic response to allergen. *J Allergy Clin Immunol* 1989;**83**:233.

20 Pauwels R, Joos G, van der Straeten M. Bronchial responsiveness is not bronchial responsiveness is not bronchial asthma. *Clin Allergy* 1988;**18**:317–21.

21 Hargreave FE, Dolovich J, O'Byrne PM, Ramsdale EH, Daniel EE. The origin of airway hyperresponsiveness. *J Allergy Clin Immunol* 1986;**78**:825–32.

22 Dolovich J, Hargreave FE, O'Byrne PM, Ruhno J, Newhouse MT. Asthma terminology; troubles in wordland. *Am Rev Respir Dis* 1986;**134**:1102.

23 Hargreave FE, Woolcock AJ. *Airway responsiveness; measurement and interpretation.* Mississauga: Astra Pharmaceuticals Canada 1985.

24 Hargreave FE, Sterk PJ, Ramsdale EH, Dolovich J, Zamel N. Inhalation challenge tests and airway responsiveness in man. *Chest* 1985;**87**:S202–6.

25 Hargreave FE, Fink JN, Cockcroft DW, *et al.* Workshop 4; The role of bronchoprovocation. *J Allergy Clin Immunol* 1986;**78**:517–24.

26 Hargreave FE. Inhalation provocation tests. In; Lessof MH, Lee TH, Kemeny DM, eds. *Allergy: immunological and clinical aspects.* 2nd edition. Chichester: John Wiley 1987:289–303.

27 Anderson SA, Schoeffel RE. The inhalation of ultrasonically nebulized aerosols as a provocation test for asthma. In; Hargreave FE, Woolcock AJ, eds. *Airway responsiveness; measurement and interpretation.* Mississauga: Astra Pharmaceuticals Canada 1985:39–50.

28 Boulet L-P, Legris C, Thibault L, Turcotte H. Comparative bronchial responses to hyperosmolar saline and methacholine in asthma. *Thorax* 1987;**42**:953–8.

29 Adelroth E, Morris MM, Hargreave FE, O'Byrne PM. Airway responsiveness to leukotrienes C_4 and D_4 and to methacholine in patients with asthma and normal controls. *N Engl J Med* 1986;**315**:480–4.

30 Thomson NC, Roberts R, Bandouvakis J, Newball H, Hargreave FE. Comparison of bronchial responses to prostaglandin F_{2a} and methacholine. *J Allergy Clin Immunol* 1981;**68**:392–8.

31 Hardy CC, Robinson S, Tattersfield AE, Holgate ST. The bronchoconstrictor effect of inhaled prostaglandin D_2 in normal and asthmatic men. *N Engl J Med* 1984;**311**:209–13.

32 Joos G, Pauwels R, van der Straeten M. Effect of inhaled substance P and neurokinin A on the airways of normal and asthmatic subjects. *Thorax* 1987;**48**:779–83.

33 Cushley MJ, Holgate ST. Adenosine-induced bronchoconstriction in asthma; role of mast cell-mediator release. *J Allergy Clin Immunol* 1985;**75**:272–8.

34 Mann JS, Holgate ST, Renwick AG, Cushley MJ. Airway effects of purine nucleosides and nucleotides and release with bronchial provocation in asthma. *J Appl Physiol* 1986;**62**:1667–76.

35 Foresi A, Chetta A, Corbo GM, Cuomo A, Olivieri D. Provocative dose and dose–response curve to inhaled propranolol in asthmatic patients with bronchial hyperresponsiveness to methacholine. *Chest* 1987;**92**:455–9.

36 Fuller RW, Dixon CMS, Cuss FMC, Barnes PJ. Bradykinin-induced broncho-constriction in humans. *Am Rev Respir Dis* 1987;**135**:176–80.

37 Du Toit JI, Woolcock AJ, Salome CM, Sundrum R, Black JI. Characteristics of bronchial responsiveness in smokers with chronic airflow limitation. *Am Rev Respir Dis* 1986;**134**:498–501.

38 Barnes PJ, Brown MJ, Silverman M, Dollery CT. Circulating catechol-amines in exercise and hyperventilation induced asthma. *Thorax* 1981;**36**:435–40.

39 Jackson PJ, Manning PJ, O'Byrne PM. New role for histamine H$_2$ receptors in asthmatic airways. *Am Rev Respir Dis* 1988;**138**:784–8.

40 Bascom R, Bleecker ER. Bronchoconstriction induced by distilled water. Sensitivity in asthmatics and relationship to exercise-induced bronchospasm. *Am Rev Respir Dis* 1986;**134**:248–53.

41 Hargreave FE, Ramsdale EH, Pugsley SO. Occupational asthma without bronchial hyperresponsiveness. *Am Rev Respir Dis* 1984;**130**:513–5.

42 Hargreave FE, Gibson PG, Girgis-Gabardo A, Morris MM, Denburg J, Dolovich J. Asthmatic airway inflammation without airway hyperresponsiveness to methacholine. *J Allergy Clin Immunol* 1989;**83**:245.

43 Ramsdale EH, Roberts RS, Morris MM, Hargreave FE. Differences in respon-siveness to hyperventilation and methacholine in asthma and chronic bronchitis. *Thorax* 1985;**40**:422–6.

44 Taylor RG, Joyce H, Gross E, Holland F, Pride NB. Bronchial reactivity to inhaled histamine and annual rate of decline in FEV$_1$ in male smokers and ex-smokers. *Thorax* 1985;**40**:9–16.

45 Lim TK, Taylor RG, Watson A, Joyce H, Pride NB. Changes in bronchial responsiveness to inhaled histamine over four years in middle aged male smokers and ex-smokers. *Thorax* 1988;**43**(Suppl.8):599–604.

46 Woolcock AJ, Cheung W, Salome CM. Relationship between bronchial responsiveness to propranolol and histamine. *Am Rev Respir Dis* 1986;**133**:A177.

47 Cockcroft DW. Measurement of airway responsiveness to inhaled histamine or methacholine; method of continuous aerosol generation and tidal breath-ing inhalation. In; Hargreave FE, Woolcock AJ, eds. *Airway responsiveness; measurement and interpretation*. Mississauga: Astra Pharmaceuticals Canada 1985:22–8.

48 Fabbri LM, Mapp CE, Hendrick DJ. Standardization of the dosimeter method for measurement of airway responsiveness in man. In; Hargreave FE, Woolcock AJ, eds. *Airway responsiveness; measurement and interpretation*. Mississauga: Astra Pharmaceuticals Canada 1985:29–34.

49 Ryan G, Dolovich MB, Roberts RS *et al*. Standardization of inhalation provocation tests; two techniques of aerosol generation and inhalation compared. *Am Rev Respir Dis* 1981;**123**:195–9.

50 Yan K, Salome C, Woolcock AJ. Rapid method for measurement of bronchial responsiveness. *Thorax* 1983;**38**:760–5.

51 Woolcock AJ, Salome CM, Yan K. The shape of the dose–response curve to histamine in asthmatic and normal subjects. *Am Rev Respir Dis* 1984;**130**:71–5.

52 Macklem PT. Bronchial hyporesponsiveness. *Chest* 1985;**87**(Suppl.5):S158–9.

53 James AL, Pare PD, Hogg JC. The mechanics of airway narrowing in asthma. *Am Rev Respir Dis* 1989;**139**:242–6.

54 Kern RA. Dust sensitization in bronchial asthma. *Med Clin North Am* 1921;**5**:751–8.

55 Voorhorst R, Spieksma FThM, Varekamp N, *House dust atopy and the house dust mite Dermatophagoides pteronyssinus (Troussart, 1877)*. Leiden: Stafleu's Scientific Pub 1969.

56 Ohman JL, Lorusso JR, Lewis S. Cat allergen content of commercial house dust extracts; Comparison with dust extracts from cat-containing environ-ment. *J Allergy Clin Immunol* 1987;**79**:955–9.

57 Pollart Sm, Reid MJ, Fling JA, Chapman MD, Platts-Mills TAE. Epidemiology of emergency room asthma in northern California; Association with IgE antibody to rye grass pollen. *J Allergy Clin Immunol* 1988;**82**:224–30.

58 Reid MJ, Moss RB, Hsu Y-P, Kwasnicki JM, Commerford TM, Nelson BL. Seasonal asthma in northern California; Allergic causes and efficacy of immunotherapy. *J Allergy Clin Immunol* 1986;**78**:590–600.

59 Bruce CA, Rosenthal RR, Lichtenstein LM, Norman PS. Diagnostic tests in ragweed-allergic asthma. A comparison of direct skin tests, leukocyte histamine release, and quantitative bronchial challenge. *J Allergy Clin Immunol* 1974;**53**:230–9.

60 Platts-Mills TAE, Chapman MD, Dust mites; Immunology, allergic disease, and environmental control. *J Allergy Clin Immunol* 1987;**80**:755–75.

61 Pepys J. Skin tests in diagnosis. In; Gell PGH, Coombs RRA, Lachmann PJ, eds. *Clinical aspects of immunology*, 3rd edition. Oxford: Blackwell Scientific Publications 1975:55–80.

62 Chapman MD, Rowntree S, Mitchell EB, Di Prisco de Fuenmajor MC, Platts-Mills TAE. Quantitative assessments of IgG and IgE antibodies to inhalant allergens in patients with atopic dermatitis. *J Allergy Clin Immunol* 1983;**72**:27–33.

63 Marsh DG, Goodfriend L, King TP, Lowenstein H, Platts-Mills TAE. Allergen nomenclature. *Clin Allergy* 1988;**18**:201–9.

64 Chapman MD, Heymann PW, Wilkins SR, Brown MJ, Platts-Mills TAE. Monoclonal immunoassays for the major dust mite (*Dermatophagoides*) allergens, *Der p* I and *Der f* I, and quantitative analysis of the allergen content of mite and house dust extracts. *J Allergy Clin Immunol* 1987;**80**:184–94.

65 Gleich GJ, Yunginger JW. Standardization of allergens. In; Rose NR, Friedman H, eds. *Manual of clinical immunology*. American Society for Microbiology 1976:575.

66 Cockcroft DW, Ruffin RE, Frith PA *et al*. Determinants of allergen-induced asthma; dose of allergen, circulating IgE antibody concentration, and bronchial responsiveness to inhaled histamine. *Am Rev Respir Dis* 1979;**120**:1053–8.

67 Arlian LG, Bernstein IL, Gallagher JS. The prevalence of house dust mites Dermatophagoides spp. and associated environmental conditions in homes in Ohio. *J Allergy Clin Immunol* 1982;**69**:527–32.

68 Tovey E, Vandenberg R. Mite allergen content in commercial extracts and bed dust determined by radioallergosorbent tests. *Clin Allergy* 1979;**9**:253–62.

69 Chapman MD, Aalberse RC, Brown MJ, Platts-Mills TAE, Monoclonal antibodies to the major feline allergen *Fel d* I. II. Single step affinity purification of *Fel d* I, N-terminal sequence analysis, and development of a sensitive two-site immunoassay to assess *Fel d* I exposure. *J Immunol* 1988;**140**:812–8.

70 Chapman MD, Platts-Mills TAE. Purification and characterization of the major allergen from *Dermatophagoides pteronyssinus*-antigen P_1. *J Immunol* 1980;**125**:587–92.

71 Chua KY, Stewart GA, Thomas RJ *et al*. Sequence analysis of cDNA coding for a major house dust mite allergen, *Der p* I; homology with cysteine proteases. *J Exp Med* 1988;**167**:175–82.

72 Pollart SM, Platts-Mills TAE, Chapman MD. Identification, quantification and purification of cockroach (CR) allergens using monoclonal antibodies (mAb). *J Allergy Clin Immunol* 1989;**83**:293.

73 Lind P, Schou C, Lowenstein H, Lockey RF. Characterization of cockroach extracts and purification of a cross-reacting, acidic allergen. *J Allergy Clin Immunol* 1988;**81**:269.

74 Heymann PW, Chapman MD, Aalberse RC, Fox JW, Platts-Mills TAE. Purification of *Der f* II and *Der f* III from pyroglyphid mites; Applications of monoclonal antibodies in structural and immunochemical analyses. *J Allergy Clin Immunol* 1988 (in press).

75 Tovey ER, Chapman MD, Wells CW, Platts-Mills TAE. The distribution of dust mite allergen in the houses of patients with asthma. *Am Rev Respir Dis* 1981;124:630–5.

76 Swanson MC, Agarwal MK, Reed CE. An immunochemical approach to indoor aeroallergen quantitation with a new volumetric air sampler; studies with mite, roach, cat, mouse, and guinea pig antigens. *J Allergy Clin Immunol* 1985;76:724–9.

77 Findlay SR, Stotsky E, Leitermann K, Hemady Z, Ohman JL Jr. Allergens detected in association with airborne particles capable of penetrating into the peripheral lung. *Am Rev Respir Dis* 1983;128:1008–12.

78 Van Metre TE, Marsh DG, Adkinson NF et al. Dose of cat (Felis domesticus) allergen I (*Fel d* I) that induces asthma. *J Allergy Clin Immunol* 1986;78:62–75.

79 Tovey ER, Chapman MD, Platts-Mills TAE. Mite faeces are a major source of house dust allergens. *Nature* 1981;289:592–3.

80 Luczynska CM, Chapman MD, Platts-Mills TAE. Aerodynamic size and airborne levels of cat allergen (*Fel d* I); relevance to asthma. *J Allergy Clin Immunol* 1988;81:310.

81 Dust mite allergens and asthma—a world wide problem. *J Allergy Clin Immunol* 1989;83:416–27.

82 Van Bronswijk JEMH, Bischoff E, Schirmacher W et al. Evaluating mite allergenicity of house dust by guanine quantification. *J Med Entomol* (in press).

83 Korsgaard J. Mite asthma and residency. A case-control study on the impact of exposure to house dust mites in dwellings. *Am Rev Respir Dis* 1983;128:231–5.

84 Green WF, Woolcock AJ, Stuckey M, Sedgwick C, Leeder SR. House dust mites and skin tests in different Australian localities. *Aust NZ J Med* 1986;16:639–43.

85 Dowse GK, Turner KJ, Stewart GA, Alpers MP, Woolcock AJ. The association between *Dermatophagoides* mites and the increasing prevalence of asthma in village communities within the Papua New Guinea highlands. *J Allergy Clin Immunol* 1985;75:75–83.

86 Stewart GA, Dowse GK, Turner KJ, Alpers MP, Nisbet A. Isotype specific immunoglobulin responses to the house dust mite *Dermatophagoides pteronyssinus* and the purified allergen *Der p* I in asthmatic and control subjects from the Eastern Highlands of Papua New Guinea. *Clin Allergy* 1988;18:235–43.

87 Smith TF, Kelly LB, Heymann PW, Wilkins SR, Platts-Mills TAE. Natural exposure and serum antibodies to house dust mite of mite-allergic children with asthma in Atlanta. *J Allergy Clin Immunol* 1985;76:782–8.

88 Platts-Mills TAE, Hayden ML, Chapman MD, Wilkins SR. Seasonal variation in dust mite and grass pollen allergens in dust from the houses of patients with asthma. *J Allergy Clin Immunol* 1987;79:781–91.

89 Platts-Mills TAE, Tovey ER, Mitchell EB, Moszoro H, Nock P, Wilkins SR. Reduction of bronchial hyperreactivity during prolonged allergen avoidance. *Lancet* 1982;ii:675–8.

90 Chan-Yeung M, Lam S. Occupational asthma. *Am Rev Respir Dis* 1986;133:686–703.

91 Cartier A, Malo J-L, Forest F et al. Occupational asthma in snow crab-processing workers. *J Allergy Clin Immunol* 1984;74:261–9.

92 Lichtenstein LM, Holtzman NA, Burnett LS. A quantitative *in vitro* study of the chromatographic distribution and immunoglobulin characteristics of human blocking antibody. *J Immunol* 1968;101:317–24.

93 Platts-Mills TAE, von Maur RK, Ishizaka K, Norman PS, Lichtenstein LM. IgA and IgE anti-ragweed antibodies in nasal secretions. Quantitative measurements of antibodies and correlation with inhibition of histamine release. *J Clin Invest* 1986;57:1041–50.

94 Ishizaka K, Ishizaka T. Immunology of IgE-mediated hypersensitivity. In: Middleton E Jr, Reed CE, Ellis E, eds. *Allergy, Principles and Practice*, 2nd edition. St Louis: CV Mosby Company 1983:43.

95 Conroy MC, Adkinson NF Jr, Lichtenstein LM. Measurement of IgE on human basophils; relation to serum IgE and anti-IgE-induced histamine release. *J Immunol* 1977;**118**:1317–21.

96 Lichtenstein LM, MacGlashan DW Jr. The concept of basophil releasability. *J Allergy Clin Immunol* 1986;**77**:291–4.

97 Hunt KJ, Valentine MD, Sobotka AK, Benton AW, Amodio FJ, Lichtenstein LM. A controlled trial of immunotherapy in insect hypersensitivity. *N Engl J Med* 1978;**299**:157–61.

98 Sampson HA, Albergo R. Comparison of results of skin tests, RAST, and double-blind placebo-controlled food challenges in children with atopic dermatitis. *J Allergy Clin Immunol* 1984;**74**:26–33.

99 Howarth PH, Durham SR, Kay AB, Holgate ST. The relationship between mast cell-mediator release and bronchial reactivity in allergic asthma. *J Allergy Clin Immunol* 1987;**80**:703–11.

100 Howarth PH, Pao GJ-K, Church MK, Holgate ST. Exercise- and isocapnic hyperventilation-induced bronchoconstriction in asthma; relevance of circulating basophils to measurements of plasma histamine. *J Allergy Clin Immunol* 1984;**73**:391–9.

101 Marone G, Poto S, Celestino D, Bonini S. Human basophil releasability. III. Genetic control of human basophil releasability. *J Immunol* 1986;**137**:3588–92.

102 Marone G, Columbo M, Soppelsa L, Condorelli M. The mechanism of basophil histamine release induced by pepstatin A. *J Immunol* 1984;**133**:1542–6.

103 Marone G, Findlay SR, Lichtenstein LM. Modulation of histamine release from human basophils *in vitro* by physiological concentrations of zinc. *J Pharmacol Exp Ther* 1981;**217**:292–8.

104 Bazaral M, Orgel HA, Hamburger RN. Genetics of IgE and allergy; Serum IgE levels in twins. *J Allergy Clin Immunol* 1974;**54**:288–304.

105 Gerrard J, Rao D, Morton N. A genetic study of immunoglobulin E. *Am J Hum Genet* 1978;**30**:46–58.

106 Hopp RJ, Bewtra AK, Watt GD. Nair NM, Townley RG. Genetic analysis of allergic disease in twins. *J Allergy Clin Immunol* 1984;**73**:265–70.

107 Dvorak AM, Galli SJ, Schulman ES, Lichtenstein LM, Dvorak HF. Basophil and mast cell degranulation. Ultrastructural analysis of mechanisms of mediator release. *Fed Proc* 1983;**42**:2510–5.

108 Marone G. The role of basophils and mast cells in the pathogenesis of pulmonary diseases. *Arch Allergy Appl Immunol* 1985;**76**(Suppl.1):70–82.

109 Peachell PT, Columbo M, Kagey-Sobotka A, Lichtenstein LM, Marone G. Adenosine potentiates mediator release from human lung mast cells. *Am Rev Respir Dis* 1988;**138**:1143–51.

110 Tung R, Lichtenstein LM. *In vitro* histamine release from basophils of asthmatic and atopic individuals in D_2O. *J Immunol* 1982;**128**:2067–72.

111 Kazimierczak W, Plaut M, Knauer KA, Meier HL, Lichtenstein LM. Deuterium-oxide-induced histamine release from basophils of allergic subjects. I. Responsiveness to deuterium oxide requires an activation step. *Am Rev Respir Dis* 1984;**129**:592–6.

112 Marone G, Giugliano R, Lembo G, Ayala F. Human basophil releasability. II. Changes in basophil releasability in patients with atopic dermatitis. *J Invest Dermatol* 1986;**87**:19–23.

113 Busse WW, Swenson CA, Sharpe G, Koschat M. Enhanced basophil histamine release to concanavalin A in allergic rhinitis. *J Allergy Clin Immunol* 1986;**78**:90–7.

114 Casolaro V, Galeone D, Giacummo A, Sanduzzi A, Melillo G, Marone G. Human basophil/mast cell releasability. V. Functional comparisons of cells obtained from peripheral blood, lung parenchyma and from bronchoalveolar lavage in asthmatics. *Am Rev Respir Dis* 1989 (in press).

115 Marone G, Casolaro V, Ayala F, Melillo G, Condorelli M. The concept of releasability in allergic disorders. In; Melillo G, Norman PS, Marone G, eds. *Clinical Immunology*, Volume 2. Toronto: BC Decker 1989 (in press).

116 Findlay SR, Lichtenstein LM. Basophil 'releasability' in patients with asthma. *Am Rev Respir Dis* 1980;**122**:53–9.

117 Lampl KL, Lichtenstein LM, Schleimer RP. *In vitro* resistance to dexamethasone of basophils from patients receiving long-term steroid therapy. *Am Rev Respir Dis* 1985;**132**:1015–8.

118 Gaddy JN, Busse WW. Enhanced IgE-dependent basophil histamine release and airway reactivity in asthma. *Am Rev Respir Dis* 1986;**134**:969–74.

119 Neijens HJ, Raatgeep HC, Degenhart HJ, Kerrebijn KF. Release of histamine from leukocytes and its determinants *in vitro* in relation to bronchial responsiveness to inhaled histamine and exercise *in vivo*. *Clin Allergy* 1982;**12**:577–86.

120 Neijens HJ, Raatgeep RE, Degenhart HJ, Duiverman EJ, Kerrebijn KF. Altered leukocyte response in relation to the basic abnormality in children with asthma and bronchial hyperresponsiveness. *Am Rev Respir Dis* 1984;**130**:744–7.

121 Plaut M, Kazimierczak W, Lichtenstein LM. Abnormalities of basophil 'releasability' in atopic and asthmatic individuals. *J Allergy Clin Immunol* 1986;**78**:968–73.

122 Agius RM, Godfrey RC, Holgate ST. Mast cell and histamine content of human bronchoalveolar lavage fluid. *Thorax* 1985;**40**:760–7.

123 Casale TB, Wood D, Richerson HB *et al*. Elevated bronchoalveolar lavage fluid histamine levels in allergic asthmatics are associated with methacholine bronchial hyperresponsiveness. *J Clin Invest* 1987;**79**:1197–203.

124 Rankin JA, Kaliner M, Reynolds HY. Histamine levels in bronchoalveolar lavage from patients with asthma, sarcoidosis, and idiopathic pulmonary fibrosis. *J Allergy Clin Immunol* 1987;**79**:371–7.

125 Gravelyn TR, Pan PM, Eschenbacher WL. Mediator release in an isolated airway segment in subjects with asthma. *Am Rev Respir Dis* 1988;**137**:641–6.

126 Wenzel SE, Fowler AA, Schwartz LB. Activation of pulmonary mast cells by bronchoalveolar allergen challenge. *Am Rev Respir Dis* 1988;**137**:1002–8.

4: Physiology

J. M. **Drazen**, C. Hirschman, P. T. Macklem,
R. Pauwels, S. Permutt & C. Persson

Asthma is clearly associated with airway inflammation, but the
evidence associating asthma with inflammation, although com-
pelling, is circumstantial. It has yet to be established if the
inflammation observed in asthmatic syndromes is the cause,
direct or indirect, of the altered airway responsiveness characteristic of the disease. In this chapter the mechanisms associated
with inflammatory processes which might influence airway
responsiveness will be reviewed and the supporting evidence considered.

The response of asthmatic subjects to inhaled bronchoactive
agonists has at least two distinct components which distinguish it
from the response of normal subjects. In asthmatics, the airways
respond to inhaled smooth muscle agonists at doses which have
little or no effect in normal subjects, and the maximal response
observed (if there is a maximum) is much greater than that in
normal subjects.[1,2] These two distinguishing features may have
distinct aetiologies.[3] Any association between airway inflammation and hyperresponsiveness should provide an explanation for
both of these features. Most studies referred to in this chapter,
however, deal with the association between airway inflammation
and the sensitivity of the airways to a particular dose or concentration of an agonist rather than the maximal response achieved.

Firstly, alterations at the level of contractile elements themselves will be looked into. Specifically, is there evidence to support
a role for altered smooth muscle function as a result of inflammatory processes? Next, the way in which inflammatory mediators
could alter airway responsiveness will be considered: how such
mediators could act to alter the state of airway responsiveness.
Three broad categories of mediators—lipids, peptides, and adenosine—will be considered. Mechanisms linking the effects of mediators or other physical processes, including airway fluid balance in
altered airway responses, will be examined. Their integration in
animal models, and evidence and conjecture on the important
mechanisms will also be discussed. It should be stated at the
outset that although animal models have been used to study
airway hyperresponsiveness (BHR), it is not at all clear if these
models are an accurate representation of the hyperresponsiveness
of asthma. This chapter is not meant to be an exhaustive review,

but rather to highlight the mechanisms whereby inflammation could alter airway responsiveness.

INFLAMMATION AND AIRWAY CONTRACTILE TISSUES

Muscular constriction within the airway walls is thought to be an important mechanism of obstruction in various airway diseases. Little or no information exists on how inflammation itself affects the response of isolated contractile tissues. Indeed, airway smooth muscle removed from subjects with BHR is not hyperresponsive to contractive agonists compared with muscle obtained from normal subjects.[4-11] There may be diminished responsiveness to β-agonists of smooth muscle from asthmatic subjects *in vitro*,[11,12] but this is controversial.[13] Because airway tissues removed from subjects with asthma are likely to be inflamed[14] this suggests, but by no means proves, that inflamed and normal airway smooth muscle are the same. There is some evidence, however, to suggest that smooth muscle removed from animals which have been subjected to allergic sensitisation may be different from smooth muscle removed from normal animals.[15-17] To the extent that the sensitisation process is an inflammatory one, these data suggest that such tissues are physiologically different from normal tissues. These findings are not universal, however, as noted by Mansour and Daniel,[18] who suggest that specific aspects of the sensitisation process are critical in achieving this altered smooth muscle state.

In guinea-pigs, sensitisation to ovalbumin is accompanied by an increase in the resting membrane potential of about 11 mV in airway smooth muscle cells. The membrane potential is further altered after 'boosting' sensitised animals. These changes have been attributed to an increase in the activity of the electrogenic sodium pump.[15,16]

Tracheal smooth muscle from actively sensitised dogs exhibits a greater maximal response, an increased velocity of shortening, and responds at a lower dose of histamine than tracheal smooth muscle from normal dogs.[19-21] The former properties seem to be related to an enhanced activity of early cross bridge cycling.[22] This finding, together with the demonstration that tracheal smooth muscle from sensitised animals has increased adenosine triphosphatase (ATPase) activity,[23] suggests that more energy is available to sustain the enhanced rate of cycling of these cross bridges in sensitised tissues. The histamine hyperresponsiveness of tissues from actively sensitised animals has been attributed to a parasympathetic mechanism because it is atropine labile.[21] The mechanism of this response may be an alteration in acetylcholine release or breakdown in sensitised as opposed to non-sensitised tissues, as inhibitors of acetylcholinesterase can induce a state in non-sensitised tissues similar to that observed in sensitised tissues.[24] How the altered histamine response is linked to the early cross bridge cycling, if at all, is unclear.

At present, the associations between the sensitisation process and airway inflammation are not known, and future research in this area should include pathological examination of the tissues to determine the extent and nature of any inflammatory response. The inflammation induced by 'booster' injections, for example, may serve as an inflammatory stimulus leading to the observed effects. On the other hand, the two may be unrelated.

MEDIATORS OF INFLAMMATION AND ALTERED AIRWAY RESPONSES

Many different chemically distinct mediators are produced by inflammatory cells: the abilities of the mediators to alter the state of the airways by producing smooth muscle constriction or by altering fluid balance, represent powerful mechanisms whereby inflammation could alter airway responsiveness. In addition to the direct effects of constriction or altered airway fluid balance, these two effects could be interactive. For example, altered fluid balance could change the elastic properties of the airways and thus alter the load against which airway smooth muscle must act. Among the possible important mediators in asthma are three major classes of mediators; lipids, peptides, and adenosine.

Lipid mediators

There are two principal classes of lipid mediators—the eicosanoids and ether-induced phospholipids. The former class includes the prostaglandins, thromboxanes, and leukotrienes, while the major phospholipid mediator is platelet activating factor (PAF).

Eicosanoids

The sources, metabolism, pharmacology and physiology of the eicosanoids have been exhaustively reviewed,[25-28] and so attention will be focussed on the possible role that eicosanoids may have in inducing a state of heightened airway responsiveness.

The ability of the prostaglandins, thromboxanes and leukotrienes to induce BHR *in vivo* has been shown in two ways. In the first type of study subthreshold doses of eicosanoids (which do not cause bronchoconstriction) are given immediately before, or at the same time as each dose of the bronchoconstrictor agonist being tested. Walters *et al.*[29] and Heaton *et al.*,[30] showed that when inhaled by healthy subjects, PGF_2 decreases, by two to threefold, the provocative dose of histamine required to cause a 20% decrease in specific airways conductance (sGaw) (PD$_{20}$sGaw). Fuller *et al.*[31] showed that PGD$_2$ caused roughly a twofold reduction in the dose of histamine or methacholine needed to decrease sGaw by 35%. Using LTD$_4$, Barnes *et al.*[32] induced a sevenfold decrease in the PD$_{20}$sGaw for PGF$_2$. The thromboxane mimetic U-46619 and PGF$_2$ both decreased the concentration of inhaled acetylcholine in aerosol form required to cause an increase in pulmonary resistance (R$_L$) of 5 cmH$_2$O/l/s.[33,34] Subthreshold doses of LTD$_4$ in aerosol form sensitised the airways of rhesus monkeys to subsequent doses of LTD$_4$ or PAF.[35]

A potential complication of this type of experiment is that the methods used to measure airway smooth muscle tone are indirect. Subthreshold doses of bronchoconstrictor agonists may induce contraction of airway smooth muscle not evidenced by measurements of sGaw or R$_L$. Furthermore, it has been argued that small changes in baseline airway calibre may influence the subsequent responses to contractile agonists. In general, the approach to this problem has been to show that subthreshold doses of other bronchoconstrictor agonists do not provoke similar changes in airway responsiveness. Nevertheless, it could be argued that this type of experiment can not distinguish a supra-additive interaction, or synergism, between the eicosanoid and other specific bronchoactive mediators, from induction of increased airway responsiveness, which is known not to be mediator specific.

In the second type of study the eicosanoid is administered and airway responsiveness determined after allowing time for the effects of the eicosanoid to dissipate, as determined by normalisation of the pulmonary function which is used as the outcome indicator. Using this approach, Kern *et al.*[36] showed that inhalation of a dose of LTD$_4$ in normal subjects, which caused a 50% decrease in the maximal expiratory flow at 30% of the vital capacity measured on a partial flow–volume curve (V$_{30}$P), resulted in a twofold decrease in the concentration of methacholine required to elicit a 30% change in V$_{30}$P. In contrast, inhalation of methacholine rather than LTD$_4$ had the opposite effect. Similar results have been obtained in dogs[37] and guinea-pigs[38,39] after inhalation of LTB$_4$, LTC$_4$, or LTD$_4$. In dogs, inhalation of an aerosol form of LTB$_4$ (10 μM), which had no effect on pulmonary resistance, caused an increase in airway responsiveness, which persisted as long as three hours after inhalation of the leukotriene.[37] Munoz *et al.*[40] have shown that injection of U-46619 into the tracheal circulation of dogs potentiates subsequent isometric force generation of an isolated tracheal segment in response to stimulation of the vagus nerves. While the contraction induced by U-46619 subsides in less than one minute, the potentiation of responses to vagal stimulation continues for as long as one hour. A similar effect occurs after the administration of PGF_2, but the effect is smaller in magnitude and of shorter duration.[41] Each of these studies has the same drawback—that is, that the test used to confirm the dissipation of the effects of the eicosanoid may be insufficiently sensitive to perform that task.

The effects of eicosanoids on airway smooth muscle responsiveness can also be observed *in vitro*. Orehek *et al.*[42] reported that PGF_2 enhanced contraction of the trachea in the guinea-pig induced by acetylcholine and histamine. LTD_4 in the trachea of dogs[43] and LTE_4 in isolated guinea-pig trachea[44] have both been reported to increase the responsiveness to histamine. Fennessey *et al.*[38] and Lee *et al.*[44] however, were not able to show that LTD_4 behaved in this way in the trachea of guinea-pigs.

An alternative method of implicating eicosanoids in altered airway responsiveness is to examine the effects of interventions known to increase airway responsiveness in the presence or absence of agents that inhibit the metabolism of arachidonic acid by the cyclo-oxygenase or lipoxygenase pathways. Indomethacin and the thromboxane synthetase inhibitor, OKY-046, both inhibit BHR induced by ozone in dogs.[45,46] In guinea-pigs, the combined cyclo-oxygenase and lipoxygenase inhibitor BW755C and the leukotriene antagonist FPL55712 are effective blockers of this type of BHR.[47] Indomethacin also prevents the increased airway sensitivity to histamine that is induced in man by influenza vaccination,[48] and the increased airway responsiveness associated with inhalation of PAF in dogs.[49] In sheep both indomethacin and the leukotriene antagonist FPL57231 block the increase in airway responsiveness induced by antigens that is observed in animals with late reactions to antigen.[50] It is important to note, however, that in most asthmatics cyclo-oxygenase inhibitors do not alter airway responsiveness.

Taken together, these data suggest that eicosanoids can alter airway responses and responsiveness, but it is not clear if they can mediate changes in airway responsiveness similar to those observed in hyperresponsiveness states in man.

Platelet activating factor

Platelet activating factor (PAF), or 1-o-alkyl, 2-acetyl, *sn*3-phosphorocholine, is a mediator derived from the plasma membrane which can be produced by a variety of inflammatory cells including eosinophils and various mononuclear cells. A recent review covers in detail the biochemistry, pharmacology and physiology of PAF.[51] What is of greatest interest is its ability to induce a state of BHR in man: when PAF is inhaled by healthy volunteers acute airway obstruction ensues; this resolves over a few hours.[52,53] This is succeeded, however, by BHR which may persist for days to weeks.[52] There is uncertainty as to the mechanism(s) which provoke this hyperresponsive state: it is known that it is not a result of the secondary synthesis of cyclo-oxygenase products, or enhanced parasympathetic tone, but may be related to release of endogenous histamine.[54] Because studies in animals show that PAF is a potent chemotactic factor for eosinophils, the recruitment of this inflammatory cell to the airways may very well be of importance in the observed response.

Physiology

Peptide mediators

Peptide mediators, which function as circulating hormones, local regulators, or neurotransmitters are synthesised and secreted by endocrine cells and nerves. The presence of more than 10 peptides has been shown in mammalian lungs by radioimmunoassay or immunocytochemistry (Table 4.1).[55,56] Some peptides have been localised to isolated mucosal endocrine cells or neuroepithelial bodies; others are present within pulmonary nerves, and are therefore called neuropeptides. The existence in the airways of nerves containing peptides is supported by electron microscopic studies: axon profiles with a predominance of large, granular, or opaque vesicles (LGV) (80–120 nm) have been found in the airways of animals and man.[57] These are believed to contain peptides.

Vasoactive intestinal polypeptide and peptide histidine isoleucine

Vasoactive intestinal polypeptide (VIP) is a 28 amino acid peptide, originally discovered in lung extracts,[58] which is known to be present in human airway nerves.[59] The main pharmacological effects of this peptide are smooth muscle relaxation, vasodilatation and stimulation of exocrine gland secretion. Nerve fibres immunoreactive to VIP have been found within the airway smooth muscle, the walls of pulmonary and bronchial vessels, and around submucosal glands of the tracheobronchial wall.

Peptide histidine isoleucine (PHI) contains 27 amino acids, is homologous to VIP, and exerts various biological effects similar to those of VIP. It has been detected by immunochemical methods in the upper respiratory tract of various animals. Its distribution is similar to that of VIP and it elicits a dose-dependent relaxation of isolated airway smooth muscle which is quantitatively similar to VIP.[60] A related peptide, peptide histidine methionine (PHM), is probably the human form of PHI.[61] PHM is a potent relaxant of human bronchi *in vitro*.[62]

An infusion of VIP given to asthmatic volunteers caused bronchodilatation.[63] This effect, however, is probably partially mediated by a reflex release of catecholamines. Inhalation of VIP

Table 4.1 Regulatory peptides within the lung

	Localisation	Effect of stimulation
Calcitonin	EC	?
Calcitonin gene-related peptide (CGRP)	NF/EC	Vasodilatation/potentiation of action substance P/bronchoconstriction?
Cholecystokinin	Only dosage by RIA	?
Enkephalins	EC	Stimulation of J-receptors/inhibition of cholinergic neurotransmitters
Galanin	N/NF	?/contraction of gastrointestinal smooth muscle
Gastrin releasing peptide (GRP)/bombesin	EC/NF	Lung maturation/bronchoconstriction/mitogen for small cell carcinoma
Neurokinins	NF	See substance P
Neuropeptide Y (NPY)	N + NF	Modulation of sympathetic airway innervation?
Peptide histidine isoleucine (PHI)	N + NF	See VIP
Somatostatin	N/EC	Inhibitory neurotransmitter?
Substance P	NF	Bronchoconstriction/submucosal gland secretion/mast cell secretion/increase of vasopermeability/ mediator of NANC nerves?
Vasoactive intestinal peptide (VIP)	N + NF	Bronchodilatation/pulmonary vasodilatation/bronchial secretion/mediator of NANC?

EC, endocrine cells; N, neurones; NANC, non-adrenergic non-cholinergic; NF, nerve fibres; RIA, radioimmunoassay.

has not been shown to consistently induce bronchodilatation. VIP afforded some protection against bronchoconstriction induced by histamine, although it was less effective than salbutamol.[64]

Substance P and related tachykinins

Substance P is an undecapeptide with amidated C-terminal (Table 4.2). Substance P is widely distributed in the central and peripheral nervous system. Several peptides structurally related to substance P have been extracted from the skin of amphibians (physalaemin, kassinin) and the salivary gland of octopods (eledoisin). They are all deca, undeca or dodecapeptides with a similar, amidated C-terminal sequence (Table 4.2). They are called

Table 4.2 Amino acid sequence of tachykinins

Mammalian	
Substance P	ARG –PRO– LYS –PRO–GLN–GLN–*PHE*–PHE–*GLY*–*LEU*–*MET*–NH$_2$
Neurokinin A (substance K)	HIS – LYS –THR–ASP– SER –*PHE*–VAL–*GLY*–*LEU*–*MET*–NH$_2$
Neurokinin B (neuromedin K)	ASP–MET– HIS – ASP–PHE–*PHE*–VAL–*GLY*–*LEU*–*MET*–NH$_2$
Neuropeptide K	ASP– ALA – ASP – SER – SER – ILE –GLU– LYS –GLN–VAL–ALA– LEU – LEU
	LYS – HIS – SER – ILE –GLN–GLY – HIS –GLY –TYR– LEU –ALA–LYS
	ARG – HIS – LYS –THR–ASP– SER –*PHE*–VAL–*GLY*–*LEU*–*MET*–NH$_2$
Amphibian	
Kassinin	ASP– VAL –PRO– LYS – SER –ASP–GLN–*PHE*–VAL–*GLY*–*LEU*–*MET*–NH$_2$
Physalaemin	pGLU–ALA–ASP –PRO–ASN– LYS –*PHE*–TYR–*GLY*–*LEU*–*MET*–NH$_2$
Molluscan	
Eledoisin	pGLU–PRO– SER – LYS –ASP–ALA–*PHE*– ILE –*GLY*–*LEU*–*MET*–NH$_2$

tachykinins because they contract smooth muscle rapidly. Three tachykinin peptides have been identified in human airways-substance P, substance K (or neurokinin A) and an N-terminal extended form of neurokinin A called neuropeptide K.[65] Single nerve fibres or, less frequently, small bundles of nerve fibres containing these tachykinins, are present beneath and within the airway epithelium, around blood vessels and submucosal glands, within the bronchial smooth muscle layer and around local tracheobronchial ganglion cells. These nerve fibres are found in and around bronchi, bronchioles, and more distal airways, occasionally extending into the alveoli.

The main physiological effects of substance P and tachykinins are dilatation of vascular smooth muscle and constriction of airway smooth muscle.[66] They also stimulate exocrine gland secretion, increase microvascular permeability and cause histamine to be released from mast cells. Whereas inhalation of substance P does not cause any change in sGaw, the inhalation of neurokinin A, at rather high concentrations, results in a significant decrease in sGaw in mild asthmatics, but not in normal volunteers.[67]

Substance P may have a role in the regulation of bronchial secretion and mucociliary clearance. Nerve fibres immunoreactive to substance P are present around submucosal glands.[68] In investigations on human nasal mucosa, however, the topical administration of substance P, at doses that produced systemic vascular effects, had no effect on the rates of mucociliary transport and nasal secretion.[69]

Antidromic stimulation of sensory nerves (C-fibre afferents) produces vasodilatation (in skin, dental pulp, and nasal mucosa) and an increase in vascular permeability to plasma proteins (in skin and respiratory tract). These responses, also known as 'neurogenic inflammation', are assumed to be caused by mediator release from the peripheral endings of C-fibres.[70] Neurogenic inflammation has been described in the airways of rodents.[71] Electrical stimulation of the vagus nerves caused an atropine-resistant extravasation of Evans blue in rat trachea, indicating an increased vascular permeability. Cigarette smoke and light mechanical or local chemical irritation by ether, formalin, bradykinin or capsaicin also induced an increase in vascular permeability.[72] The increase in permeability was reduced in animals pretreated with a substance P antagonist.[73] Substance P (or a related tachykinin) might, therefore, have a role in neurogenic airway inflammation in airways of rodents.

Tachykinins are susceptible to degradation by endogenous enkephalinase or neutral metalloendopeptidase (EC.3.4.24.11). The biological activity of various tachykinins is enhanced in the presence of the enkaphalinase-inhibitors phosphoramidon or thiorphan.[74-78] Enkephalinase is present on the cell membranes of airway mucosal glands, epithelium, smooth muscle and nerves, and may therefore have an important regulatory role in the function of neuropeptides both in normal subjects and asthmatic patients. Indeed, regulation of the degradation of peptide mediators by various enzymes represents a principal mechanism whereby inflammation could influence the response to tachykinins. An inflammatory response that decreases expression of neutral endopeptidase will magnify the response to a stimulus which releases tachykinins.

Calcitonin gene-related peptide

Calcitonin gene-related peptide (CGRP) is a recently discovered neuropeptide containing 37 amino acids that is derived from the same gene as calcitonin.[79] In the peripheral nervous system CGRP is present in sensory neurons and nerve fibres where it is co-

localised with the tachykinins.[65] The biological actions of CGRP
include contraction of airway smooth muscle and relaxation of
vascular smooth muscle. Immunoreactivity to CGRP has been
shown in the mammalian and human lungs.[80,81] Nerve fibres
with immunoreactivity to CGRP are present in the tracheobronchial wall, beneath and within the airway epithelium, in vascular
and non-vascular smooth muscle, and sometimes close to small
glands. A few endocrine-like cells containing CGRP-like immunoreactivity have also been described in the tracheal epithelium.
Nerve fibres immunoreactive to substance P and CGRP and with a
similar distribution are located around blood vessels and smooth
muscle of the lower respiratory tract. Although it does not
influence the airway tone of rodents,[80] CGRP was reported to
have a potent contractile effect on isolated tissue from human
airways.[82] CGRP itself does not increase vascular permeability,
but it potentiates the protein leakage induced by substance P and
neurokinin A in rat and rabbit skin.[83] The coexistence of CGRP
with substance P, and the finding that CGRP is a potent inhibitor
of substance P degradation, suggest that CGRP can modulate the
actions of substance P.[84]

Bombesin—gastrin releasing peptide

Bombesin is a tetradecapeptide isolated from the skin of the frog
Bombina bombina. It has potent biological actions in mammals
such as release of gastrin and other gut hormones, stimulation of
the exocrine pancreas, and contraction of smooth muscle. Bombesin was found to be a potent bronchoconstrictor in anaesthetised
guinea-pigs.[85] Gastrin releasing peptide (GRP) contains 27 amino
acids. It has a C-terminal end with nine out of 10 amino acid
residues identical with bombesin and has similar biological
actions. GRP is regarded as the mammalian counterpart of
bombesin.[86] Immunocytochemical methods have localised bom-
besin-like immunoreactivity to mucosal endocrine cells (single
cells or groups of cells).[87] The presence in the respiratory tract of
nerve fibres immunoreactive to GRP was reported recently.[88]
These fibres were mainly distributed around blood vessels and
seromucous glands; scattered fibres were found in the smooth
muscle of the tracheal wall.

Neuropeptide Y

Neuropeptide Y (NPY) is a neuropeptide comprising 36 amino
acids.[89] It coexists with norephinephrine in sympathetic nerve
fibres in various vascular areas.[90] In the airways, immunoreactivity to NPY has been found in nerve fibres running in the
adventitia of blood vessels and in smooth muscle. The distribution

of NPY in the respiratory tract was similar to that of sympathetic nerve fibres.[88] NPY is a vasoconstrictor and modulates adrenergic neural effects.[90] Its role in the airways has not yet been examined.

Other peptides in airways

Galanin contains 29 amino acids;[91] immunoreactivity to galanin has been detected in the trachea, bronchus and major intra-pulmonary airways of various animal species. Nerve fibres positive for galanin have been detected predominantly in smooth muscle, as well as around seromucous glands and in the adventitia of blood vessels.[92] Its function in the airways is unknown at present. Calcitonin and leu-enkephalin have been localised to mucosal endocrine cells.[93] Somatostatin and cholecystokinin are present in the lung in very low concentrations.[94] The exact role of these peptides in the lung remains to be defined.

Adenosine

Adenosine, the main storage form of intracellular energy, is a purine nucleoside that is formed during the metabolism of adenosine triphosphate (ATP); it is broken down to adenosine monophosphate (AMP) when energy is required.[95] The AMP leaking out of the cell is metabolised by 5-nucleosidase into adenosine. Another possible source of adenosine is the nucleosides derived from digested nucleoproteins. ATP is also present in the nerve endings and is thought to act as a co-transmitter.[96] The released ATP may be rapidly transformed into adenosine. It may be expected that under conditions of high metabolic demand, cells and tissues release more adenosine than usual. Tissue concentrations of adenosine in animal lungs are increased by stimuli such as hypoxia[97] and antigen–IgE interaction.[98]

A possible role for adenosine in asthma was first suggested after the observation that therapeutic concentrations of theophylline effectively antagonised the activity of adenosine at the receptor level.[99,100] Further supporting evidence in favour of a pathogenetic role is derived from the following observations. The inhalation of adenosine produces a concentration-dependent bronchoconstriction in asthmatics but not in healthy people.[101] The fact that adenosine does not affect healthy volunteers may be due to the limited solubility of the substance—that is, an insufficient concentration to induce bronchoconstriction in healthy people with a lower non-specific bronchial responsiveness than that of asthmatics. It has also been shown that adenosine is a potent and rapidly acting stimulant of airway secretion.[102]

After allergen challenge, asthmatics show a biphasic increase in plasma adenosine concentration, while bronchial challenge with methacholine causes only one peak.[103] The initial increase in plasma adenosine after antigen challenge has been attributed to IgE-induced activation of mast cells and other inflammatory cells resident in the airways. The *in vitro* release of adenosine from mast cells has been documented in mice and rats.[104] Rat serosal mast cells release adenosine when challenged with either antigen (cells sensitised to IgE), compound 48/80, or the calcium ionophore A23187. Mast cells derived from mouse bone marrow have been shown to release adenosine when challenged with calcium ionophore. The *in vitro* release of adenosine from actively sensitised rat lung by antigen and compound 48/80 has been reported.[98] Hypoxia caused nearly a 10-fold increase in the pulmonary adenosine concentration in dogs.[97] Thus adenosine is likely to be present in inflammatory states.

Adenosine has been shown to enhance the release of preformed mediators from mast cells and basophils. For example, adenosine caused roughly a threefold increase in the rate of histamine release from isolated rat peritoneal mast cells stimulated with the calcium ionophore.[105] Similarly, adenosine potentiated the antigen-induced histamine release from chopped lung tissue, prepared from actively sensitised guinea-pigs.[106] Peters *et al.*[107] observed that adenosine enhanced histamine release induced by anti-IgE from dispersed human lung mast cells at low concentrations, but inhibited release at high concentrations. Hughes *et al.*[108] showed that the effect of adenosine on IgE-dependent release of histamine from human lung mast cells relied on the timing of the adenosine addition. When added to the dispersed lung mast cells up to five minutes before the immunological challenge, adenosine inhibited the release of histamine; when adenosine was added less than five minutes before challenge it caused a small potentiation.[109] A similar influence of the timing of adenosine administration has been shown *in vitro* in basophils in man.[110]

Another argument used in favour of a possible role for adenosine in asthma is the anti-asthmatic effect of theophylline, a known antagonist of adenosine under experimental conditions. Both oral and inhaled theophylline have also been shown to inhibit the bronchoconstriction induced by adenosine in asthmatic subjects.[101,111,112] This argument lost some of its strength when enprofylline, a xanthine with a poor adenosine-antagonist effect, was reported to be a more potent anti-asthmatic drug than theophylline.[113,114]

The mechanism of the bronchoconstriction induced by adenosine has been studied in a rat model.[115] Study of the potency of various adenosine analogues suggested that the bronchial adenosine receptor belongs to the A2 type. The bronchoconstriction caused by adenosine was inhibited by atropine, methysergide, sodium cromoglycate, nedocromil sodium and ketotifen. The observations in the rat model match closely those made in asthmatic patients. The bronchoconstriction induced by adenosine in asthmatics was inhibited by sodium cromoglycate,[101] nedocromil sodium,[116] atropine,[117] and the anti-histaminic drug terfenadine,[118] suggesting that the same mechanism as that in the rat model may be involved. Adenosine may therefore have a role in asthma both as a mediator released from nerve endings and as a positive feedback mechanism which provokes further mediator release. If the findings in dogs are applied to man it suggests that hypoxia should exacerbate asthma; this does not seem to be the case.

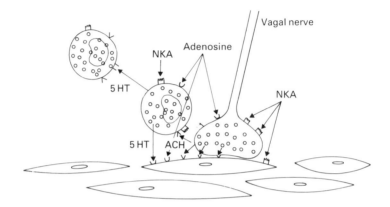

Fig 4.1 Potential relationships among vagal nerve fibres, mast cells (shown as round cells with 5HT, ACH, adenosine, and NKA receptors) and smooth muscle cells in asthmatic conditions.

Pharmacological studies in rats and man suggest that bronchoconstriction induced by adenosine is caused by stimulation of the adenosine receptors present on postganglionic vagal nerve endings and on mast cells. It is the synergism between the released acetylcholine and mast cell mediators that causes the bronchoconstriction. The adenosine released from mast cells may also further enhance the release of mediators from other mast cells. Other compounds also exert a synergistic effect between mast cells and vagal nerve endings; neuropeptides have been shown to be capable of using the same pathway for their bronchoconstrictor effects in the airway.[119] These mechanisms are illustrated in Figure 4.1: they may constitute a general pathway which may explain some of the controversial observations in asthma concerning the possible role of mast cells and nervous reflexes.

AIRWAY LIQUID IN LUNG DISEASE

One of the principal links between mediators and BHR is an airways epithelial surface containing greater than normal quantities of secretion. For many decades it has been accepted that airways in asthmatic patients may contain abnormal amounts of secretion. In 1932 Florey et al.[120] made some classic observations on cholinergic stimulation of mucus secretion. These workers also made an interesting remark about the source of fluid in inflamed airways, which was not, or only marginally, reduced by large doses of atropine: 'the bulk of fluid collected', is the 'product of vascular transudation rather than secretion from glands'. This information was omitted from their summary and, hence, has gone unnoticed. In 1949, Ingelstedt and Ivstam showed that the mucosal surface liquid in inflamed nasal airways in man was mostly a 'plasma exudate'.[121]

It is only in the past few years that plasma exudation and its potential roles in obstructive airway disease are beginning to receive due attention.[122] Contributing to this revival of a humoral role for asthma (dating back to Galen and Aeretus) is the understanding that active and reversible processes are involved in plasma exudation across airway endothelial–epithelial barriers, and that exuded plasma and its derived peptides and other contents may contribute to airway disease in ways other than by just the production of a degree of oedema in the mucosa.

Asthma and chronic bronchitis are both characterised as inflammatory airway diseases, with hypersecretion as one of the important symptoms.[123,124] Airway epithelial and glandular secretory processes have been examined extensively for many years and several excellent reviews describe the recent progress in the neural control, structural and molecular biology, and pharmacology of airway secretions.[125–131] A potential role for inflammation in hypersecretion has been particularly addressed. Despite a wealth of published reports on the subject, the role of bronchial secretions in the pathogenesis of obstructive airway diseases has been difficult to define.

Sputum production is increased especially in severe asthma.[132,133] Clinical improvement is associated with a reduced sputum production, in particular during treatment with anti-inflammatory drugs including glucocorticoids, cromoglycate, and terbutaline.[133–138] A consistent effect seems to be a reduction of the plasma exudate component of the sputum. Keal specifically looked for changes in secretory indices during treatment with glucocorticoids.[135] An increase, rather than a reduction, in sputum volume was observed, and Keal suggested that the effect of treatment with steroids 'lies in the reduction of transudate rather than any change in mucosal gland secretion'.[135] This suggestion was supported by Moretti et al., who analysed various markers of secretion and plasma proteins in sputum from 19 subjects with asthmatic bronchitis.[138] Thus two weeks of treatment with glucocorticoids reduced albumin and IgG concentrations to one-fifth and one-third, respectively, of starting values; the concentrations of fucose and N-acetylneuraminic acid remained virtually unchanged.[138]

If sputum production is reduced, an unchanged amount of a secretory product per unit of sputum produced also indicates an overall reduced secretion. The major reduction, however, seems to be in the amount of plasma exudation in the sputum. If the concentration of albumin in asthmatic sputum represented only undiluted plasma, this volume would constitute less than 10% of the sputum volume.[139,140] A larger volume of vessel fluid, however, is likely to accompany the exuded plasma—for example, the inflammatory breakdown of extravasated proteins will increase the number of molecules and, hence, interstitial osmotic pressure, thus promoting transudation.[141] A more diluted exudate—that is, a transudate—may be a large component of airway luminal liquids in asthma. Quantitative data on the composition of this lining fluid are sparse.

In human airways, the presence of glucocorticoids has been shown to reduce baseline secretion, but even large concentrations of these drugs had only marginal effects on mucus secretion induced by histamine and 5-monohydroxyeicosatetraenoic acid.[142] There is abundant experimental support for the prevention of plasma leakage by anti-asthma drugs, in particular glucocorticoids.[143] Serum is a potent stimulus of glycoprotein secretion in the airways.[130] Hence, reduction *in vivo* of mucus secretion induced by glucocorticoids may be secondary to inhibition of plasma leakage. The possibility of a pathogenetic role in asthma of that component of airway 'hypersecretion', which, by definition, is not a secretion but a plasma exudate/transudate, is supported by the composition of airway liquids in asthma, and by the effects of drugs targeted on that composition.

PLASMA EXUDATION IN ASTHMA

Exposure of the airway mucosa to a wide range of inflammatory stimuli thought to be involved in asthma produces prompt leakage of plasma not only into the airway wall, but also into the lumen.[143,144] Even at therapeutic threshold concentrations there was a correlation between plasma leakage into the airway wall and lumen (Erjfalt & Persson 1989, personal communication). Hence, it should be possible to examine the occurrence of plasma exudation in asthma by analysing sputum and mucus plugs, and by direct sampling of airway liquids. Such techniques have shown that plasma proteins are abundant in the airways of asthmatics.[139,143,145,146] It has been suggested that this feature distinguishes asthma not only from the normal healthy state but also from other airway diseases.[139,147] Airway plasma exudation,

however, is not pathognomonic to asthma. Plasma exudation is a
cardinal sign of an ongoing inflammatory process.[148] Thus, it
occurs in chronic bronchitis and cystic fibrosis as well as in
asthma, which is consistent with the inflammatory nature of
these diseases.[104,140,149]

Despite the limitations inherent in the bronchoalveolar lavage
(BAL) procedure—it involves additional drug treatment, cannot
be performed frequently to follow time courses, and is much more
specific for alveolar lining fluid than airway liquids—this technique has provided interesting information on plasma leakage in
asthma, especially at induced exacerbations. Lam et al.[150] obtained bronchial lavage fluids in control subjects and patients
with western red cedar asthma 24–48 hours after provocation
with plicatic acid. In the ordinary large volume lavage liquids, no
difference in plasma proteins could be shown between asthmatics
and normal controls, tallying with the hypothesis that asthma is
an airway and not an alveolar disease. Using a small volume
lavage in a large bronchus, Lam et al. also managed to obtain
relatively enriched airway fluid samples.[150] They showed a 10-
fold increase in albumin and IgG concentrations in asthmatics
compared with controls, suggesting that plasma exudation was
confined to the bronchial microcirculation. Fabbri et al. sampled
bronchial lavage fluid in asthmatics two and eight hours after
provocation with toluene diisocyanate (TDI).[151] Those responding to TDI with a late phase reaction had raised albumin levels in
the bronchial lavage liquids at both time points, suggesting that
the late reaction is preceded by, and associated with, an inflammatory process. In unsensitised guinea-pigs, topical exposure to
TDI induces dose-dependent plasma leakage into the airway
lumen. The leakiness is induced promptly, shows a peak at five
hours, and is maintained for at least 18 hours (Erjefalt & Persson,
unpublished observations). Immediate and late phase airway
responses stimulated by IgE are associated with clinically important plasma leakage in the airways of guinea-pigs.[152,153] Allergen
provocation of asthmatic bronchi has yielded inconsistent data on
mucosal appearance of exuded plasma proteins such as albumin
and fibrinogen,[154] but the inconsistencies may be due to the BAL
sampling procedure.

Nasal and tracheobronchial endothelial–epithelial barriers also
seem to show evidence of inflammatory plasma exudation.[155]
Exacerbation of symptoms of infection in the nasal airways, and
exposure to allergens or cold dry air are associated with plasma
exudation and activation of mediators of the exuded plasma
protein system.[121,156–159] Furthermore, in patients with atopic
rhinitis, natural exposure to allergens during a pollen season is
associated with plasma exudation in the airways and the development of symptoms (Pipkorn et al., unpublished observations).

Glucocorticoids, and, apparently, also xanthines, reduce both symptoms and plasma exudation in nasal airways of patients with allergic rhinitis.[160–162]

Studies of the nasal airways in man may also serve to illustrate that plasma exudation is a harmless reversible process. Svensson *et al.*[163] examined the effects of three repeated nasal challenges with histamine at 30 minute intervals (in 12 normal subjects), and compared these with the same procedure on another day. Nasal lavages were performed every 10 minutes to recover the mucosal surface liquids. Histamine considerably increased the concentrations of plasma proteins and plasma derived mediators, such as the bradykinins, in the lavage fluids. The plasma protein tracers and kinins returned to baseline within 30 minutes of provocation. Furthermore, the exudation was also reversible in the sense that repeated provocations with histamine were as effective as the first provocation.[163] Histamine is but one example of an abundance of proposed mediators of asthma, which, in addition to producing bronchoconstriction in animals and man, are potent inducers of plasma leakage into the airway wall and lumen.[143]

Plasma exudation in the pathogenesis of asthma

Plasma exudation is not only a sign of ongoing inflammation in asthma but may play a large part in its pathogenesis as well. An immediate consequence of tracheobronchial exudation is airway oedema. Oedema is also consistently cited in airway disease in asthma, but has, presumably due to technical difficulties, only received qualitative support for a definite role from the results of biopsies and post-mortem examinations.[145] Unlike luminal mucous material, the airway oedema is not moved away from critical sites of resistance. It can be deformed by constriction of deeper lying airway smooth muscle but resists compression and, therefore, exaggerates the reduction in airway lumen that occurs during bronchoconstriction. Moreno *et al.*[164] made quantitative associations between the narrowing of airway smooth muscle and the effects of incompressible wall material on the availability of lumen for airflow. The interfacial tension between airway liquid in asthma and the luminal air may be raised resulting in an additional source of inward recoil.[165] The effects of altered surface tension would only be of importance in smaller airways, but none the less could serve as an amplifier of smooth muscle responses. Airway oedema could also serve to 'uncouple' airway smooth muscle from the elastic load imposed by the parenchyma; if this occurred the smooth muscle could narrow further in the presence of oedema than it could in its absence of oedema.[3,166] Thus both plasma exudation and airway oedema might be substantial factors in BHR.[165,167]

When plasma enters the airway lumen there are potential negative consequences which could contribute to airway obstruction. Mucociliary transport could be reduced by a rapid exudation leading to an increase in periciliary fluid layer with the attendant decrease in fluid clearance.[168] It has been suggested that the oedema and the transepithelial passage of plasma contribute to, or cause, sloughing of epithelium.[145] Plasma proteins increase mucus production,[130] may prevent its normal hydration,[169] could increase interfacial tension between airway liquid and luminal air,[170] and increase its viscosity by mucin–albumin complexes[171] and by activation of the coagulation system with fibrin formation.[172]

Exuded plasma proteins, in particular in an inflamed airway, can also be harmful. The kinin, complement, clotting, fibrinolysis, and other systems may be activated to produce a wide variety of inflammatory and bronchoactive mediators. These, and other defined, or as yet unknown, factors of exuded plasma may cause further recruitment, priming and activation of inflammatory cells.[143] Hence, both physical and physiological aspects suggest that plasma exudation needs to be considered as a contributory factor in BHR in asthma.

Mechanisms of airway plasma exudation

Physiologically, fluid equilibrium in a tissue is maintained by a balance between the hydrostatic pressure in the capillary bed, which tends to drive fluid out of the vascular compartment, and the counteracting force of the transmural colloid osmotic pressure gradient. The vascular leakage of large molecules, which is an active process under physiological and pharmacological control, is generally referred to as increased vascular permeability.[173,174]

Proposed bronchoconstrictor mediators of asthma (amines, peptides, lipid products, etc.) have, with few exceptions, the additional capacity of increasing microvascular permeability and hence inducing plasma exudation. A mediator released by neurogenic stimuli, such as substance P, causes vascular and mucosal permeability in rodents when its degradation is inhibited,[175] but its inflammatory action in human airways remains unconfirmed. Because asthma is an airway and not an alveolar disease the distribution of the profuse microvascular networks, belonging to the systemic tracheobronchial circulation, coincides with the distribution of asthma. Furthermore, the pulmonary microvessels, in contrast to the bronchial venules, are resistant to the vascular leakage effect of many proposed mediators of asthma.[176]

The vascular target cells, responsible for increased permeability to macromolecules in inflammation, are the endothelial cells of postcapillary venules (8–30 μm in diameter).[174,177] They also have an intriguing organisation of filaments and myoid proteins that could exert contractile activity. Majno and Palade originally suggested that the mediator-induced deformation of endothelial cells, which produced the gaps, was due to a contractile effect.[177] Although there is no direct proof of the validity of this hypothesis, it has been widely accepted.

Normally, the epithelial lining is a tight barrier, but an inflammatory increase in epithelial permeability to macromolecules as a result of stimulus may be as sudden as the change in vascular permeability. Ultrastructural alterations in the epithelium are probably associated with a bulk flow of macromolecules, except that the dominating pathway must be between epithelial cells. It is important to recognise that the inflammatory epithelial permeability may be largely one-directional. Passage of extravasated plasma macromolecules into the lumen does not necessarily mean that luminal macromolecules can freely enter airway tissues (Erjefalt & Persson 1989, personal communication). Indeed, it has been difficult to prove that asthmatic bronchi absorb inhaled factors to an abnormally large extent.

Hogg[178] suggested that inflammation may open up epithelial tight junctions, but they could not show a correlation between numbers of open junctions and the inflammatory state. Hogg and Walker[179] suggested that permeability may increase at corners where three epithelial cells meet and perhaps around goblet cells that have emptied their contents. Persson and Erjefalt[144] suggested that paracellular routes must be involved because large volumes of plasma exudate/transudate rapidly entered the airway lumen, and after its entry the epithelium appeared intact and was not sloughed off. It has also been shown that plasma tracers appear promptly on the mucosal surface of tracheobronchial airways after a large variety of mucosal provocations: mediators such as histamine, bradykinin, PAF, a neurogenic stimulus, an allergen-induced reaction stimulated by IgE, and effects of an occupational asthma agent. Such mucosal challenges have produced immediate plasma leakage, but biphasic responses with a late phase leakage and sustained plasma leakage have also been recorded. All agents produced concentration-dependent responses, and with all responses—even the threshold effects—there was an excellent correlation between plasma exuded into the interstitium of the airway wall and that appearing on the mucosal surface (Erjefalt & Persson 1989, personal communication).

The closest microvessels, which are abundant just beneath the epithelium, are probably affected by the mucosal provocations and leakage of plasma. The subepithelial interstitium is then endowed with exuded plasma, and the negative surface charges, and other factors in this environment, activate the exuded plasma protein systems. This activation produces a large number of inflammatory peptides, and the increased number of molecules increase the osmotic load. The serous membrane of the epithelium will therefore be under attack by the exudate, with the likely result of a build-up of interstitial pressure. This pressure increase, perhaps together with mediator-induced destabilisation of the epithelium, will cause the epithelial cells to separate transiently, thus permitting passage of interstitial plasma along the pressure gradient into the lumen. This hypothesis is supported by the finding of only a small increase in absorption of luminal macro-molecules during exudation (Erjefalt & Persson 1989, personal communication). Interestingly, Nordin[180] has reported high interstitial osmotic pressure in the mucosa of rat trachea inflamed by intubation, and Man et al.[181] showed that an osmotic load produced noticeable ultrastructural changes in the epithelium, but only when that challenge was applied to the serous membrane.

Although airway responsiveness may be altered by changing the contractile properties of airway smooth muscle, changes in contractility do not always account for the excessive narrowing of the airway. The role of mediators released from autonomic nerve endings and inflammatory cells cannot be ignored, nor can plasma exudation and oedema. These factors have the potential to alter responsiveness by several possible mechanisms which could be interrelated in complex ways.

MECHANICS OF BRONCHOCONSTRICTION INFLUENCED BY INFLAMMATION

In this section, the way in which inflammation might alter the structure of the airways so that an identical response of the smooth muscle to a bronchoconstrictive stimulus could produce a hyperconstrictive response will be considered. The constriction of small intrapulmonary airways seems to be responsible for the increased residual volume and decreased vital capacity of the asthmatic attack.[182,183] There are two principal sites where the effects of products of inflammation result, by and large, in tissue oedema. These are:

1 Between the surface of the airway lumen and the smooth muscle at the base of the airway wall.

2 Between the surrounding lung tissue and the smooth muscle and elastic elements of the airway wall.[184]

Using simple geometric arguments Moreno et al. showed that the proportion of airway wall area to total airway cross-sectional area profoundly influences the change in airway resistance (Raw) for the same degree of muscle shortening.[164] If the proportion is increased by mucosal oedema or mucosal infiltration, their analysis shows how such changes could, 'produce trivial alterations in baseline Raw but profoundly affect maximal response'. A small increase in wall thickness, while causing only a small decrease in radius in the relaxed state, could lead to complete closure in the contracted state, thus causing an infinite increase in resistance in that airway, at the degree of muscle shortening that would otherwise have minimal effect.

The limitation of the analysis of Moreno *et al.* is that the degree of shortening is not constant for the same degree of muscle activation, but depends on the load against which the muscle is working. In the lung, changes in pulmonary volume can have a profound influence on airway smooth muscle load. The relationships between wall tension, airway radius, and the baseline distending pressure (P_{tm}), under equilibrium conditions, have been analysed by Burton,[185,186] and his analysis has been extensively applied to blood vessels, but less frequently to airways.[187] Burton used the Laplace equation for the relationship between wall tension, transmural pressure, and radius. He considered the wall tension to be the sum of the passive tension (smooth muscle relaxed) and the tension produced by the contracted muscles. The passive tension is a function of length (radius) and the elastic properties of the wall. Burton assumed that the active smooth muscle tension was essentially unaffected by the radius. While this is not strictly so, that component of the active tension which changes with radius has only a small effect on the relationship between transmural pressure and radius. It can therefore be shown that the change in airway radius per unit change in active muscle tension is negatively correlated with P_{tm}.

When Burton's analysis is applied to a thin-walled tube that has no passive tension and zero transmural pressure at a radius less than a specific length (r_o), active muscle tension will produce closure of the tube at transmural pressures below a value determined by the ratio of the active tension to r_o. The transmural pressure below which closure occurs is the critical closing pressure (P_c). Gunst and co-workers[188,189] found that canine intrapulmonary airways, less than 0.5 cm in diameter, when dissected from the surrounding lung tissue, developed closing pressures in excess of 30 cmH$_2$O when stimulated with acetylcholine. Murtagh *et al.*[190] found that small airways within gas-free canine lobes, when exposed to methacholine, could not be inflated with pressures below 50 cmH$_2$O. In the studies by Gunst and Stropp, no lung parenchyma was present,[188] and in the studies of Murtagh *et al.* the lungs had no elastic recoil. Thus in both studies the effect of radial traction from the surrounding lung tissue on the airways was absent. In spite of the high closing pressures produced by cholinergic stimulation *in vitro*, airway closure does not occur *in vivo* after maximal responses to cholinergic stimuli, as evidenced by the rather trivial increase in residual volume in dogs and non-asthmatic subjects after provocation with such stimuli.

These data suggest that the lung parenchyma have an important role. In particular, the effective pressure at the external surface of an intrapulmonary airway is determined by the gas pressure of the surrounding alveoli and the stress at the surface produced by the radial traction.[191,192] The gas pressure of the surrounding alveoli pushes towards the airway, and the radial traction pulls outward. In the static state, the pressure within the airway is equal to the surrounding alveolar pressure, so the entire distending pressure of the airway is produced only by the radial traction. With normal airways and lung tissue, inflation of the lung is uniform (homogeneous), and the radial traction produces a stress at the outer surface of the airway roughly equal to the pleural pressure. Thus the effective P_{tm} of an intrapulmonary airway under homogeneous inflation is equal to the alveolar pressure minus the pleural pressure (static transpulmonary pressure or elastic recoil pressure (P_L)). It can, therefore, be inferred that the radius of an intrapulmonary airway would be the same, whether in the lung or excised, when the P_{tm} of the excised airway is equal to the P_L.

Insofar as the effective transmural pressure of an intrapulmonary airway is equal to the P_L, the same degree of smooth muscle tension would produce a greater change in radius at a low lung volume rather than at a high lung volume. Furthermore, at high lung volume the radius in the relaxed state would be greater. Thus, the proportional change in resistance produced by a given change in muscle tension could be very small at high lung volume and very large at low lung volume. This could result in a constrictor agonist producing an increase in resistance at low lung volume which could not be detected at high lung volume. Ding *et al.* found that in normal subjects exposed to inhaled methacholine, the maximum increase in pulmonary resistance, while breathing 0.5 l below functional residual capacity, was much greater than the increase while breathing 0.5 l above functional residual capacity.[3] They could not, however, find a difference in response at low concentrations of methacholine. Pride *et al.* found exaggerated muscle relaxation at low lung volumes: at low lung volumes isoproterenol resulted in an increase in expiratory flow, but there was no change at high lung volume during forced expiration at the same driving pressure.[187]

There is a body of evidence to suggest that induced bronchoconstriction reaches a maximum in normal subjects.[193-195] If the maximum response of the smooth muscle is of the same order *in vivo* as it is *in vitro*, and if the P_{tm} of the intrapulmonary airways was indeed equal to P_L, airway closure would prevent ventilation at a P_L of less than 30 cmH$_2$O, a level close to total lung capacity. While this may happen in severely asthmatic patients, normal dogs and healthy subjects are not forced to breath at lung volumes anywhere near total lung capacity. Thus, either the *in vivo* response of the smooth muscle is less than the *in vitro* response, or the P_{tm} of the constricted airway is greater than the P_L.

There are strong reasons to believe that the latter is true—that is, that the P_{tm} of the constricted airway is considerably greater than the P_L. As the airway constricts from smooth muscle contraction, the forces pulling outward on the airway are acting over a smaller surface area. Because the stress from radial traction is the force per unit surface area, the outward acting stress is increased by a factor equal to the ratio of the relaxed to the contracted radius. The outward acting stress is further increased by an increase in the radial tissue forces due to the stretch of the tissue elements pulling against the contracted airway. This increase in P_{tm}, or distending pressure, is a remarkably effective negative feedback mechanism: the greater the constriction, the greater the P_{tm} response to P_L, and the greater the load against which the smooth muscle must work.

Closure of an airway will still occur if active tension is present at zero cross-sectional area, but the P_L required to prevent closure will be considerably less than the P_c. Gunst and Stropp have provided experimental support for these inferences.[188] They assumed that the maximum *in vivo* response to cholinergic stimulation is the development of a P_c of 30 cmH$_2$O. They used this assumption in a theoretical model of the interaction between intrapulmonary airways and the surrounding lung tissue forces to predict that airway closure with a P_c of 30 cmH$_2$O could be prevented by a P_L of only 10 cmH$_2$O. In tests of this theory, exposure of excised canine lobes to methacholine aerosol caused complete airway closure at low lung volumes, but the closure could be overcome by increasing P_L to levels between 7.5 and 10 cmH$_2$O.

During severe asthmatic attacks, the patient is often breathing near total lung capacity with a P_L approaching 30 cmH$_2$O. Asthmatic subjects, unlike healthy subjects, often lack a demonstrable maximum response to inhaled bronchoconstrictors. This could be explained by a decrease in the interdependence between the constricted intrapulmonary airways and the surrounding lung tissue forces. It is tempting to speculate that the major difference between normal and asthmatic subjects depends on the effectiveness of the forces of lung recoil to be transmitted to the airways from the surrounding lung tissue.

If inflammatory products result in changes which increase the cross-sectional area of the airway wall but do not alter the elastic properties of the wall, the P_{tm} will be decreased, and there will be less of an increase in P_{tm} resulting from a given degree of smooth muscle activation. Rather small increases in external radius, either from peribronchial oedema or inflammatory infiltration of the airway wall, can be shown to have a great effect on the P_L required to overcome airway closure. Thus the outward extension of the airway wall from its normal 'rest configuration' resulting from the effects of inflammatory reactions, would cause a decrease in P_{tm} because of a decrease in radial stress from the tissue elements. Clearly, a process whose primal locus was external to the lumen of the airway could narrow the airway lumen through loss of elastic recoil.

If the products of an inflammatory response simply resulted in thickening of the airway wall at a locus internal to the airway this would narrow the airway but would not alter the forces of interdependence. In contrast, if the normal airway interfacial tension between luminal liquid and air were fouled in such a way that luminal surface tension increased, this additional inward recoil force would 'pull against' the forces of interdependence and tend to narrow the airway. In both of these cases, as well as in the external wall swelling case noted above, a zero cross-sectional area would be achieved at a smaller degree of smooth muscle activation than in the normal case. As a result, a higher P_L would be required to overcome airway closure for the same degree of active smooth muscle tension.

An increase in the level of P_L required to overcome airway closure at the same active muscle tension can result in alterations similar to those observed in asthma. If the maximum level of smooth muscle tension that can be achieved in healthy subjects and asthmatics is the same, and this maximal tension is responsible for the dose–response curve plateau in healthy subjects, and if the level of P_L below which closure occurs is low in healthy subjects (close to or below the P_L at functional residual capacity), but high in asthmatics (close to the P_L at total lung capacity), the plateau in response will not be observed in the asthmatic—despite similar smooth muscle function. Furthermore, once an airway is closed, it can be opened during spontaneous respiration only by an increase in P_L. Even if the asthmatic is forced to breathe at a P_L sufficient to keep the airways open, there is still likely to be an increase in resistance which can account, in part, for decreased maximum expiratory flow rates.

Reduction of maximum expiratory flow rates, commonly observed in asthma, is also closely related to the P_{tm} at airway closure.[187,196] As expiratory airflow increases at constant P_L the radius of the airway decreases due to a decrease in P_{tm}. The decrease in radius during forced expiration is somewhat analogous to the decrease in radius during smooth muscle contraction. In both situations, the forces of constriction are buffered by the increase in the outward stress, and in both situations the response is maximum when the P_{tm} reaches a critical level. In the case of active smooth muscle tension in the static state, the P_{tm} cannot fall below P_c, and this occurs at airway closure. In the case of forced expiration at constant P_L, expiratory flow cannot increase above a specific level (flow limitation) due to the formation of a choke point within the airway. When flow limitation is present the P_{tm} immediately upstream from the choke point is constant and its level is highly correlated with P_L.

The size of the airways affected (small vs large), and the locus within the wall where inflammatory swelling occurs, would be expected to influence the characteristics of the hyperresponsiveness. If rather large intrapulmonary airways have swollen due to the products of inflammation extending toward the lumen, there should be an increase in sensitivity—that is, a detectable response at a lower dose of agonist. The maximum response would not be affected. Furthermore, there should be a high level of correlation between the sensitivity and the depression of baseline pulmonary function. These are the characteristics of the hyperresponsiveness in cigarette smokers with mild chronic bronchitis,[197] and in dogs exposed to ozone.[198] If the inflammation were within small peripheral airways, the hyperresponsiveness would not be well correlated with baseline pulmonary function, because changes in resistance in small airways can be very extensive before there are clinically important changes in conventional measurements of pulmonary function,[199] but such changes might be detected by an increase in airway closure (increased closing volume). If the locus of swelling in the small airways was toward the lung parenchyma, the response to a bronchoconstrictor agonist would be exaggerated, and the enhanced response could be detected with a change in both FEV_1 and FVC. Thus an increased sensitivity and maximum response could be present with little alteration in baseline pulmonary function. These are the characteristics of the hyperresponsiveness in mild asthma.[195] James *et al.*[200] recently presented evidence of structural alteration in the peripheral airways in asthmatic patients. There is also functional evidence for peripheral airway effects in asthmatics with near normal baseline function. When the resistance to collateral flow of such subjects was measured with the wedged bronchoscope technique there was a sixfold increase in the resistance to airflow in the small airways compared with normal subjects.[201] Furthermore, there was a significant negative correlation in asthmatic subjects between their peripheral resistance and the PD_{20} to methacholine determined on another day (Wagner *et al.*, unpublished observations).

CHAPTER 4
Physiology

ANIMAL MODELS OF HYPERRESPONSIVENESS

Because airway tissue cannot easily be obtained from healthy subjects, investigators have turned to experimental models of inflammation and BHR to appreciate fully the association between these two components of the asthmatic response. The general approach has been to examine airways before and after an intervention. In such cases the degree of inflammation measured, either histologically or by analysis of cells in the BAL fluid, is related to the development of BHR. These models fall into three major categories. Most commonly, animals are exposed once to ozone, antigen, viruses, endotoxin or chemicals. In the second approach, animals are exposed over a prolonged period to irritant stimuli. The third approach involves animal models of persistent BHR treated with known inhibitors of inflammation.

Acute exposure models

Studies using a variety of inflammatory stimuli originally pointed to a causal relationship between polymorphonuclear leucocytes in the lung and the development of BHR. Inhalation of C5a in rabbits is associated with increased airway reactivity to histamine and airway inflammation characterised by influx of polymorphonuclear leucocytes at four hours.[202] Sensitised dogs exposed to ragweed antigen show increased airway reactivity to acetylcholine and increased numbers of polymorphonuclear leucocytes and eosinophils in the BAL fluid.[203] Similarly, Principal ponies, which develop heaves on exposure to hay (presumably by an allergic mechanism), show increased numbers of polymorphonuclear leucocytes in BAL fluid[204] and BHR to histamine.[205] BHR to inhaled histamine is seen in sheep five hours after the intravenous administration of endotoxin,[206] and occurs when lymphocytes and polymorphonuclear leucocytes are sequestered in the lung.[207] Polymorphonuclear leucocytes (and lymphocyte) depletion with hydroxyurea significantly attenuated the hyperreactivity,[207,208] again suggesting an important association between airway inflammation and reactivity.

Subsequent studies, however, have suggested that the association between the development of inflammation (the presence of polymorphonuclear leucocytes in lung) and the development of changes in airway reactivity is unlikely to be causal. Among the models used to study acute airway responsiveness the dog model has been most extensively studied.

Dogs exposed to ozone (1–2.2 ppm for up to two hours) develop increases in airway reactivity to acetylcholine aerosols at one hour after exposure; in some animals this may persist for 24 hours. Airway reactivity does return to normal within one week after exposure.[209,210] Dogs that show increased BHR also develop a pronounced and reversible increase in the number of polymorphonuclear leucocytes in the airway epithelium[210] and increased numbers of polymorphonucelar leucocytes and epithelial cells in the BAL fluid.[211] Pretreatment with hydroxyurea, which depletes polymorphonuclear leucocytes and probably has other effects, prevented the increase in BHR after exposure to ozone,[212] implicating polymorphonuclear leucocytes. Moreover, in dogs pretreated with indomethacin, exposure to ozone was associated with an influx of polymorphonuclear leucocytes into the airways, but increases in airway reactivity failed to develop.[45] Similarly, pretreatment with a thromboxane synthetase inhibitor prevented the increase in airway reactivity induced by ozone, again without altering polymorphonuclear leucocyte influx.[46] The findings of these three studies suggest that products, derived from cyclooxygenase, of inflammatory cells (largely thromboxane) are necessary for the development of BHR following exposure to ozone in dogs. Although dogs exposed to ozone develop BHR, the alterations in pulmonary mechanics do not mimic the changes observed in asthma. In particular, there is a shift toward increased sensitivity to inhaled mediators but there is no change in the plateau response.[198]

Exposure to ozone in guinea-pigs suggests that factors other than the influx of polymorphonuclear leucocytes are involved in the development of BHR. Exposure to ozone in this model increases airway reactivity to intravenous acetylcholine for between two hours and three days. Although epithelial damage is observed at two hours when there is BHR, polymorphonuclear leucocytes influx into the airway occurs four hours after the development of BHR, and persists long after BHR has resolved.[213] Moreover, polymorphonuclear leucocyte depletion by cyclophosphamide fails to inhibit the increase in airway reactivity provoked by ozone.[214] Similarly, Hulbert *et al.*[215] showed that in guinea-pigs exposed to cigarette smoke, BHR to histamine precedes the migration of polymorphonuclear leucocytes into the airway epithelium. These data suggest that the appearance of polymorphonuclear leucocytes is a consequence of the initial ozone insult rather than the cause of the increased airway reactivity. The events leading to tissue oedema, or tissue oedema itself, may be responsible for the increased reactivity because of increased airway permeability or increased reactivity based on the locus of inflammatory changes.

Finally, the genetic make-up of the test animals seems to be crucial to the development of hyperresponsiveness. It has been shown that among three types of rats that developed impressive polymorphonuclear leucocyte influx one and a half hours after inhalation of endotoxin, only two of the strains became hyperreactive.[216] Similarly, Folkerts *et al.*[217] found a pronounced polymorphonuclear leucocyte influx into the lungs of guinea-pigs exposed to endotoxin with no increased airway reactivity to histamine. These studies, again, suggest that a positive association between airway reactivity and inflammation is less clear than that suggested by the original ozone studies done on dogs.

Acute exposure models—late antigen response

Several studies in animal models have shown an association between inflammatory cell infiltration in the airways (polymorphonuclear leucocytes, eosinophils, or mast cells), the late constrictor response to antigen, and increases in airway reactivity. Aerosol challenge with *Ascaris* antigen produces acute bronchoconstriction in sheep sensitive to it.[218] In some sheep, a second bronchoconstrictor response occurs six to eight hours later, and in these sheep (dual responders) increased BHR to cholinergic agonists is seen.[219] Although both acute responders and dual responders show increased polymorphonuclear leucocytes in the BAL fluid seven to eight hours after challenge, only the dual responders show increased eosinophils in the BAL fluid at that time.[220] Prevention of the acute response by pretreatment with cromolyn,[219] aminophylline,[220] or β-adrenergic agonist[220] protects against development of the delayed response. Pretreatment with corticosteroids or LY 171883 (a leukotriene D_4 receptor antagonist) prevents the late response.[220] Inhalation of leukotriene D_4 itself induces both acute and delayed bronchoconstriction in dual, but not single, responder sheep.[221] Taken together, these studies suggest that lipoxygenase products released during acute exposure to antigen during waking hours have a role in the subsequent development of the late response and, by inference, the increased airway reactivity and inflammation.

Larson *et al.*[222] developed a rabbit model of the late asthmatic response by immunising neonatal animals to extracts of antigens such as alternaria or ragweed. Although these animals developed both IgG and IgE antibodies, the late bronchoconstriction seemed to be IgE, and not IgG, dependent.[223] Histological examination of the lungs of these animals showed interstitial oedema of the large airways within 15 to 30 minutes without pronounced cellular infiltration; most of the cells present were polymorphonuclear leucocytes. At six hours (the time of the late response), oedema and a mixed cellular infiltrate of polymorphonuclear leucocytes, eosinophils, and mononuclear leucocytes were found in both large and small airways. Forty-eight hours after antigen challenge, the oedema had subsided and cellular infiltrates were largely mononuclear in character. Eighty percent of the granulocytes present were eosinophils;[222] within several days, histological examination showed that the lung had returned to normal.[222] In this same model airway reactivity to histamine has increased three days after antigen challenge when few polymorphonuclear leucocytes are found in the lung and returned to baseline within a week.[224] Immune rabbits, made neutropenic by administration of nitrogen mustard, showed no late response when challenged with antigen,[225] but when treated with nitrogen mustard and transfused with a neutrophil-rich population of white cells, they developed late phase reactions when challenged with antigen.[222] Airway reactivity to histamine increases only in the granulocytopenic rabbits transfused with neutrophil-rich populations of white cells at the time of antigen exposure,[222] suggesting that, in rabbits, the initiation of late response and the initial development of BHR depend in some way on the presence of circulating polymorphonuclear leucocytes.

Mongrel dogs,[226,227] guinea-pigs,[228,229] and rats[230] have also been used as models of late phase reactions, but concurrent studies of airway reactivity in these models have not yet been completed. It is interesting to note that, in guinea-pigs sensitised to ovalbumin, its inhalation produces two late phase increases in airway tone, at 17 and at 72 hours.[229] Although polymorphonuclear leucocytes are seen early on, by six hours, it is eosinophils and not polymorphonuclear leucocytes which predominate in the BAL fluid and histologically in tracts between smooth muscle layers and in the epithelium.[228,229] The role of eosinophils in the perpetuation of BHR in late phase reactions to antigen remains to be determined.

Inhalation of relatively high concentrations of TDI (2 ppm) in guinea-pigs is associated with BHR to acetylcholine after two and six hours, but not 24 hours after exposure. The numbers of polymorphonuclear leucocytes in the epithelium of these animals, however, is increased only after two hours. Guinea-pigs exposed to only 1 ppm show increased numbers of polymorphonuclear leucocytes after two hours, but do not develop BHR.[231] Further studies in this model by another group using 3 ppm of TDI, show that pretreatment with cyclophosphamide had no effect on either the incidence, or the degree, of airway reactivity to acetylcholine, suggesting that, at least in guinea-pigs, BHR after exposure to TDI is independent of circulating or airway polymorphonuclear leucocytes.[232] It is interesting to note that exposure to TDI is also associated with loss of ciliated epithelium and disruption of the

Chronic exposure studies

In contrast to acute exposure to antigen, ozone, or TDI, which
cause transient increases in airway reactivity, chronic exposure to
sulphur dioxide (SO_2) or cigarette smoke is associated with
inflammation and decreased airway reactivity to challenge aerosols. Dogs chronically exposed to 200 ppm SO_2 for two hours a
day, four to five days a week for 1–2 months, show lung disease
consistent with persistent inflammation of airway glands and air
spaces. This is characterised by infiltration of polymorphonuclear
leucocytes and mononuclear cells[232] and decreased, not increased, airway reactivity to bronchoconstrictor aerosols.[234] Exposure to only 50 ppm SO_2 for a similar time period produces little
evidence of airway inflammation and no changes in airway
reactivity to histamine or methacholine aerosols in this same
model.[235] More recent studies fail to show an association between
the onset of inflammation (measured by increases in polymorphonuclear leucocytes in BAL fluid) and airway reactivity to
methacholine aerosols.[236] Notably, airway reactivity to intravenously administered methacholine is not changed by chronic
exposure to SO_2, suggesting that the decreased reactivity to
aerosols observed during persistent pulmonary inflammation in
dogs exposed to SO_2 is not due to altered contractile state of the
airway muscle, but reflects an inhibitory influence of the muco-
epithelial barrier.

Similar results have been obtained after chronic exposure to
cigarette smoke in baboons. Such exposure is associated with
small decreases in airway reactivity to methacholine, but inflammatory changes in the airway were not documented.[237] Moreover, dogs repeatedly exposed to nitric acid aerosols show airway
inflammation and decreased airway reactivity to histamine.[238]

Animal models with natural hyperresponsiveness

A different way of addressing the association between airway
reactivity and inflammation is to manipulate animals with naturally occurring hyperreactivity with agents thought to initiate the
inflammatory process, and to examine the temporal course of
changes in airway reactivity and cell populations in BAL fluid.
Basenji greyhound dogs have persistent airway hyperreactivity to
aerosol challenge, including methacholine and citric acid.[239] This
model also shows increased percentages of luminal mast cells,
lymphocytes[240] and eosinophils in the BAL fluid (Hirschman *et
al.*, unpublished observations). Daily treatment with methyl-
prednisoline, 2 mg/kg for six weeks, decreases airway reactivity to

methacholine, and abolishes reactivity to citric acid aerosols. This is associated with pronounced decreases in eosinophils in circulating and BAL fluids.[241] Although the mechanisms by which glucocorticoids exert their effects in this model are not known, it is likely that part of the action is through their anti-inflammatory actions.

CONCLUSIONS

Data from isolated systems suggest many possible ways in which inflammation and hyperresponsiveness could be associated, but different animal models of inflammation and airway reactivity have shown that a causal relationship between the two is complex. Most of the studies are descriptive, and a temporal relationship between one cell type and changes in airway reactivity provides a rather simplistic approach. Association does not imply causation. Perhaps we need to characterise better which markers of inflammation are critical. The mobilisation of one cell type (such as polymorphonuclear leucocytes or eosinophils) is just as likely to be a consequence of an, as yet, unidentified event(s) which leads to altered airway responses, rather than a cause of airway reactivity.

A major problem in understanding the association (if any) between BHR and airway inflammation is that it requires a multidisciplinary interrelated approach. Bronchoconstriction is a mechanical event and, therefore, must be described in terms of mechanics. On the other hand, it can be caused by neural and chemical mediators, so that an understanding of the neurophysiological and biochemical events is essential. A knowledge of cell biology to understand which cells may release specific mediators, what attracts these cells to the airways in the first place, and what biochemical and mechanical effects of these mediators are, is equally necessary. Too often, individual researchers have worked alone on their own speciality without collaborating with or even seriously trying to understand the insights of an investigator in a different speciality. A truly interdisciplinary approach, where concerted efforts are made by all groups to understand the approaches of the others and to collaborate with jointly planned, executed, analysed, and interpreted research will be necessary before the association between asthma and airway inflammation can be clarified.

REFERENCES

1 Woolcock AJ, Peat JK, Salome CM. Prevalence of bronchial hyperresponsiveness and asthma in a rural adult population. *Thorax* 1987;42:361–8.
2 Woolcock AJ, Yan K, Salome CM. Effects of therapy on bronchial hyperresponsiveness in the long-term management of asthma. *Clin Allergy* 1988;18:165–76.

3 Ding DJ, Martin JG, Macklem PT. Effects of lung volume on maximal methacholine-induced bronchoconstriction in normal humans. *J Appl Physiol* 1987;**62**:1324–30.

4 Vincenc KS, Black JL, Yan K, Armour CL, Donnelly PD, Woolcock AJ. Comparison of *in vivo* and *in vitro* responses to histamine in human airways. *Am Rev Respir Dis* 1983;**128**:875–9.

5 Armour CL, Black JL, Berend N, Woolcock AJ. The relationship between bronchial hyperresponsiveness to methacholine and airway smooth muscle structure and reactivity. *Respir Physiol* 1984;**58**:223–33.

6 Armour CL, Lazar NM, Schellenberg RR *et al*. A comparison of *in vivo* and *in vitro* human airway reactivity to histamine. *Am Rev Respir Dis* 1984;**129**:907–10.

7 Schellenberg RR, Foster A. *In vitro* responses of human asthmatic airway and pulmonary vascular smooth muscle. *Int Arch Allergy Appl Immunol* 1984;**75**:237–41.

8 Roberts JA, Raeburn D, Rodger IW, Thomson NC. Comparison of *in vivo* airway responsiveness and *in vitro* smooth muscle sensitivity to methacholine in man. *Thorax* 1984;**39**:837–43.

9 Roberts JA, Rodger IW, Thomson NC. Airway responsiveness to histamine in man; effect of atropine on *in vivo* and *in vitro* comparison. *Thorax* 1985;**40**:261–7.

10 Taylor SM, Pare PD, Armour CL, Hogg JC, Schellenberg RR. Airway reactivity in chronic obstructive pulmonary disease. Failure of *in vivo* methacholine responsiveness to correlate with cholinergic, adrenergic, or nonadrenergic responses *in vitro*. *Am Rev Respir Dis* 1985;**132**:30–5.

11 Cerrina J, Ladurie LRM, Labat C, Raffestin B, Bayol A, Brink C. Comparison of human bronchial muscle responses to histamine *in vivo* with histamine and isoproterenol agonists *in vitro*. *Am Rev Respir Dis* 1986;**134**:57–61.

12 Goldie RG, Spina D, Henry PJ, Lulich KM, Paterson JW. *In vitro* responsiveness of human asthmatic bronchus to carbachol histamine, β-adrenoceptor agonists and theophylline. *Br J Clin Pharmacol* 1986;**22**:669–76.

13 DeJongste JC, Sterk PJ, Willems LNA, Mons H, Timmers MC, Kerrebijn KF. Comparison of maximal bronchoconstriction *in vivo* and airway smooth muscle responses *in vitro* in nonasthmatic humans. *Am Rev Respir Dis* 1988;**138**:321–6.

14 Laitinen LA, Heino M, Laitinen A, Kava T, Haahtela T. Damage of the airway epithelium and bronchial reactivity in patients with asthma. *Am Rev Respir Dis* 1985;**131**:599–606.

15 Souhrada M, Souhrada JF. Sensitization-induced sodium influx in airway smooth muscle cells of guinea pigs. *Respir Physiol* 1985;**60**:157–68.

16 Souhrada M, Souhrada JF. Alterations of airway smooth muscle cell membrane by sensitization. *Pediatr Pulmonol* 1985;**1**:207–14.

17 Stephens NL. Airway smooth muscle and disease workshop: structure and mechanical properties. *Am Rev Respir Dis* 1987;**136**:1–7.

18 Mansour S, Daniel EE. Responsiveness of isolated tracheal smooth muscle from normal and sensitized guinea pigs. *Can J Physiol Pharmacol* 1987;**65**:1942–50.

19 Antonissen LA, Mitchell RW, Kroeger EA, Kepron W, Tse KS, Stephens NL. Mechanical alterations of airway smooth muscle in a canine asthmatic model. *J Appl Physiol* 1979;**46**:681–7.

20 Antonissen LA, Mitchell RW, Kroeger EA, Kepron W, Stephens NL, Bergen J. Histamine pharmacology in airway smooth muscle from a canine model of asthma. *J Pharmacol Exp Ther* 1980;**213**:150–5.

21 Mitchell RW, Antonissen LA, Kepron W, Kroeger EA, Stephens NL. Effect of atropine on the hyperresponsiveness of ragweed-sensitized canine tracheal smooth muscle. *J Pharmacol Exp Ther* 1986;**236**:803–9.

22 Stephens NL, Morgan G, Kepron W, Seow CY. Changes in cross-bridge properties of sensitised airway smooth muscle. *J Appl Physiol* 1986;**61**:1492–8.

23 Kong SK, Shiu RP, Stephens NL. Studies of myofibrillar ATPase in ragweed-sensitized canine pulmonary smooth muscle. *J Appl Physiol* 1986;**60**:92–4.

24 Mitchell RW, Kroeger EA, Kepron W, Stephens NL. Local parasympathetic mechanisms for ragweed-sensitized canine trachealis hyperresponsiveness. *J Pharmacol Exp Ther* 1987;**243**:907–14.

25 Drazen JM, Austen KF. Leukotrienes and airway responses. *Am Rev Respir Dis* 1987;**136**(4):985–98.

26 Hanley SP. Prostaglandins and the lung. *Lung* 1986;**164**:65–77.

27 Holgate ST, Twentyman OP, Rafferty P *et al*. Primary and secondary effector cells in the pathogenesis of bronchial asthma. *Int Arch Allergy Appl Immunol* 1987;**82**(3–4):498–506.

28 Shore SA, Austen KF, Drazen JM. Eicosanoids and airway responses in cell biology of the lung. In: D Massoro ed. New York: Marcel Dekker 1989 (in press).

29 Walters EH, Parrish RW, Bevan C, Smith AP. Induction of bronchial hypersensitivity: evidence for a role for prostaglandins. *Thorax* 1981;**36**:571–4.

30 Heaton RW, Henderson AF, Dunlop LS, Costello JF. The influence of pretreatment with prostaglandin F_2 on bronchial sensitivity to inhaled histamine and methacholine in normal subjects. *Br J Dis Chest* 1984;**78**:168–73.

31 Fuller RW, Dixon CMS, Dollery CT, Barnes PJ. Prostaglandin D_2 potentiates airway responsiveness to histamine and methacholine. *Am Rev Respir Dis* 1986;**133**:252–4.

32 Barnes N, Watson A, Kkoulouris N, Piper PJ, Costello J. Effect of preinhalation of leukotriene D_4 on sensitivity to inhaled prostaglandin F_2. *Thorax* 1984;**39**:697.

33 Seltzer J, Bigby BG, Stulbarg M *et al*. O_3-induced change in bronchial reactivity to methacholine and airway inflammation in humans. *J Appl Physiol* 1986;**60**:1321–6.

34 O'Byrne PM, Aizawa H, Bethel RA, Chung KF, Nadel JA, Holtzman MJ. Prostaglandin F_x increases responsiveness of pulmonary airways in dogs. *Prostaglandins* 1984;**28**:537–43.

35 Patterson R, Bernstean PR, Harris KE, Krell RD. Airway responses to sequential challenges with platelet-activating factor and leukotriene D_4 in rhesus monkeys. *J Lab Clin Med* 1984;**104**:340–5.

36 Kern R, Smith LJ, Patterson R, Krell RD, Bernstein PR. Characterization of the airway response to inhaled leukotriene D_4 in normal subjects. *Am Rev Respir Dis* 1986;**133**:1127–32.

37 O'Byrne PM, Leikauf GD, Aizawa H *et al*. Leukotriene B_4 induces airway hyperresponsiveness in dogs. *J Appl Physiol* 1985;**59**:1941–6.

38 Fennessy MR, Stewart AG, Thompson DC. Aerosolized and intravenously administered leukotrienes: effects on the bronchoconstrictor potency of histamine in the guinea pig. *Br J Pharmacol* 1986;**87**:741–9.

39 Thorpe JE, Murlas CG. Leukotriene B_4 potentiates airway muscle responsiveness *in vivo* and *in vitro*. *Prostaglandins* 1986;**31**:899–908.

40 Munoz NM, Takanobu T, Murphy TM *et al*. Potentiation of vagal contractile response by thromboxane mimetic U-46619. *J Appl Physiol* 1986;**61**:1173–9.

41 Creese BR, Bach MK. Hyper-reactivity of airways smooth muscle produced *in vitro* by leukotrienes. *Prost Leuk Med* 1983;**11**:161–9.

42 Orehek J, Douglas JS, Bouhuys A. Contractile responses of the guinea pig trachea *in vitro*: modification by prostaglandin synthesis-inhibiting drugs. *J Pharmacol Exp Ther* 1975;**194**:554–64.

43 Leff AR, Munoz NM, Tallet J, Cavigelli M, David AC. Augmentation of parasympathetic contraction in tracheal and bronchial airways by PGF_2 in situ. *J Appl Physiol* 1985;**58**:1558–64.

44 Lee TH, Austen KF, Corey EJ, Drazen JM. Leukotriene E$_4$-induced airway hyperresponsiveness of guinea pig tracheal smooth muscle to histamine and evidence for three separate sulfidopeptide leukotriene receptors. *Proc Natl Acad Sci USA* 1984;**81**:4922–5.

45 O'Byrne PM, Walters EH, Aizawa J, Fabbri LM, Holtzman MJ, Nadel JA. Indomethacin inhibits the airway hyperresponsiveness but not the neutrophil influx induced by ozone in dogs. *Am Rev Respir Dis* 1984;**130**:220–4.

46 Aizawa H, Chung KF, Leikauf GD *et al.* Significance of thromboxane generation in ozone-induced airway hyperresponsiveness in dogs. *J Appl Physiol* 1985;**59**:1918–23.

47 Lee HKI, Murlas C. Ozone-induced bronchial hyperreactivity in guinea pigs is abolished by BW755C or FPL55712 but not by indomethacin. *Am Rev Respir Dis* 1985;**132**:1005–9.

48 Walters EH. Effect of inhibition of prostaglandin synthesis on induced bronchial hyperresponsiveness. *Thorax* 1983;**38**:195–9.

49 Chung KF, Aizawa H, Becker AB, Frick O, Gold WM, Nadel JA. Inhibition of antigen-induced airway hyperresponsiveness by a thromboxane sythetase inhibitor (OKY-046) in allergic dogs. *Am Rev Respir Dis* 1986;**134**(2):258–61.

50 Lanes S, Stevenson JS, Codias E *et al.* Indomethacin and FPL-57231 inhibit antigen-induced airway hyperresponsiveness in sheep. *J Appl Physiol* 1986;**61**:864–72.

51 Braquet P, Touqui L, Shen TY, Vargaftig BB. Perspectives in platelet-activating factor research. *Pharmacol Rev* 1987;**39**:97–145.

52 Cuss FM, Dixon CM, Barnes PJ. Effects of inhaled platelet activating factor on pulmonary function and bronchial responsiveness in man. *Lancet* 1986;ii:189–92.

53 Rubin AH, Smith LJ, Patterson R. The bronchoconstrictor properties of platelet-activating factor in humans. *Am Rev Respir Dis* 1987;**136**:1145–51.

54 Smith LJ, Rubin AH, Patterson R. Mechanism of platelet activating factor-induced bronchoconstriction in humans. *Am Rev Respir Dis* 1988;**137**(5):1015–19.

55 Polak JM, Bloom SR. Regulatory peptides of the gastrointestinal and respiratory tracts. *Arch Int Pharmacodyn Ther* 1986;**280**(Suppl.):16–49.

56 Lundberg JM, Saria A. Polypeptide-containing neurons in airway smooth muscle. *Am Rev Physiol* 1987;**49**:557–72.

57 Laitinen A, Partanen M, Hervonen A, Laitinen LA. Electron microscopic study on the innervation of the human lower respiratory tract: evidence of adrenergic nerves. *Eur J Respir Dis* 1985;**67**:209–15.

58 Said SI, Mutt V. Long acting vasodilator peptide from lung tissue. *Nature* 1969;**224**:699–700.

59 Uddman R, Alumets J, Densert O, Hakanson R, Sunderl F. Occurrence and distribution of VIP nerves in the nasal mucosa and tracheobronchial wall. *Acta Otolaryngol* 1978;**86**:443–8.

60 Christofides ND, Yiangou Y, Piper PJ *et al.* Distribution of peptide histidine isoleucine in the mammalian respiratory tract and some aspects of its pharmacology. *Endocrinology* 1984;**115**:1958–63.

61 Itoh N, Obata K, Yanaihara N, Okamoto H. Human preprovasoactive intestinal polypeptide contains a novel PHI-27-like peptide, PMH-27. *Nature* 1983;**304**:547–9.

62 Palmer JB, Cuss FM, Barnes PJ. VIP and PHM and their role in nonadrenergic responses in isolated human airways. *J Appl Physiol* 1986;**61**:1322–8.

63 Morice A, Unwin RJ, Sever PS. Vasoactive intestinal peptide causes bronchodilatation and protects against histamine induced bronchoconstriction in asthmatic subjects. *Lancet* 1983;ii:1225–7.

64 Barnes PJ, Dixon CMS. The effect of inhaled vasoactive intestinal peptide on bronchial reactivity to histamine in humans. *Am Rev Respir Dis* 1984;**130**:162–6.

65 Martling CR. Sensory nerves containing tachykinins and CGRP in the lower airways. *Acta Physiol Scand* 1987;**130**(Suppl. 563):1–57.

66 Nilsson G, Dahlberg K, Brodin E, Sundler F, Strandberg K. Distribution and constrictor effect of substance P in guinea pig tracheabronchial tissue. In: Von Euler US, Pernow B eds. *Substance P*. New York: Raven Press 1977:75–81.

67 Joos G, Pauwels R, Van Der Straeten M. The effect of inhaled substance P and neurokinin A on the airways of normal and asthmatic subjects. *Thorax* 1987;**42**:779–83.

68 Lundberg JM, Hokfelt T, Martling R, Saria A, Cuello AC. Substance P immunoreactive sensory nerves in the lower respiratory tract of various mammals including man. *Cell Tissue Res* 1984;**235**:251–61.

69 Karlsson G, Pipkorn U, Andreasson L. Substance P and human nasal mucociliary activity. *Eur J Clin Pharmacol* 1986;**30**:355–7.

70 Foreman JC, Jordan C. Neurogenic inflammation. *Trends Pharmacol Sci* 1984;**5**:116–19.

71 Lundberg JM, Saria A. Capsaicin sensitive vagal neurons involved in control of vascular permeability in rat trachea. *Acta Physiol Scand* 1982;**115**:521–3.

72 Lundberg JM, Saria A. Capsaicin induced desensitization of airway mucosa to cigarette smoke, mechanical and chemical irritants. *Nature* 1983;**101**:251–3.

73 Lundberg JM, Saria A, Brodin E, Rosell S, Folkers K. A substance P antagonist inhibits vagally induced increase in vascular permeability and bronchial smooth muscle contraction in the guinea pig. *Proc Natl Acad Sci USA* 1983;**80**:1120–4.

74 Sekizawa K, Tamaoki J, Graf PD, Basbaum CB, Borson DB, Nadel JA. Enkephalinase inhibitor potentiates mammalian tachykinin-induced contraction in ferret trachea. *J Pharmacol Exp Ther* 1987;**243**:1211–17.

75 Thompson JE, Sheppard D. Phosphoramidon potentiates the increase in lung resistance mediated by tachykinins in guinea pigs. *Am Rev Respir Dis* 1988;**137**:337–80.

76 Shore SA, Stimler-Gerard NP, Coats SR, Drazen JM. Substance P-induced bronchoconstriction in the guinea pig. Enhancement by inhibitors of neutral metalloendopeptidase and angiotensin-converting enzyme. *Am Rev Respir Dis* 1988;**137**:331–6.

77 Black JL, Johnson PRA, Armour CL. Potentiation of the contractile effects of neuropeptides in human bronchus by an enkephalinase inhibitor. *Pulm Pharmacol* 1988;**1**:21–3.

78 Joos GF, Pauwels RA, Van Der Straeten M. The mechanism of tachykinin-induced bronchoconstriction in the rat. *Am Rev Respir Dis* 1988;**137**:1038–44.

79 Rosenfeld MG, Mermod JJ, Amara SG *et al*. Production of a novel neuropeptide encoded by the calcitonin gene via tissue specific RNA processing. *Nature* 1983;**304**:129–35.

80 Lundberg JM, Franco-Cerceda A, Hua X, Hokfelt T, Fischer JA. Coexistence of substance P and calcitonin gene related peptide like immunoreactivities in sensory nerves in relation to cardiovascular and bronchoconstrictor effects of capsaicin. *Eur J Pharmacol* 1985;**108**:315–19.

81 Uddman R, Luts A, Sundler F. Occurrence and distribution of calcitonin gene-related peptide in the mammalian respiratory tract and middle ear. *Cell Tissue Res* 1985;**241**:551–5.

82 Barnes PJ. Neuropeptides in the airways: functional significance. In: Kay AB ed. *Asthma—clinical pharmacology and therapeutic progress*. Oxford: Blackwell Scientific Publications 1986:58–72.

83 Brain SD, Williams TJ. Inflammatory oedema induced by synergism between calcitonin gene-related peptide (CGRP) and mediators of increased vascular permeability. *Br J Pharmacol* 1985;**86**:855–60.

84 Le Greves P, Nyberg F, Terenius L, Hokfelt T. Calcitonin gene-related peptide is a potent inhibitor of substance P degradation. *Eur J Pharmacol* 1985;**115**:309–11.

85 Impiccatore M, Bertaccini G. The bronchoconstrictor action of the tetradeca-peptide bombesin in the guinea pig. *J Pharm Pharmacol* 1973;**25**:872–5.

86 Brown M, Marki W, Rivier J. Is gastrin releasing peptide mammalian bombesin? *Life Sci* 1980;**27**:125–8.

87 Wharton J, Polak JM, Bloom SR *et al*. Bombesin like immunoreactivity in the lung. *Nature* 1978;**273**:769–70.

88 Uddman R, Moghimzadeh E, Sundler F. Occurrence and distribution of GRP-immunoreactive nerve fibres in the respiratory tract. *Arch Otorhinolaryngol* 1984;**239**:145–51.

89 Tatemoto K, Carliquist M, Mutt V. Neuropeptide Y—a novel brain peptide with structural similarities to peptide YY and pancreatic polypeptide. *Nature* 1982;**296**:659–60.

90 Lundberg JM, Terenius L, Hokfelt T *et al*. Neuropeptide Y (NPY) like immunoreactivity in peripheral noradrenergic neurons and effects of NPY on sympathetic function. *Acta Physiol Scand* 1982;**116**:477–80.

91 Tatemoto K, Rokaeus A, Jornvall M, McDonald TJ, Mutt V. Galanin a novel biologically active peptide from porcine intestine. *FEBS Lett* 1983;**164**:124–8.

92 Cheung A, Polak JM, Bauer FE *et al*. Distribution of galanin immunoreactivity in the respiratory tract of pig, guinea-pig, rat and dog. *Thorax* 1985;**40**:889–96.

93 Gosney JR, Sissons MCJ, O'Malley JA. Quantitative study of endocrine cells immunoreactive for calcitonin in the normal adult human lung. *Thorax* 1985;**40**:866–9.

94 Ghatei MA, Sheppard MN, Henzen-Logman S, Blank MA, Polak JM, Bloom SR. Bombesin and vasoactive intestinal polypeptide in the developing lung: marked changes in acute respiratory distress syndrome. *J Clin Endocrin Metab* 1983;**57**:1226–32.

95 Fox IH, Kelley WN. The role of adenosine and 2'deoxyadenosine in mammalian cells. *Am Rev Biochem* 1978;**47**:655–86.

96 Burnstock G. Purines as cotransmitters in adrenergic and cholinergic neurones. *Prog Brain Res* 1986;**68**:193–203.

97 Mentzer RM, Rubio R, Berne RM. Release of adenosine by hypoxic canine lung tissue and its possible role in pulmonary circulation. *Am J Physiol* 1975;**229**:1625–31.

98 Fredholm BB. Release of adenosine from rat lung by antigen and compound 48/80. *Acta Physiol Scand* 1981;**111**:507–8.

99 Fredholm BB, Brodin K, Strandberg K. On the mechanism of relaxation of tracheal muscle by theophylline and other cyclic nucleotide phosphodiester-ase inhibitors. *Acta Pharmacol Toxicol* 1979;**45**:336–44.

100 Fredholm BB. Are methylxanthine effects due to antagonism of endogenous adenosine. *Trends Pharmacol Sci* 1980;**1**:129–32.

101 Cushley MJ, Holgate ST. Adenosine induced bronchoconstriction in asthma: role of mast cell mediator release. *J Allergy Clin Immunol* 1985;**75**:272–8.

102 Johnson HG, McNee MLO. Adenosine induced secretion in the canine trachea: modification by methylxanthines and adenosine derivatives. *Br J Pharmacol* 1985;**86**:63–7.

103 Mann JS, Holgate ST, Renwick AG, Cushley MJ. Airway effects of purine nucleosides and nucleotides and release with bronchial provocation in asthma. *J Apply Physiol* 1986;**61**:1667–76.

104 Marquardt DL, Gruber HE, Wasserman SI. Adenosine release from stimulated mast cells. *Proc Natl Acad Sci USA* 1984;**81**:192–6.

105 Marquardt DL, Parker CW, Sullivan TJ. Potentiation of mast cell mediator release by adenosine. *J Immunol* 1978;**120**:871–8.

106 Welton AF, Simko BA. Regulatory role of adenosine in antigen induced

histamine release from the lung tissue of actively sensitized guinea pigs. *Biochem Pharmacol* 1980;**29**:1085–92.

107 Peters SP, Schulman ES, Schleimer RP, Macglashan DW Jr, Newball HH, Lichtenstein LM. Dispersed human lung mast cells. Pharmacologic aspects and comparison with human tissue fragments. *Am Rev Respir Dis* 1982;**126**:1034–9.

108 Hughes PJ, Holgate ST, Church MK. Adenosine inhibits and potentiates IgE-dependent histamine release from human lung mast cells by an A2-purinoceptor mediated mechanism. *Biochem Pharmacol* 1984;**33**:3847–52.

109 Church MK, Hughes PJ. Adenosine potentiates immunological histamine release from rat mast cells by a novel cyclic AMP independent cell-surface action. *Br J Pharmacol* 1985;**85**:3–5.

110 Church MK, Holgate ST, Hughes PJ. Adenosine inhibits and potentiates IgE-dependent histamine release from human basophils by an A_2-receptor mediated mechanism. *Br J Pharmacol* 1983;**80**:719–26.

111 Mann JS, Holgate ST. Specific antagonism of adenosine induced bronchoconstriction in asthma by oral theophylline. *Br J Clin Pharmacol* 1985;**19**:85–92.

112 Pauwels R. The role of adenosine in bronchial asthma. *Bull Eur Physiopathol Respir* 1987;**23**:203–8.

113 Persson CGA, Carlsson JA, Erjefalt I. Differentiation between bronchodilatation and universal adenosine antagonism among xanthine derivatives. *Life Sci* 1982;**30**:2181–98.

114 Pauwels R, Van Renterghem D, Van Der Straeten M, Johannesson N, Persson CGA. The effect of theophyllline and enprofylline on allergen-induced bronchoconstriction. *J Allergy Clin Immunol* 1985;**76**:583–90.

115 Pauwels R, Van Der Straeten M. An animal model for adenosine-induced bronchoconstriction. *Am Rev Respir Dis* 1987;**23**:203–8.

116 Crimi N, Palermo F, Oliveri R, Cacipardo B, Vancheri G, Mistretta A. Adenosine induced bronchoconstriciton—comparison between nedocromil sodium and sodium cromoglycate. *Eur J Respir Dis* 1986;**69**(Suppl. 147):258–62.

117 Okayama M, Ma JY, Hataoka I *et al.* Role of vagal nerve on adenosine induced bronchoconstriction in asthma. *Am Rev Respir Dis* 1986;**133**(Suppl.):A93.

118 Rafferty P, Beasley R, Southgate P, Holgate ST. The role of histamine in allergen and adenosine-induced bronchoconstriction. *Int Arch Allergy Appl Immunol* 1987;**82**(3–4):292–4.

119 Joos GFP, Pauwels RAR, Van Der Straeten M. The role of neuropeptides as neurotransmitters of non-adrenergic, non-cholinergic nerves in bronchial asthma. *Bull Eur Physiopathol Respir* 1988;**23**:619–37.

120 Florey H, Carleton HM, Wells AQ. Mucus secretion in the trachea. *Br J Exp Pathol* 1932;**13**:269–84.

121 Ingelstedt S, Ivstam B. The source of nasal secretion in infectious allergic and experimental conditions. *Acta Otolaryngol* 1949;**37**:451–56.

122 Persson CGA. Role of plasma exudation in asthmatic airways. *Lancet* 1986;**2**:1125–9.

123 Pride NB. Epidemiology of bronchial hypersecretion: recent studies. *Eur J Respir Dis* 1987;**71**(Suppl.153):13–18.

124 Dunnell MS, Mossarella GR, Anderson JA. A comparison of quantitative anatomy of the bronchi in normal subjects, in status asthmaticus, in chronic bronchitis and in emphysema. *Thorax* 1969;**24**:176–9.

125 Lopez-Vidreri MT, Reid L. Chemical markers of mucous and serum glycoproteins and their relations to viscosity in mucoid and purulent sputum from various hypersecretory diseases. *Am Rev Respir Dis* 1978;**117**:465–77.

126 Sturgess JM. Structure of human airway mucosa. *Sem Respir Med* 1984;**5**:301–7.

127 Nadel JA, Holtzmann MJ. Regulation of airway responsiveness and secretion: role of inflammation. In: Kay AB, Austen KF, Lichtenstein LM eds. *Asthma.* London: Academic Press 1984:129–53.

128 Kaliner M, Shelhamer JH, Borson B, Nadel J, Patow C, Marom Z. Human respiratory mucus. *Am Rev Respir Dis* 1986;**134**:612–21.

129 Marin MG. Pharmacology of airway secretion. *Pharmacol Rev* 1986;**38**:273–89.

130 Richardson PS, Peatfield AC. The control of airway mucus secretion. *Eur J Respir Dis* 1987;**153**(Suppl.):43–51.

131 Basbaum C, Carlson D, Davidson E, Verdugo P, Gail DG. Cellular mechanisms of airway secretion. *Am Rev Respir Dis* 1988;**137**:479–85.

132 Salter HH. On asthma: its pathology and treatment, 2nd edition. London: Churchill 1968.

133 Turner-Warwick M, Openshaw P. Sputum in asthma. *Postgrad Med J* 1987;**63**(Suppl.1):79–82.

134 Bordley JE, Carey RA, Harvey AM *et al.* Preliminary observations on the effect of adrenocorticotrophic hormone (ACTH) in allergic diseases. *Bull John Hopkins Hosp* 1949;**85**:396–8.

135 Keal EE. Biochemistry and rheology of sputum in asthma. *Postgrad Med J* 1971;**47**:171–7.

136 Heilpern S, Rebuck AS. Effect of disodium cromoglycate (Intral) on sputum protein composition. *Thorax* 1972;**27**:726–8.

137 Sadoul P, Puchelle E, Zahan JM, Jaquot J, Aug F, Polu J-M. Effect of turbutaline on mucociliary transport and sputum properties in chronic bronchitis. *Chest* 1981;**80**(Suppl.):885–9.

138 Moretti M, Giannico G, Marchioni CF, Bisetti A. Effects of methylprednisolone on sputum biochemical components in asthmatic bronchitis. *Eur J Respir Dis* 1984;**66**:365–70.

139 Brogan TD, Ryley HC, Neale L, Yassa J. Relation between sputum sol phase composition and diagnosis in chronic chest diseases. *Thorax* 1971;**26**:418–23.

140 Honda I, Shimura S, Sasaki T, Sasaki H, Takishima T, Nakamura M. Airway mucosal permeability in chronic bronchitis and bronchial asthmatics with hypersecretion. *Am Rev Respir Dis* 1988;**137**:866–71.

141 Florey HW. *General Pathology*, 4th edition. London: Lloyd-Luke 1970.

142 Maron Z, Shelhamer J, Alling D, Kaliner M. The effects of corticosteroids on mucous glycoprotein secretion from human airways *in vitro. Am Rev Respir Dis* 1984;**129**:62–5.

143 Persson CGA. Plasma exudation and asthma. *Lung* 1988;**166**:1–23.

144 Persson CGA, Erjefalt I. Inflammatory leakage of macromolecules from the vascular compartment into the tracheal lumen. *Acta Physiol Scand* 1986;**126**:615–6.

145 Dunhill MS. The pathology of asthma. In: Middleton E, Reed CE, Ellis EF eds. *Allergy principles and practice II*. St Louis: CV Mosby 1978:678–86.

146 Guirgis HA, Townley RG. Biochemical study on sputum in asthma and emphysema. *J Allergy Clin Immunol* 1973;**51**:86.

147 Sanerkin NG, Evans DMP. The sputum in bronchial asthma: pathopneumonic patterns. *J Pathol Bacteriol* 1965;**89**:535–54.

148 Cohnheim J. *Volesungen uber Allgemeine Pathologie I*. Berlin: August Hirschwald 1882:232–367.

149 Brogan TD, Ryley HC, Neale L, Yassa J. Soluble proteins of bronchopulmonary secretions from patients with cystic fibrosis, asthma, and bronchitis. *Thorax* 1975;**30**:72–9.

150 Lam S, Leriche JC, Kijek K, Phillips RT. Effect of bronchial lavage volume on cellular and protein recovery. *Chest* 1985;**88**:856–9.

151 Fabbri LM, Broschetto P, Zocca E *et al.* Bronchoalveolar neutrophilia during TDI-induced late asthmatic reactions. *Am Rev Respir Dis* 1987;**136**:36–42.

152 Persson CGA, Erjefalt I, Andersson P. Leakage of macromolecules from guinea pig tracheobronchial microcirculation. Effects of allergen, leukotrienes, tachykinins, and anti-asthma drugs. *Acta Physiol Scand* 1986;**127**:95–106.

153 Andersson P, Persson CGA. Developments in anti-asthma glucocorticoids. In: O'Donnell SR, Persson CGA eds. *Directions for antiasthma drugs.* Basel: Birkenhauger 1988:223–44.

154 Fick RB, Metzger WJ, Richerson HB *et al.* Increased bronchovascular permeability after allergen exposure in sensitive asthmatics. *J Appl Physiol* 1987;**63**:1147–55.

155 Persson CGA, Pipkorn U. Similarities between asthma and rhinitis; vascular-epithelial leakage of plasma. In: Dahl R, Mygind N, Pipkorn U eds. *Rhinitis and asthma, similarities and dissimilarities.* Kopenham: Munksgaard 1989 (in press).

156 Rossen RD, Butler WT, Cate TR, Szwed CF, Couch RB. Protein composition of nasal secretion during respiratory virus infection. *Proc Soc Exp Biol Med* 1965;**119**:1169–79.

157 Dolovich J, Back NH, Arbesman CE. Kinin-like activity in nasal secretions of allergic patients. *Int Arch Allergy Appl Immunol* 1970;**38**:337–44.

158 Baumgarten CR, Togias AG, Nacliero RM, Lichtenstein LM, Norman PS, Proud D. Influx of kininogens into nasal secretions after antigen challenge of allergic individuals. *J Clin Invest* 1985;**76**:191–7.

159 Togias AG, Proud D, Lichtenstein LM *et al.* The osmolarity of nasal secretions increases when inflammatory mediators are released in response to inhalation of cold, dry air. *Am Rev Respir Dis* 1988;**137**:625–9.

160 Pipkorn U, Proud C, Schleimer RP *et al.* Effect of systemic glucocorticoid treatment on human nasal mediator release after antigen challenge. *J Allergy Clin Immunol* 1986;**77**(Suppl.):180.

161 Naclerio RM, Bartenfelder D, Proud D *et al.* Theophylline reduces the response to nasal challenge with antigen. *Am J Med* 1985;**79**(Suppl. 6A):43–7.

162 Persson CGA. Xanthines as airway antiinflammatory drugs. *J Allergy Clin Immunol* 1988;**81**:615–17.

163 Svensson C, Pipkorn U, Baumgarten CR, Alkner U, Persson CGA. Histamine induces reversible and reproducible macromolecular flow across vascular-mucosal barriers of human airways. *Thorax* 1989 (in press).

164 Moreno RH, Hogg JC, Pare PD. Mechanics of airway narrowing. *Am Rev Respir Dis* 1986;**133**:1171–80.

165 Yager D, Butler J, Bastacky J *et al.* Amplification of airway constriction due to liquid-filling of airway interstices. *J Appl Physiol* 1989 (in press).

166 Macklem PT. Bronchial hyporesponsiveness. *Chest* 1987;**91**:189S–91S.

167 Hutt G, Wick H. Bronchial-lumen und Atemwiderstand. *Z Aerosol Forsch Ther* 1956;**5**:131–40.

168 Wanner A. Mucociliary function in bronchial asthma. In; Weiss EB, Segal MS, Stein M eds. *Bronchial asthma* 2nd edition. Boston: Little & Brown 1985:270–9.

169 Aitken ML, Verdugo P. Donnan mechanism of mucus hydration: effect of soluble proteins. *Am Rev Respir Dis* 1986;**133**:A294.

170 Ikegami M, Jobe A, Berry D. A protein that inhibits surfactant in respiratory distress syndrome. *Biol-Neonate* 1986;**50**(3):121–9.

171 List SJ, Findlay BP, Forstner GG, Forstner JF. Enhancement of the viscosity of mucin by serum albumin. *Biochem J* 1978;**175**:565–71.

172 Hirsch SR. *The role of mucus in asthma.* Park Ridge: American College of Chest Physicians 1975:351–63.

173 Zweifach BW. Microvascular aspects of tissue injury. In: Zweifach BW, Grant L, McCluskey RT eds. *The inflammatory process,* 2nd edition, New York: Academic Press 1973:3–46.

174 Persson CGA, Svensjo E. Vascular responses and their suppression: drugs interfering with venular permeability. In: Bonta IL, Parnham MJ eds. *Handbook of inflammation.* Volume 5: *The pharmacology of inflammation.* Amsterdam: Elsevier 1985:61–81.

175 Persson CGA, Erjefalt I. Non-neural and neural regulation of airway micro-

vascular leakage of macromolecules. In: Kaliner MA, Barnes P eds. *Neural regulation of the airways in health and disease. Lung biology in health and disease.* New York: Marcel Dekker 1988:523–50.

176 Hurley JV. *Acute inflammation,* 2nd edition. Edinburgh: Churchill Livingstone 1983.

177 Majno G, Palade GE. Studies on inflammation I. *J Biophys Biochem Cytol* 1961;**11**:571–605.

178 Hogg JC. Bronchial mucosal permeability and its relationship to airway hyperreactivity. *J Allergy Clin Immunol* 1981;**67**:421–5.

179 Hogg JC, Walker DC. Pathology of the airway epithelium in asthma. *Clin Respir Physiol* 1986;**22**(Suppl. 7):12–19.

180 Nordin U. The trachea and cuff-induced tracheal injury. *Acta Otolaryngol* 1977;**345**(Suppl.):1–71.

181 Man SFP, Thompson ABR, Hulbert W, Park DKS, Hogg JC. Asymmetry of canine tracheal epithelium: osmotically induced changes. *J Appl Physiol* 1984;**57**:1338–46.

182 Permutt S. Physiologic changes in the acute asthmatic attack. In: Austen KF, Lichtenstein LM eds. *Asthma, physiology, immunopharmacology and treatment.* New York: Academic Press 1974:15–270.

183 Woolcock AJ, Permutt S. Bronchial hyperresponsiveness. In: Fishman AP ed. *Handbook of physiology: The respiratory system III.* American Physiological Society 1986:727–36.

184 Hogg JC, Pare PD, Moreno R. The effect of submucosal edema on airways resistance. *Am Rev Respir Dis* 1987;**135**:S54–6.

185 Burton AC. On physical equilibrium of small blood vessels. *Am J Physiol* 1951;**164**:319–29.

186 Burton AC. Relation of structure to function of tissues of walls of blood vessels. *Physiol Rev* 1954;**34**:619–42.

187 Pride NB, Permutt S, Riley RL, Bromberger-Barnea B. Determinants of maximal expiratory flow from the lungs. *J Appl Physiol* 1967;**23**:646–62.

188 Gunst SJ, Stropp JQ. Pressure-volume and length-stress relationships in canine bronchi *in vitro*. *J Appl Physiol* 1988;**64**:2522–53.

189 Gunst SJ, Warner DO, Wilson TA, Hyatt RE. Parenchymal interdependence and airway response to methacholine in excised dog lobes. *J Appl Physiol* 1986;**65**:2490–7.

190 Murtagh PS, Proctor DF, Permutt S, Kelly B, Evering S. Bronchial closure with mecholyl in excised dog lobes. *J Appl Physiol* 1971;**31**:409–15.

191 Mead J, Takishima T, Leith D. Stress distribution in lungs: a model of pulmonary elasticity. *J Appl Physiol* 1970;**28**:596–608.

192 Elad D, Kamm RD, Shapiro AH. Tube law for the intrapulmonary airway. *J Appl Physiol* 1988;**65**:7–13.

193 Michoud MC, LeLorier J, Amyot R. Factors modulating the inter individual variability of airway responsiveness to histamine: the influence of H_1 and H_2 receptors. *Bull Eur Physiopathol Respir* 1981;**17**:807–21.

194 Sterk PJ, Daniel EE, Zamel N, Hargreave FE. Limited bronchoconstriction to methacholine using partial flow–volume curves in nonasthmatic subjects. *Am Rev Respir Dis* 1985;**132**:272–7.

195 Woolcock AJ, Salome CM, Yan K. The slope of the dose–response curve to histamine in asthmatic and normal subjects. *Am Rev Respir Dis* 1984;**130**:71–5.

196 Dawson SV, Elliott EA. Wave-speed limitation on expiratory flow—a unifying concept. *J Appl Physiol* 1977;**43**:498–515.

197 Ramsdale EH, Morris MM, Roberts RS, Hargreave FE. Bronchial responsiveness to methacholine and cold air in patients with chronic airflow limitation compared to asthma. *Am Rev Respir Dis* 1984;**129**(Suppl.):A251.

198 Kariya ST, Shore SA, Skornik WA, Anderson K, Ingram RH Jr., Drazen JM. Methacholine-induced bronchoconstriction in dogs; effects of lung volume and ozone exposure. *J Appl Physiol* 1988;**6**:2679–86.

199 Macklem PT. Obstruction on small airways. A challenge to medicine. *Am J Med* 1972;**52**:721–4.

200 James A, Pare P, Hogg J. The mechanics of airway narrowing in asthma. *Am Rev Respir Dis* 1989;**139**:242–6.

201 Wagner EM, Weinmann GG, Liu MC, Walden SM, Bleecker ER. Comparison of peripheral airway resistive properties in normal and asthmatic subjects. *Am Rev Respir Dis* 1988;**137**:378.

202 Irvin CG, Berend N, Henson PM. Airway hyperreactivity and inflammation produced by aerosolization of human C5A des arg. *Am Rev Respir Dis* 1986;**134**:777–83.

203 Chung KF, Becker AB, Lazarus SC, Frick OL, Nadel JA, Fold WM. Antigen induced airway hyperresponsiveness and pulmonary inflammation in allergic dogs. *J Appl Physiol* 1985;**58**:1347–53.

204 Derkson FJ, Scott JS, Miller DC, Slocombe RF, Robinson NE. Bronchoalveolar lavage in ponies with recurrent airway obstruction (heaves). *Am Rev Respir Dis* 1985;**132**:1066–70.

205 Derkson FJ, Robinson NE, Armstrong PJ, Stick JA, Slocombe RF. Airway reactivity in ponies with recurrent airway obstruction (heaves). *J Appl Physiol* 1985;**58**:598–604.

206 Hutchinson AA, Hinson JM, Brigham KL, Snapper JR. Effect of endotoxin on airway responsiveness to aerosol histamine in sheep. *J Appl Physiol* 1983;**54**:1463–8.

207 Meyrick B, Brigham KL. Acute effects of *E. coli* endotoxin on the pulmonary microcirculation of anaesthetized sheep. Structure: function relationships. *Lab Invest* 1983;**48**:458–70.

208 Hinson JM, Hutchinson AA, Brigham KL, Meyrick BD, Snapper JR. Effects of granulocyte depletion on pulmonary responsiveness to aerosol histamine. *J Appl Physiol* 1984;**56**:411–17.

209 Holtzman MJ, Fabbri LM, Skoogh BE *et al.* Time course of airway hyper-responsiveness induced by ozone in dogs. *J Appl Physiol* 1983;**55**:1232–6.

210 Holtzman MJ, Fabbri LM, O'Byrne PM *et al.* Importance of airway inflammation for hyperresponsiveness by ozone. *Am Rev Respir Dis* 1983;**127**:686–90.

211 Fabbri LM, Aizawa H, Alpert SE *et al.* Airway hyperresponsiveness and changes in cell counts in bronchoalveolar lavage after ozone exposure in dogs. *Am Rev Respir Dis* 1984;**129**:288–91.

212 O'Byrne PM, Walthers EH, Gold BD *et al.* Neutrophil depletion inhibits airway hyperresponsiveness induced by ozone exposure. *Am Rev Respir Dis* 1984;**130**:214–19.

213 Murlas CG, Roum JH. Sequence of pathologic changes in the airway mucosa of guinea pigs during ozone-induced bronchial hyperreactivity. *Am Rev Respir Dis* 1985;**131**:314–20.

214 Murlas C, Roum JH. Bronchial hyperreactivity occurs in steroid-treated guinea pigs depleted of leukocytes by cyclophosphamide. *J Appl Physiol* 1985;**58**:1630–7.

215 Hulbert WM, McLean T, Hogg JC. The effect of acute airway inflammation on bronchial reactivity in guinea pigs. *Am Rev Respir Dis* 1985;**132**:7–11.

216 Pauwels R, Peleman R, Van Der Straeten M. Airway inflammation and non-allergic bronchial responsiveness. *Eur J Respir Dis* 1986;**68**(Suppl. 144):137–62.

217 Folkerts G, Henricks PAJ, Nijkamp FP. Inflammatory reactions in the respiratory airways of the guinea pig do not necessarily induce bronchial hyperreactivity. *Agents Actions* 1988;**23**:94–6.

218 Wanner A, Mezez RJ, Reinhart M, Eyre P. Antigen induced bronchospasm in conscious sheep. *J Appl Physiol* 1979;**47**:917–22.

219 Abraham WM, Delehunt JC, Yerger L, Marchette B. Characterization of a late phase pulmonary response after antigen challenge in allergic sheep. *Am Rev Respir Dis* 1983;**128**:839–44.

220 Abraham WM. The importance of lipoxygenase products of arachidonic acid in allergen induced late responses. *Am Rev Respir Dis* 1987;**135**:S49–S53.

221 Abraham WM, Russi E, Wanner A, Delehunt JC, Yerger LD, Chapman GA. Production of early and late pulmonary responses with inhaled leukotriene D$_4$ in allergic sheep. *Prostaglandins* 1985;**29**:715–26.

222 Larson GL, Wilson MC, Clark RAF, Behrens B. The inflammatory reaction in the airways in an animal model of the late asthmatic response. *Fed Proc* 1987;**46**:105–12.

223 Beherens BL, Clark RAF, Marsh W, Larson GL. Modulation of the late asthmatic response by antigen specific immunoglobulin G in an animal model. *Am Rev Respir Dis* 1984;**130**:1134–9.

224 Marsh WR, Irvin CG, Murphy KR, Behrens BL, Larson GL. Increases in airway reactivity and inflammatory cells in bronchoalveolar lavage after the late asthmatic response in an animal model. *Am Rev Respir Dis* 1985;**131**:875–9.

225 Murphy KR, Wilson MC, Irwin CG *et al.* The requirement for polymorpho-nuclear leukocytes in the late asthmatic response and heightened airway reactivity in an animal model. *Am Rev Respir Dis* 1986;**134**:62–8.

226 Turner CR, Spannhake EW. The late asthmatic response in the canine peripheral lung. *FASEBJ* 1988;**2**:A1698.

227 Sasaki H, Yanai S, Shimura S *et al.* Late asthmatic response to Ascaris antigen challenge in dogs treated with metyrapone. *Am Rev Respir Dis* 1987;**136**:1459–65.

228 Dunn CJ, Elliott GA, Oostveen JA, Richards IM. Development of a prolonged eosinophil-rich inflammatory leukocyte infiltration in the guinea pig asth-matic response ovalbumin inhalation. *Am Rev Respir Dis* 1988;**137**:541–7.

229 Hutson PA, Church MK, Clay TP, Miller P, Holgate ST. Early and late phase bronchoconstriction after antigen-challenge of nonanesthetized guinea pigs. *Am Rev Respir Dis* 1988;**137**:548–57.

230 Blythe S, England D, Esser B, Junk P, Lemanske RF. IgE antibody mediated inflammation of rat lung; histological and bronchoalveolar lavage assess-ment. *Am Rev Respir Dis* 1986;**134**:1246–51.

231 Gordon T, Sheppard D, McDonald DM, Distefano S, Saypenski L. Airway hyperresponsiveness and inflammation induced by toluene diisocyanate in guinea pigs. *Am Rev Respir Dis* 1985;**132**:1106–12.

232 Seltzer J, Scanlon PD, Drazen JM, Ingram RH, Reid L. Morphologic correla-tions of physiologic changes caused by SO$_2$-induced bronchitis in dogs. The role of inflammation. *Am Rev Respir Dis* 1984;**129**:790–7.

233 Abulas W, Brooks SM, Murlas CG, Miller ML, McKay RT. Toluene diisocyan-ate-induced airway hyperreactivity in guinea pigs depleted of granulocytes. *J Appl Physiol* 1988;**64**:1773–8.

234 Drazen JM, O'Cain CF, Ingram RH. Experimental induction of chronic bronchitis of dogs. Effects on airway obstruction and responsiveness. *Am Rev Respir Dis* 1982;**126**:75–9.

235 Scanlon PD, Seltzer J, Ingram RH, Reid L, Drazen JM. Chronic exposure to sulfur dioxide. Physiologic and histologic evaluation of dogs exposed to 50 or 15 ppm. *Am Rev Respir Dis* 1987;**135**:831–9.

236 Shore SA, Kariya ST, Anderson K *et al.* Sulfur dioxide-induced bronchitis in dogs. Effects on airway responsiveness to inhaled and intravenously admin-istered methacholine. *Am Rev Respir Dis* 1987;**135**:840–7.

237 Roehrs JD, Rogers WR, Johanson WG. Bronchial reactivity to inhaled methacholine in cigarette smoking baboons. *J Appl Physiol* 1981;**50**:754–60.

238 Fujita M, Schroeder MA, Hyatt RE. Canine model of chronic bronchial injury. *Am Rev Respir Dis* 1988;**137**:429–34.

239 Hirshman CA, Malley A, Downes H. The Basenji-greyhound dog model of asthma. Reactivity to *Ascaris suum*, citric acid and methacholine. *J Appl Physiol* 1980;**49**:953–7.

240 Hirshman CA, Austin DR, Klein W, Hanifin JM, Hulbert W. Increased metachromatic cells and lymphocytes in bronchoalveolar lavage fluid of dogs with airway hyperreactivity. *Am Rev Respir Dis* 1986;**133**:482–7.

241 Darowski MJ, Hannon VW, Rennie L, Hirshman CA. Inflammatory mediators and airway hyperresponsiveness in the Basenji-greyhound dog. *Am Rev Respir Dis* 1988;**137**:A378.

5: Cellular Mechanisms

A. B. Kay, P. M. Henson, G. W. Hunninghake, C. Irvin,
L. M. Lichtenstein & J. A. Nadel

Bronchial hyperresponsiveness (BHR) is the increased reactivity of the airways to a wide variety of pharmacological and physical agents. It is a cardinal feature of the disease known as 'bronchial asthma' (which is probably not a single disease entity but a spectrum of disorders characterised by widespread narrowing of the airways which reverses spontaneously or with treatment). Although hyperresponsiveness underlies much of the symptomatology of asthma, that is, wheeziness provoked by exercise, exposure to cold air, fumes, smokes and sprays, as well as nocturnal and early morning symptoms, it is also observed in other conditions, albeit to a lesser extent. For instance, there is a transient increase in BHR in normal subjects after upper respiratory tract infections (URTI), as well as in those with allergic rhinitis at the height of the pollen season. Hyperresponsiveness is also a feature of some patients with chronic obstructive airways disease and cystic fibrosis, although the mechanisms here may be different. Most cases of bronchial asthma of any severity have appreciable BHR. In fact, for the present purposes it will be assumed that in studies of asthma, where the clinical features were well documented, hyperresponsiveness was present even though a formal measurement of methacholine or histamine PC_{20} might not have been performed. In this chapter we attempt to: review the evidence that inflammation is an important aetiological component of BHR; discuss the role of individual inflammatory cells as well as the mediators they elaborate; and mention the microvasculature changes that accompany inflammation, although this is also dealt with elsewhere.[1]

It is worth emphasising at the outset that asthma (and the attendant BHR) can be studied in several different ways and that the information derived from one model, that is, asthma provoked in the clinical laboratory, might not necessarily be applicable to the alterations which exist in, for example, persistent ongoing asthma in its mild or severe form. In appropriate subjects asthma can be provoked by specific agents (such as allergen inhalation) or non-specifically by exercise or exposure to cold air. The responses observed may either be immediate, delayed ('late phase' reactions) or both (dual responders). There is no evidence that a common mechanism exists to explain airway narrowing in asthma elicited in the clinical laboratory or the disease as it exists in its natural form. This adds considerably to the complexities involved in studying asthma and hyperresponsiveness. Furthermore, there may indeed be differences between BHR that might be induced or enhanced by inflammatory responses and that which may result from permanent changes in the structure of the airways.

WHAT IS INFLAMMATION?

Inflammation is the response of vascularised tissue to injury and it serves to resolve and repair the effect of damage. The factors that initiate inflammation, like those of cell injury, are diverse and include infectious agents (bacteria, viruses and parasites), physical agents (burns, radiation and trauma), chemical agents (drugs, toxins and industrial agents), and ischaemic injury to tissues and immunological reactions such as allergy and autoimmunity. The histopathological features of inflammation consist of changes in vascular blood flow and calibre of small blood vessels followed by alterations in vascular permeability and accompanied by a series of changes involving white cells. Acute inflammation is of short duration and is characterised by exudation of fluid with plasma proteins (oedema) and leucocyte emigration, with granulocytes being prominent. By contrast, chronic inflammation is of longer duration, again generally with granulocyte emigration, but also with a dense infiltration of lymphocytes and monocytes/macrophages together with proliferation of blood vessels and connective tissue. In certain specialised circumstances, such as allergy and asthma, eosinophils are often found in particularly large numbers. Both acute and chronic inflammation are associated with some degree of fibrin deposition with platelet adherence and the release of platelet products.

Basophils are also inflammatory cells which are prominent in certain forms of delayed-type hypersensitivity and are also found in the upper airways in allergic rhinitis. At present there is no conclusive evidence that basophils participate in pathological processes in the lung. Thus the cells migrating from the blood vessels which have been clearly identified in airway inflammation include neutrophils, eosinophils, lymphocytes and monocytes. Platelets may contribute to the reaction, but whether they can emigrate actively from the blood remains controversial. Certain resident tissue cells such as mast cells and epithelial cells also probably participate, as do fibroblasts. Inflammation at mucosal surfaces has two additional important features; (i) mucus hypersecretion; and (ii) shedding or denudation of the airway epithelial surface.

It is very unlikely that one cell, or one mediator, will explain totally the mechanisms of hyperreactivity, but rather that the combined effects of a number of cells and mediators are required for the observed effects.

Pathological evidence for inflammation in asthma

Until recently, studies of the pathology of asthma were largely confined to tissues taken from patients who had died in status asthmaticus. With the advent of bronchoscopy and bronchial biopsy in asthma a number of reports of pathological findings in more moderate forms of the disease are beginning to appear. In asthma deaths certain features seem to be typical. These include intense infiltration of eosinophils and deposition of eosinophil products in and around the bronchial epithelium.[2,3] Large numbers of lymphocytes and macrophages are also common and neutrophils are usually present. There is marked hyperaemia and dilatation of blood vessels and considerable mucus hypersecretion with plugging of the small airways. Shedding of epithelial cells is a common finding and appears as clumps in the sputum (Creola bodies). Other important features include thickening of the basement membrane, and goblet cell hyperplasia. Conspicuous in the pathological descriptions of asthmatic airways is the hyperplastic increase in smooth muscle.[2-5] Apart from these structural changes, the occurrence of functional changes in smooth muscle contractility is controversial.

What remain unclear are the dynamics of this process. For instance, what is the sequence of cell emigration and is it different from the sequence observed in inflammatory processes in other parts of the body? How does this inflammatory process resolve? What is the sequence of the structural changes? Do the airways of asthmatics all look the same or are the lesions heterogeneous?

Microvascular leakage

It is virtually certain that microvascular leakage occurs in asthma of any severity not only because of the histopathological findings but because sputum[6,7] and bronchoalveolar lavage (BAL) fluid from asthmatics have been shown to contain elevated concentrations of albumin[8,9] The amount of albumin in BAL fluid is also increased after exposure to inhaled antigen.[10] Many of the mediators implicated in asthma are known to cause microvascular leakage at postcapillary venules. These include histamine, bradykinin, sulphidopeptide leukotrienes and platelet activating factor (PAF).[11-14] In addition, stimulation of the vagus nerve or injection of capsaicin, via release of sensory neuropeptides such as substance P, causes microvascular leakage in rodents.[15] Furthermore, mediators which increase bronchial blood flow might be expected to exaggerate leakage in asthmatic airways. Oedema, due to increased capillary permeability, may have several sequelae relevant to asthma. These include a contribution to narrowing of small airways, epithelial shedding, the formation of mucus plugs, inhibition of mucociliary clearance and, by providing a rich source of plasma proteins, substrate for complement-derived anaphylatoxins and kinins. To the extent that oedema represents an alteration in permeability, it may also contribute directly to alterations in responsiveness by allowing greater (or different) agonist penetration to the smooth muscle.

CELLS AND MEDIATORS

General

From the points raised above it can be seen that the contribution of inflammation to asthma and BHR is currently an area of intense scientific interest. Inevitably this has led to a polarisation of viewpoints as to the importance of a given cell type or mediator in the process. These different perspectives represent a healthy approach to developing a real understanding of the pathogenesis of the disease since they promote discussion and innovative experimentation, and create important challenges for the investigator. A particular case in point is the importance of neutrophils vs eosinophils in the inflammatory processes that lead to alteration in calibre or responsiveness of the airways, or both. The way in which each of these cell types contributes to the lesions needs to be resolved experimentally, but at this point the evidence for one, the other, both, or neither is far from complete. The problem is further confounded by the difficulty of performing definitive experiments in man. The evidence provided below from experimental animals is certainly important, but must be interpreted with caution until it can be confirmed in human asthma. Caution must also be imposed on observations in the human setting.

1 The presence of a given cell or mediator is certainly a prerequisite for its involvement, but the converse does not follow. The presence of neutrophils in the airways does not necessarily demonstrate a role for them in the pathogenesis; it could just as easily indicate that the cell was involved in regulating the severity or extent of the effect. This also applies to eosinophils and monocytes.

2 To date our experimental approaches to the airways of the asthmatic have, by necessity, represented only static snapshots of a highly dynamic process. Until rates and timing of influx and

egress (removal) of inflammatory cells are determined, the total load of a given cell within the inflammatory reaction cannot be determined. This might be particularly important with respect to granulocytes as they can discharge mediators and effector molecules very rapidly after stimulation.

3 The state of activation of cells in a lesion is generally not known. It is certainly conceivable that granulocytes may be found in the airways that are no more activated than was required for their accumulation at the site. In other circumstances the cells may be, or could have been, stimulated to a greater degree, which could result in a significant release of inflammatory materials.[16] Some inflammatory cells also seem to exist in at least two states with regard to activation. Upon exposure to certain molecules, e.g. PAF or tumour necrosis factor (for neutrophils) or interferon-γ (IFN-γ) (for macrophages), which by themselves do not initiate a complete activation, the cells are nevertheless primed so that a subsequent stimulus produces a much larger effect.[17-19]. While it is difficult at present to evaluate the importance of this process in inflammatory reactions *in vivo*, the potential for such cells to exhibit different states of reactivity, and consequently of effect, in the airways, seems considerable.

4 The localisation of the cells or mediators may be of vital importance to the interpretation of their role in the pathophysiological processes. Thus (as mentioned below) BAL may reveal a different cellular composition than that exhibited by washing the airways alone. It seems logical to suggest that the critical site for cell and mediator action in asthma is in the tissues of the airways themselves. It is by no means clear, therefore, that BAL truly samples the appropriate sites in the airways.

5 By definition, mediators are relatively short acting. This usually means that their lifespan in tissues or body fluids is limited. Indeed, the stability of each mediator in biological fluids and in lavage varies significantly.[20] In this respect the detection of mediators in BAL may significantly misrepresent the true mix of molecules impinging on the tissues in a dynamic manner *in vivo*. This is not to belittle the importance of determining as effectively as possible what mediators can be detected in and around the lesions; rather, it is to sound a note of caution on the interpretation of such observations.

6 Similarly, the inflammatory cells themselves may be significantly modified by the environment of the airways. Structural cells may play an important role in modulating the action, especially in reducing the injurious effects of inflammatory cells (see below). These effects are probably of considerable importance in the response of the airways to an inflammatory response. They may also complicate the interpretation of studies of inflammatory cells removed from the airways which in their isolation, would

have been removed from the above-mentioned modulating influence.

7 There has been a tendency in the field of asthma and airways responses to focus on mediators that are lipid in nature as potential contributors to the pathophysiological responses. To a large extent this bias is historical, although recent experiments involving administration of such mediators to human subjects[21] provide evidence to support their *potential* involvement. The even more recent advent of relatively specific antagonists will help to delineate further the role of the different mediators, although the likelihood that many different molecules participate together or in sequence must constantly be borne in mind. The cells that are discussed below for their potential contribution to asthma and BHR, however, make and release a host of non-lipid mediators that may well play crucial roles in the process, by enhancing the overall inflammatory response, attracting specific inflammatory cells, causing the injury often associated with inflammation and possibly even by changing the smooth muscle and thus the airways calibre or responsiveness.

Neutrophils

The evidence that neutrophils by themselves play an important role in BHR associated with ongoing clinical asthma is controversial. On the one hand, a number of studies in experimental animals, as well as in control models of asthma in man, indicate that neutrophils may play a part early on in the asthma process. Neutrophils seem to be a 'normal' resident of larger airways both in normoresponsive and hyperresponsive subjects. For instance Wardlaw *et al.* found a large percentage of neutrophils in the bronchial wash of non-atopic controls and hayfever sufferers as well as in mild asthmatics.[22] The numbers were approximately equal in all groups and considerably higher than those observed in BAL fluid. In fact neutrophils accounted for almost 50% of the total cell count in bronchial washes in normal subjects. Is this a reflection of the local environment that the subjects were exposed to or is it a general finding? In any event it raises the question of an airway poised for an inflammatory response if the right trigger-factors and underlying disease susceptibility are present. A further question is whether the neutrophils in asthmatics demonstrate a different degree of activation or stimulation compared with those of normal subjects. It is relevant that scrapings from the nasal mucosa of normal subjects also contained large numbers of neutrophils (AJ Wardlaw, unpublished observations) as did normal conjunctiva.

Numerous studies indicate that peripheral blood neutrophils become 'activated' after allergen- and exercise-induced early and late phase asthmatic responses.[23-26] Activation was assessed by increased membrane expression of complement receptors and enhanced cytotoxicity for complement-coated targets. Such observations that suggest the circulating neutrophils have been exposed to some stimulus. Many of the currently known stimuli for neutrophils, however, are not specific for this cell type so that activation of other inflammatory cells may also result from the same circumstances.

Significant increases in the percentage of neutrophils in BAL and bronchial mucus have been observed in subjects experiencing late-phase reactions after bronchial challenge.[27] Comparable observations were made in BAL during late phase reactions in sensitised subjects challenged with toluene diisocyanate (TDI); it was found that increases in neutrophils, as well as eosinophils and lymphocytes were inhibited by prior administration of oral prednisolone.[9] In contrast, neutrophilia in BAL was not a feature of late reactions elicited by plicatic acid in red cedar asthma.[28]

The elaboration of a high molecular weight neutrophil chemotactic activity (HMW-NCA) in the circulation of patients after allergen- or exercise-induced early and late phase reactions is well documented.[29-32] HMW-NCA was associated with molecules with a molecular size of about 600 kD and a near neutral isoelectric point. This activity has recently been identified in the serum of asthmatics admitted to hospital with status asthmaticus.[33] The molecular size of NCA in acute severe asthma was heterogeneous, that is 800, 600 and < 20 kD. When peripheral blood mononuclear cells from patients with acute severe asthma were cultured in serum-free medium, NCA could also be detected in the supernatant.[34] Current evidence suggests that HMW-NCA may be derived from lymphocytes or monocytes or both, and that it is related to the 10 kD neutrophil chemotactic factor (now fully characterised and sequenced by several groups).[35-39] The high molecular weight of the serum factor might be an artefact of heating to $56°C$ for 30 minutes.

The accumulation of neutrophils in the airways during inflammation has the potential to result in significant tissue damage. This cell type is associated with tissue injury in many inflammatory conditions.[40] The mechanisms by which it may do this include the release of oxygen metabolites, proteases and cationic materials. The neutrophil is also a potential source of a wide variety of mediators, including potent lipid mediators such as prostaglandins, thromboxanes, leukotriene B_4 (LTB_4) and PAF which may then contribute to airway responses or exacerbate the inflammatory response, or both.

Convincing evidence suggesting that neutrophils are capable of altering airways functions comes from animal experiments. Neutrophils have been firmly implicated in ozone-induced and antigen-induced hyperreactivity in dogs,[41-45] in antigen-induced late phase and hyperresponsiveness reactions in rabbits[43,46] and in sheep exposed to both endotoxin[47,48] and antigen.[49] Rabbits show increased responsiveness when airways inflammation is induced with phlogistic fragments of C5, and this too was dependent on neutrophils.[16] The requirements for granulocytes (especially neutrophils) in these experiments has been established by association (lavage, histology), depletion studies (such as nitrogen mustard) and more convincingly, by depletion followed by selective repletion with enriched populations of purified neutrophils.[43] Furthermore, supernatants from phagocytosing neutrophils *in vitro* induced hyperreactivity when nebulised into the airways of rabbits,[50,51] but eosinophils[52] *in vitro* did not. The active agents in this model are yet to be identified. By contrast the guinea-pig may react differently.[53] Furthermore, while there was also a sevenfold increase at six hours and a 17-fold increase at 17 hours in neutrophils in BAL in a guinea-pig model of late phase and late-late phase bronchoconstriction,[54] nedocromil sodium blocked the late reaction and subsequent eosinophil infiltration in BAL but did not affect the neutrophil infiltration. This suggested that in the late phase and the late-late phase neutrophil infiltration is less critical for the development of airways obstruction in this species.[55]

Whether neutrophils participate in the functional alterations associated with asthma remains an open question. The frequent recovery of neutrophils from BAL of asthmatic patients,[56,57] the presence of neutrophils in pathological tissue sections of asthmatic airways[58,59] and the ability of human neutrophils to alter airways function[51] suggests that they probably do.

Eosinophils

There is circumstantial evidence to suggest that eosinophils are important pro-inflammatory cells in the asthma process. It is well known that a blood and sputum eosiniophilia is often, but not invariably, found in association with most forms of asthma. In a study by Durham and Kay a blood eosinophilia accompanied late phase but not single early asthmatic responses and there was an inverse correlation between the blood eosinophil count and the degree of non-specific BHR as measured by the methacholine PC_{20}.[60] The accumulation of eosinophils and eosinophil products (major basic protein (MBP), eosinophil cationic protein (ECP) and eosinophil-derived neurotoxin (EDN)) have been observed in BAL during allergen-induced late phase reactions.[27,61,62] Similar observations were made in red cedar asthma: plicatic acid inhalation elicited BAL eosinophilia together with sloughing of bronchial epithelial cells.[28] In a placebo-controlled double-blind study sodium cromoglycate was shown to suppress the local accumulation of eosinophils in bronchial mucus and BAL fluid and these reductions in lung eosinophils were related to clinical improvement.[56]

Eosinophils are also prominent in many of the histopathological sections obtained from subjects who died from asthma[2,3] In fact, the pathology is often termed 'chronic eosinophilic desquamative bronchitis'. MBP was prominent in the bronchial wall in the mucus plugs of virtually all of these patients, even though only a few intact eosinophils were observed by routine light microscopy.[63] MBP concentrations are also elevated in the sputum from asthmatics.

Eosinophil cationic protein and MBP are both cytotoxic to the respiratory epithelium[64] *in vitro* and in experimental animals, and both may contribute to the denudation of the epithelium seen in asthma. Asthmatics with BHR ($PC_{20} < 4$ mg/ml) had significant elevations in the eosinophil count and concentrations of MBP in BAL fluid.[22] Furthermore, there were significant correlations between the amount of MBP recovered and the percentage of eosinophils. These changes were even more marked when asthmatics with BHR were compared with subjects with normoreactive airways. There were inverse correlations between the PC_{20} and the percentage of eosinophils and epithelial cells and the amount of MBP in BAL. This study, and that by Lam *et al.*,[28] clearly suggested that BHR was associated with increased amounts of eosinophils and their products. This is also consistent with the suggestion that the responsiveness is secondary to epithelial cell damage mediated through eosinophil-derived granule products. This suggestion, however, presupposes that the hyperresponsiveness is caused by epithelial damage and that eosinophils have a particular ability to induce this damage. Both of these may be the case, but need to be clearly demonstrated.

In addition to the basic proteins of the eosinophil granule, membrane phospholipid-derived mediators may also play a role in the pathogenesis of asthma. Eosinophils produced considerable quantities of leukotriene C_4 (LTC_4) after ionophore-,[65-67] IgE-[68] and IgE-dependent stimuli,[69] and small elevations in LTC_4 were noted in BAL in the late phase reactions when fluid from diluent challenge was compared with that obtained from allergen challenge.[27] LTD_4, or its 30-OH-LTB_4 metabolite, were also observed in BAL from patients with symptomatic asthma.[70,71]

Eosinophils have the capacity to generate quantities of PAF, comparable to that produced by neutrophils.[72,73] PAF may be of particular relevance to asthma because of its ability to cause vasoconstriction and increased vascular permeability, to induce eosinophil chemotaxis,[74] and adherence to endothelial cells,[75] to enhance mucus secretion, and to increase BHR after inhalation in man.[21] There are no convincing studies to date, however, of PAF elaboration associated with clinical asthma (but see the cautionary comments on detection of lipid mediators in lavage mentioned above).

The mechanism of recruitment of eosinophils, in preference to neutrophils, to the asthmatic airway in man still needs to be explained. Is it merely a response to a larger stimulus, a less efficient removal process, or are the stimuli (signals) somehow different or more prolonged in comparison with those in other inflammatory reactions? PAF is a potent chemotactic factor for eosinophils but is also effective *in vitro* at evoking directional neutrophil migration. It seems likely that *in vitro* chemotaxis is not a true model of cell accumulation *in vivo* since it does not take into account the requirement for the chemoattractant to cross the vessel wall, the special requirements of cell adhesion to endothelial cells, the process of emigration itself, nor the metabolism to which any chemotactic signal might be subjected in the tissue.

It is now appreciated that T-cell-derived products which play a vital role in eosinophil maturation also effect the mature cell. For instance, both GM-CSF and interleukin-5 (IL-5) activate mature eosinophils in terms of increased cytotoxicity and oxidative metabolism and prolong the life of eosinophils *in vitro*.[76,77] Thus, lymphocyte and macrophage products or PAF, acting either alone or in combination or in sequence, might alter the inflammatory cell in such a way as to cause its adherence to blood vessel walls. Other factors such as IL-1 may alter the endothelium to render it more adherent for granulocytes.

Recruitment and activation of eosinophils is strongly inhibited by corticosteroids, an effect which could explain the efficacy of these drugs in modifying late phase bronchoconstriction, but this has to be tempered by the controversial nature of the steroid effects on BHR[78] (in contrast to the effects on the late phase asthmatic response) and the common clinical experience of asthma persisting long after the eosinophilia has been corrected.

Mast cells and basophils

In man, mast cells are located in the lumen of the airways (where they can be recovered by BAL), in the bronchial epithelium, and in the submucosa, as well as the lung parenchyma. Basophils have not been identified in bronchial disease or in any situation associated with hyperresponsiveness, although they are probably present there as they are in most other organs.

Current evidence suggests that the early allergic asthmatic reaction is predominantly mediated by mast cells. The immediate response to inhaled allergens in atopic subjects (accompanied by elevations in plasma histamine) is rapid in onset and easily reversed by inhaled β_2-adrenoceptor agonists (such as albuterol) and sodium cromoglycate.[79] (In these situations the drugs are assumed to act primarily on the mast cell, although as far as sodium cromoglycate is concerned *in vitro* data do not support this view.)[80] Corticosteroids given over a period of time also attenuate the immediate reaction,[81] possibly by depletion of mast cells in the mucosa.[82,83] Following allergen challenge in atopic individuals there was an elevation in plasma histamine[84] and in BAL,[22,85] and both histamine and mast cell tryptase in BAL.[86] This occurred within minutes of challenge and over the following few hours increased urinary secretion of a major catabolite N-methylhistamine was identified.[87] Mast cells recovered from the airways by lavage within the first 15 minutes of allergen challenge have all the morphological features of non-cytotoxic degranulation.[62,88] Human lung mast cells also elaborate LTC_4, prostaglandin D_2, PAF, various chemotactic peptides, proteolytic enzymes and proteoglycans. The pathophysiological role of these lipid mediators, proteolytic enzymes and proteoglycans, however, is as yet unknown. In ongoing, day to day asthma, there is an inverse correlation between the methacholine PC_{20} and the percentage of mast cells in BAL[22] and the amounts of histamine in BAL fluid.[85] Furthermore, asthmatics with BHR had significant increases in spontaneous histamine release from BAL mast cells.

What is the role of the mast cell in late-phase reactions, airways reactivity and ongoing asthma? Almost a decade ago it was shown that $F(ab')_2$ anti-IgE, when injected into the skin, produced a late phase reaction which had many of the histopathological features of allergen-induced late phase reaction. It was therefore hypothesised that mast cells were essential for late phase reactions and that mast cell-derived chemotactic factors accounted for the subsequent infiltration of eosinophils, neutrophils and basophils. More recently, a similar dependency on IgE was shown for the induction of an aero-allergen induced late phase response in the airways of rabbits (inflammation and bronchoconstriction).[89] But these do not prove the involvement of mast cells since the anti-IgE or antigen may also have interacted with macrophages or lymphocytes through IgE on their $Fc_\varepsilon R_2$ and these cells, in turn, may have contributed to the late phase reaction. The airways late-cell phase was induced in rabbits passively sensitised with IgE containing serum, further suggesting a so-called 'type I allergic reaction'. On the other hand, evidence is now accumulating that late phase reaction (mainly from the skin, and to the lesser extent in the lung) is associated with the presence of lymphocytes and may therefore include elements of delayed-type hypersensitivity (type IV reactions) (see under 'Lymphocytes').

Activation of mast cells as a pathogenetic mechanism of immediate bronchoconstriction is not limited to allergen exposure since there is some evidence that it is also involved in asthma provoked by exercise, cold air and hyperventilation.[90] Neverthe-less, the evidence that mast cells are involved in immediate bronchoconstriction to immunological and non-immunological stimuli is still persuasive. The evidence that mast cells play a part in the late phase reaction is debatable and there is little evidence for or against the suggestion that these cells play a pivotal role in ongoing, day to day, chronic asthma. Mast cells may be involved in inflammation in general and are found in association with a variety of pulmonary pathologies. Indeed the most dramatic increases in mast cell numbers in the lung are found in fibrotic conditions, although as noted above, the presence of these cells does not necessarily indicate what role they may have in patho-physiological processes.

Monocytes and macrophages (mononuclear phagocytes)

The majority of cells recovered from BAL in normal as well as in asthmatic subjects are macrophages. These cells contain function-al IgE receptors ($Fc_\varepsilon R_2$),[91,92] and the numbers of these IgE-bearing cells are substantially greater in atopic asthmatics than normal controls.[93] Macrophages have the capacity to produce a wide range of lipid mediators including eicosanoids from the lipoxygenase and cyclo-oxygenase pathways as well as PAF. Mononuclear phagocytes also make and secrete a vast array of proteins and peptides that have biological activities that may contribute to the airways reactions. It would be very surprising if this cell type did not participate in airways responses to inhaled allergens. Appreciable amounts of β-glucuronidase were re-covered free in BAL[94] although the macrophage is only one potential source of this marker for lysosomal enzyme secretion, and a substantial increase in the number of macrophages has been reported after allergen challenge.[62] This increase seems to be due to the migration of monocytes into the lung because it can largely be accounted for by peroxidase positive cells (a characteris-tic feature of monocytes compared with alveolar macrophages).

Lung macrophages are also activated in late phase reaction after allergen challenge as shown by an increase in the number of complement rosettes.[27] Chronic severe asthmatics who are rela-tively unresponsive to corticosteroids have increased numbers of circulating activated monocytes.[95] This was once thought to be a primary monocyte defect but this now seems to be secondary to T-lymphocyte activation.[96]

These observations provide only circumstantial support for a role for the mononuclear phagocyte in the pathogenesis of asthma. Nevertheless, the cell type is pluripotential, and is in-volved not only in most inflammatory reactions but also in the afferent arm of the immune response as well. Histologically the inflammatory lesions in asthma include mononuclear phagocytes and they may be presumed to be participating in the process. It is also worth recognising, however, the role that the mononuclear phagocyte series of cells plays in the resolution of inflammation.[97] Thus it is unclear at present whether these cells contribute actively to the pathophysiology of asthma or are involved in removing and modulating the effects of other cells and the mediators they produce, or both. Because macrophages can manifest many different functional phenotypes it is entirely possible that the airways of asthmatics may contain macrophages that are contributing to the disease as well as cells that are serving to limit the extent of the inflammation and of the pathophysiology.

Platelets

Initial experiments in rabbits and guinea-pigs suggested that platelet depletion prevented PAF-induced airway responses,[98,99] although the presence of these cells may not always be necessary.[100,101] Platelets have been reported in the lavage fluid following allergen challenge[102] and platelet-like structures have been identified histologically in the inflamed airways of guinea-pigs.[103] Unfortunately, it is not always possible to identify platelets clearly by morphological means, and specific tags (such as antibody) have not yet been used. The question of how platelets might get out of the blood vessels and through the tissues has not been addressed. The cells are only poorly phagocytic *in vitro* and have not yet been shown to have that property *in vivo*. Alternatively, the platelets might be present as a result of loss of vessel wall integrity.

In another approach to possible platelet involvement, platelet factor 4 was identified in the plasma of atopic subjects[104] but further studies have not provided confirmation[105] (and Henson *et al.*, unpublished observations). Platelets do bear the second IgE Fc receptor in a functionally active form, as shown by IgE-dependent oxidative metabolism and cytotoxicity.[106] By and large, there is no evidence that platelets play a pivotal role in human asthma and are directly concerned in BHR. The observations that suggest a role for platelets raise some important questions relating to the possible mechanisms by which they might become involved. Intravascular participation of platelets in inflammatory reactions in general and in airways inflammation in particular, seems highly likely, and the cells can release many molecules and mediators that could contribute to the process. If they migrate into the tissues themselves they would certainly represent a potentially important additional inflammatory cell, but this process needs to be formally demonstrated. In any event, one intriguing role that these cells might have is as a major source of lipid mediators. Platelets synthesise thromboxane directly upon activation. Additionally, stimulation of whole blood with phagocytic particles leads to a generation of significant amounts of thromboxane which requires both neutrophils and mononuclear cells as well as platelets for optimal production.[107] Platelets also participate in transcellular metabolism of LTC_4 in which stimulation of neutrophils leads to release of LTA_4 which is then converted to LTC_4 by the platelets.[108] This process is highly efficient and results in the production of large amounts of LTC_4, even in whole blood.[107]

Lymphocytes

An area of considerable current interest is the role of the T-lymphocyte in the regulation and expression of the inflammation associated with allergy and asthma. The T-cell-derived lymphokines, IL-4, IL-5 and IFN-γ, are intimately involved in the regulation of the IgE production.[109] Some lymphokines are active in the control of eosinophil production by the bone marrow (IL-5, GM-CSF, IL-3) and in the regulation of mast cell differentiation, others have chemotactic activity for neutrophils, eosinophils and basophil granulocytes as well as monocytes and can activate or degranulate these effector cells. T-lymphocytes also have a general role in the regulation of specific immune responses and are a possible target cell for desensitisation immunotherapy.

Direct evidence for T-lymphocyte changes in asthma and allergy come from a variety of sources. Post-mortem examination of the airways of asthmatic patients showed large numbers of lymphocytes.[2,3] Increased numbers of 'atypical intraepithelial lymphocytes' were found in an ultrastructural morphological study of bronchial biopsy specimens taken during life with subjects with mild asthma.[110,111] These lymphocytes are probably activated T-cells but formal proof of this is not yet available. Increased natural killer cell activity has been described in the peripheral blood of asthmatic patients.[112] Natural killer activity is an inducible property of T-cells and of non-T, non-B, lymphocytes and thus a non-specific indicator of lymphocyte activation.

Measurements in chronic asthmatics indicated that patients who were relatively refractory to treatment with corticosteroids had a relative decrease in the numbers of circulating T-suppressor (CD8) cells.[113] These patients also had an abnormality of T-cells grown *in vitro* (colony counts in soft agar) since, unlike T-cells from normal subjects and those responsive to corticosteroids, cell proliferation from the refractory patients was not inhibited by optimal concentrations of methylprednisolone.[114] A defect in concanavalin A-induced suppressor cell function has been described in asthma,[115-119] and successful immunotherapy was associated with an increase in the relative number of T-suppressor cells (OKT8).[120]

T-lymphocyte subset changes have also been studied using the model of bronchial allergen challenge in three separate studies.[62,121,122] The design of each of these three investigations was different, but taking them together it appears that T-lymphocytes bearing the CD4 marker (helper/inducer subset) were depleted in peripheral blood and selectively retained in the lung following challenge, but the kinetics and significance of this finding are as yet unclear. In addition, it appears that there is a difference in the profile of regulatory T-cell subsets present in BAL in asthmatics who respond with an early reaction alone, compared with the dual asthmatic (early and late phase) responders.

A recent study of cell traffic and activation in allergen-induced late phase reactions in human skin showed a lymphocyte infiltration which was almost exclusively CD4-positive (helper/inducer subset).[123] Some of these T-cells were activated in that they stained positively for the presence of IL-2 receptors. Further evidence of T-lymphocyte activation was provided by the observation that endothelial cells in the allergen challenged biopsies showed an increased density of HLA-DR (histocompatibity antigen) expression compared with control sites. This indicated local secretion of the T-lymphocyte-derived soluble inflammatory mediator, IFN-γ. In the same study it was shown that eosinophil accumulation and activation were striking features of the late phase skin reaction with numerous activated eosinophils (EG2 +) present at six hours after challenge and persisting in tissue for up to 48 hours. While the airways and the skin may not be exactly equivalent, the study certainly suggests the possibility of comparable processes in bronchial late phase responses.

Lymphocytes from the peripheral blood of patients with status asthmaticus demonstrated significant elevations of the expression of three surface proteins associated with T-lymphocyte activation (interleukin-2 receptor (IL-2R), class II HLA-DR and 'very late activation' antigen (VLA-1)), compared with control subjects (mild asthma, chronic obstructive airways disease and normal individuals).[124] Phenotypic analysis of the IL-2R positive T-lymphocytes showed that these cells were exclusively of the CD4 'helper-inducer' phenotype. The percentages of IL-2R and HLA-DR-positive (but not VLA-1–positive) lymphocytes tended to decrease as the patients were treated and improved clinically. The serum concentrations of IFN-γ and soluble IL-2R were also significantly elevated in patients with acute severe asthma as compared with all the control groups.[125] Concentrations decreased as the patients improved clinically during the first seven day period of hospital treatment. A significant correlation was observed between the degree of airways obstruction as measured by the peak expiratory flow rate and: (i) the percentages of peripheral blood T-lymphocytes expressing IL-2R; and (ii) the serum concentrations of soluble IL-2R. Taken together, therefore, these observations provide further evidence that CD4 T-lympho-cyte activation may contribute to the pathogenesis of acute severe asthma.

Epithelial cells

Loss of epithelium is a consistent finding in the airways of asthmatics. During asthma attacks, epithelial cells are desquamated and are found in the sputum as Creola bodies or Curschmann's spirals. Post-mortem examination of asthmatics shows extensive shedding of epithelial cells and severe epithelial inflammation. Even subjects with stable asthma show evidence of airway epithelial desquamation.[58]

Until recently, airway epithelial cells were considered simply to be an inert, physical lining covering the airways. It is now apparent that these cells, with their key location at the interface between the external environment and the internal milieu, have an important role in the defence of the airways, and probably in the inflammatory process.

Inflammatory cells such as neutrophils or eosinophils must migrate across the epithelium to reach the airways lumen, a site in which they are found in asthma (see above). This process is not as simple as might at first be thought. Granulocytes penetrate the junctions between the epithelial cells and once one cell has migrated there seems to be some preference for this site to be used by others. It is generally presumed that this migration is in response to chemotactic factors that themselves have crossed, and have established a gradient across, the epithelium. *In vitro*, neutrophils can be induced to cross 'tight' monolayers of epithelial cells under the influence of chemoattractants.[126] Since this process can occur without changes in the electrical properties of the monolayer it seems likely that the migrating cells can maintain a tight seal with the endothelial cells on each side, thus preventing alterations in epithelial permeability during migration.[127] On the other hand, migration of granulocytes *in vivo* is often associated with epithelial damage (see above). It seems likely therefore that different degrees, times, or locations of granulocyte stimulation are critical determinants of the degree of injury that accompanies the migratory process. A further question to be addressed is the potential role of the epithelial cell itself in the migration, and also in modulating the degree of stimulation of the inflammatory cell and the degree of ensuing injury.

Airway epithelial cells are capable of generating lipoxygenase products of arachidonic acid.[128,129] Thus human cells produce 15-hydroxyeicosatetraenoic acid (15-HETE) and 8,15-di-HETEs[129] and dog epithelial cells produce LTB_4 and selected HETEs.[128] Both LTB_4 and 8,15-di-HETEs[130,131] are chemotactic for neutrophils, and these molecules could therefore contribute to the neutrophil infiltration of the airways that occurs with viral infection,[132] ozone,[44,133] and other airway stimuli. The 15-HETEs are also of interest because they are reported to stimulate the release of mediators from mast cells.[134] They can also be converted to lipoxins, substances that contract airway smooth muscle.[135,136]

Other functions of 15-lipoxygenase have also been described. Thus 14,15-di-HETE and lipoxin A have been reported to be potent inhibitors of natural killer cell activity.[137,138] 15-HETE inhibits LTB_4 release by rabbit neutrophils[139] and LTC_4 production in the human eosinophil.[140] The biological importance of these anti-inflammatory properties is not known.

Because 15-lipoxygenase exists in the epithelial cell and produces the major mediators from this cell, the enzyme is likely to play a key role in epithelial cell biology.

The roles of 15-lipoxygenase in airway function and modification by disease are still unknown. Purification of the enzyme has been accomplished.[141] More recently molecular cloning and the primary structure of human 15-lipoxygenases has been accomplished.[142] The purification and cloning of the enzyme should prove useful in understanding its role in health and disease.

Thus epithelial cell stimulation during conditions associated with damage or by other mediators could produce lipoxygenase products which in turn stimulate other inflammatory cells. In the presence of stimulated inflammatory cells it might be important to question the possible transcellular metabolism of lipid mediator precursors,[143] leading to a different mix of products and thus of effects.

Smooth muscle modulation by airway epithelium

Airway epithelium has multiple effects on airway smooth muscle. Intact epithelium inhibits muscle tone by releasing prostaglandin E_2 (PGE_2). PGE_2 has inhibitory effects directly in the muscle and also by inhibiting vagal neural transmission.[144] Human and canine airway epithelial cells *in vitro* produce low concentrations of PGE_2, but when they are stimulated by inflammatory mediators such as bradykinin,[145] or by eosinophil MBP,[146] these cells produce large amounts of PGE$_2$ which have profound effects on smooth muscle.[147] Removal of airway epithelium is reported to produce inhibitory effects on airway smooth muscle via an unknown mechanism.[148] Contractile effects of tachykinins such as substance P are modulated by a membrane-bound enzyme, neutral endopeptidase (also called enkephalinase), which exists on airway epithelial cell membranes.[149] By cleaving and thus inactivating these neuropeptides, epithelial neutral endopeptidase limits the action of tachykinins on airway smooth muscle. Removal of airway epithelium decreases the amount of neutral endopeptidase in the airway and thus selectively increases the bronchoconstrictor effects of substance P. Although neutral endopeptidase does not affect contractions due to mediators such as acetylcholine,[149] it does cleave and thereby modulate contractions due to such peptides as bradykinin[150] and neurotensin.[151]

Epithelial glycocalyx

The luminal surface of the airway epithelium contains a glycocalyx consisting of high molecular weight glycoconjugates that contain specific types of carbohydrate chains of the poly(N-acetyllactosamine)-type.[152] These high molecular weight materials are produced and secreted by the airway epithelium and thus contribute to the luminal secretions. As with other secretions, their exact function is unknown, but they may contain binding sites for bacterial and other cells.

Under appropriate conditions, inflammatory cells such as mast cells, neutrophils, eosinophils and macrophages migrate to the airways. If these inflammatory cells adhere to airway epithelium, their actions may be increased and prolonged. Mast cells adhere to tracheal epithelial cells in culture and in tissue sections.[153] This adhesion is selective and occurs preferentially with epithelial cells, with minimal adhesion to surfaces coated with basement membrane collagen (type IV), connective tissue matrix collagen (type I) or fibronectin. Adhesion to cultured epithelial cells was a characteristic of a sub-population of mast cells, persisted for more than 48 hours, did not require energy or the presence of divalent cations, and was not mediated by a known family of leucocyte-associated adhesion glycoproteins. Adhesion was completely abolished by pretreatment of the mast cells with proteinase K or proteinase E but not with trypsin. Pretreatment of the epithelial cells with proteinases was without effect. This latter fact suggests that the epithelial adhesion molecules are not proteins. Some epithelial cells carry glycolipid receptors,[154] and the airway epithelial binding sites for mast cells might also be lipids.

The existence of a population of adherent mast cells in and on the epithelium has important clinical implications because a population of highly reactive cells are at a site where they may readily respond to inhaled materials and where their products have ready access to the structures of the epithelium and submucosa. These adhesion properties may explain the localisation of certain mast cell populations in the airway epithelium. Thus in cigarette smokers,[155] and in asthmatics,[156] intraepithelial mast cells may be selectively adherent. This selective localisation may play an important part in determining the phenotype of the intraepithelial mast cells. Adhesion may also form a microenvironment between the mast cells and epithelium by increasing local concentrations of mediators, thereby causing changes such as increased mucosal permeability to antigens and to other stimuli, increased secretions, ion transport and smooth muscle contraction, and influx of other inflammatory cells. This selectively adherent population of mast cells may differ in functional properties from non-adherent cells, such as those readily available to BAL.

Ion transport and mucus secretion

This subject has been reviewed elsewhere[157] and will only be discussed briefly. Most of the fluid and mucus present in the airway lumen is believed to be derived from airway submucosal glands and can be stimulated to secrete mucus of different chemical and viscoelastic properties by different autonomic nervous and chemical mediators.[157] Active ion transport of chloride by airway epithelial cells[158] and secondary movement of fluid[159] provide a mechanism for fine regulation of the sol layer in which the cilia move. PGE_2 produced by the epithelial cells stimulates Cl transport,[160] and various inflammatory mediators stimulate PGE_2 production, thus increasing Cl transport. Nadel *et al.*[157] have postulated that this autocrine function of the epithelium allows it to dilute inflammatory irritants in the microenvironment and thus lessen their deleterious effects.

Water is lost in the airway during breathing, and this loss is exaggerated during exercise and when breathing dry air. The water loss must first occur from the airway lumen and then from the interstitial space. Ultimately, the water loss must be made up from fluid supplied by the bronchial arteries, or hyperosmolarity of the airway tissues must occur. Because exercise-induced asthma is believed to be triggered by hyperosmolarity, knowledge of the fluid reservoirs and limitations of fluid production in airways are important to the understanding and possibly the prevention of asthmatic attacks during exercise.

In summary, the epithelium is a dynamic tissue which may have a role in defending the airways. In asthma and in other inflammatory diseases of the airways there are conspicuous alterations in the epithelium, many of which may be presumed to result from the inflammatory process itself. On the other hand, the epithelium is by no means passive and almost certainly contributes to, and modulates, the inflammation itself.

GENERAL SUMMARY

An attempt has been made to review the importance or otherwise of various inflammatory cells and mediators in the pathogenesis of BHR. The possible participation of neutrophils, eosinophils, mast cells, basophils, mononuclear phagocytes, platelets, lymphocytes and epithelial cells has been considered, particularly as products from these cell types have the potential for contributing directly to the features of bronchial asthma (and by implication to BHR). It is not possible at present to judge the importance or otherwise of each individual cell type. It seems far more likely that they act together in a complex cascade. In the absence of knowledge on the dynamics of the bronchial pathology associated with the asthma process, however, anything more than speculation is unwarranted at present. Furthermore, the heterogeneity of asthma and associated pathology is still poorly understood and so the likelihood exists that different cells and their mediators may be important in various forms of hyperresponsiveness and at different stages in its natural history.

There are several particular issues which need to be urgently addressed. These include the relevance or otherwise of clinical models of asthma and hyperresponsiveness to the natural disease and the relation between the immediate and the late phase response in provoked asthma (and, in turn, the significance of these to the hyperresponsiveness of persistent asthma). Advances in technology and the ability to probe the airways by methods such as fibreoptic bronchoscopy and mucosal biopsy, together with prospects for analysing complex biological fluids in the microenvironment of the bronchial mucosa, may pave the way to a greater understanding of asthma and hyperresponsiveness.

REFERENCES

1 Drazen JM. Physiology. In: Holgate ST ed. *The role of inflammatory processes in airway hyperresponsiveness.* Oxford: Blackwell Scientific Publications 1989:108–50.
2 Dunnill MS. The pathology of asthma with special reference to changes in the bronchial mucosa. *J Clin Pathol* 1960;13:27.
3 Dunnill MS, Massarella GR, Anderson JA. A comparison of the quantitative anatomy of the bronchi in normal subjects, in status asthmaticus, in chronic bronchitis and in emphysema. *Thorax* 1969;24:176–9.
4 Dunnill MS. The pathology of asthma. In: Middleton E Jr, Reed CE, Ellis EF, eds. *Allergy, principles and practices.* St Louis, Missouri: CV Mosby 1978:678–86.

5 Heard BE, Hossain S. Hyperplasia of bronchial muscle in asthma. *J Path* 1973;110:319.

6 Ryley HC, Brogan TD. Variation in the composition of sputum in chronic chest diseases. *Br J Exp Pathol* 1968;49:25.

7 Brogan TD, Ryley HC, Neale, L, Yassa L. Soluble proteins of bronchopulmonary secretions from patients with cystic fibrosis, asthma and bronchitis. *Thorax* 1975;30:72–9.

8 Lam S, LeRiche JC, Kijek K, Phillips RT. Effect of bronchial lavage volume on cellular and protein recovery. *Chest* 1985;88:856–9.

9 Boschetto P, Fabbri LM, Zocca E *et al.* Prednisone inhibits late asthmatic reactions and airway inflammation induced by toluene diisocyanate in sensitized subjects. *J Allergy Clin Immunol* 1987;80:261–7.

10 Fick RB Jr, Metzger WJ, Richerson HB *et al.* Increased bronchovascular permeability after allergen exposure in sensitive asthmatics. *J Appl Physiol* 1987;63:1147–55.

11 Saria A, Lundberg JM, Skofitsch G, Lembeck F. Vascular protein leakage in various tissues induced by substance P, capsaicin, bradykinin, serotonin, histamine and by antigen challenge. *Naunyn-Schmiedeberg's Arch Pharmacol* 1983;324:212–8.

12 Persson CGA. Leakage of macromolecules from the tracheobronchial circulation. *Am Rev Respir Dis* 1987;135:S71.

13 Hua X-Y, Dahlen S-E, Lundberg JM, Hammarstrom S, Hedqvist P. Leukotrienes C_4 and E_4 cause widespread and extensive plasma extravasation in the guinea pig. *Naunyn-Schmiedeberg's Arch Pharmacol* 1985;330:136–41.

14 Evans TW, Chung K, Rogers DF, Barnes PJ. Effect of platelet-activating factor on airway vascular permeability; possible mechanisms. *J Appl Physiol* 1987;63:479–84.

15 Lundberg JM, Saria A, Lundblad L *et al.* Bioactive peptides in capsaicin-sensitive C-fiber afferents of the airways; functional and pathophysiological implications. In: Kaliner MA, Barnes PJ, eds. *Neural control in health and disease.* New York: Marcel Dekker 1987:417.

16 Irvin CG, Berend N, Henson PM. Airways hyperreactivity and inflammation produced by aerosolization of human C5a des arg. *Am Rev Respir Dis* 1986;134:777–83.

17 Pabst MJ, Johnston RB Jr. Increased production of superoxide anion by macrophages exposed in vitro to muramyl dipeptide or lipopolysaccharide. *J Exp Med* 1980;151:101–14.

18 Guthrie LA, McPhail LC, Henson PM, Johnston RB Jr. The priming of neutrophils for enhanced release of superoxide anion and hydrogen peroxide by bacterial lipopolysaccharide; evidence for increased activity of the superoxide-producing enzyme. *J Exp Med* 1984;160:1656–71.

19 Riches DWH, Channon JY, Leslie CC, Henson PM. Receptor-mediated signal transduction in mononuclear phagocytes. In: Ishizaka K, Kallos P, Lachmann PJ, Waksman BH, eds. *Progress in allergy,* Volume 42. Basel: S Karger 1988:65–122.

20 Westcott JY, McDonnel TJ, Voelkel NF. Alveolar transfer and metabolism of eicosanoids in the rat lung. *Am Rev Respir Dis* 1989 (in press).

21 Cuss FM, Dixon CM, Barnes PJ. Effects of platelet activating factor on pulmonary function and bronchial responsiveness in man. *Lancet* 1986;ii:189–92.

22 Wardlaw AJ, Dunnette S, Gleich GJ, Collins JV, Kay AB. Eosinophils and mast cells in bronchoalveolar lavage in mild asthma; relationship to bronchial hyperreactivity. *Am Rev Respir Dis* 1988;137:62–9.

23 Papageorgiou N, Carroll M, Durham SR, Lee TH, Walsh GM, Kay AB. Complement receptor enhancement as evidence of neutrophil activation after exercise-induced asthma. *Lancet* 1983;ii:1220–3.

24 Moqbel R, Durham SR, Shaw RJ *et al.* Enhancement of leukocyte cytotoxicity after exercise-induced asthma. *Am Rev Respir Dis* 1986;133:609–13.

25 Carroll M, Durham SR, Walsh GM, Kay AB. Activation of neutrophils and monocytes after allergen- and histamine-induced bronchoconstriction. *J Allergy Clin Immunol* 1985;**75**:290–6.

26 Durham SR, Carrol M, Walsh GM, Kay AB. Leucocyte activation in allergen-induced late-phase asthmatic reactions. *N Engl J Med* 1984;**311**:1398–402.

27 Diaz P, Gonzalez MC, Galleguillos FR *et al.* Leucocytes and mediators in bronchoalveolar lavage during allergen-induced late-phase asthmatic reactions. *Am Rev Respir Dis* 1989 (in press).

28 Lam S, LeRiche J, Phillips D, Chan-Yeung M. Cellular and protein changes in bronchial lavage fluid after late asthmatic reaction in patients with red cedar asthma. *J Allergy Clin Immunol* 1987;**80**:44–50.

29 Atkins PC, Norman M, Weiner H, Zweiman B. Release of neutrophil chemotactic activity during immediate hypersensitivity reactions in humans. *Ann Intern Med* 1977;**86**:415–8.

30 Nagy L, Lee TH, Kay AB. Neutrophil chemotactic activity in antigen-induced late asthmatic reactions. *N Engl J Med* 1982;**306**:497–501.

31 Lee TH, Nagy L, Nagakura T, Walport MJ, Kay AB. The identification and partial characterisation of an exercise-induced neutrophil chemotactic factor in bronchial asthma. *J Clin Invest* 1982;**69**:889–99.

32 Lee TH, Nagakura T, Papageorgiou N, Iikura Y, Kay AB. Exercise induced late asthmatic reactions with neutrophil chemotactic activity. *N Engl J Med* 1983;**308**:1502–5.

33 Buchanan DR, Cromwell O, Kay AB. Neutrophil chemotactic activity in acute severe asthma ('status asthmaticus'). *Am Rev Respir Dis* 1987;**136**:1397–402.

34 Buchanan DR, Fitzharris P, Cromwell O, Kay AB. Neutrophil chemotactic activity from cultured blood mononuclear cells in acute severe asthma. *Thorax* 1987;**42**:749.

35 Yoshimura T, Matsushima K, Tanakana S *et al.* Purification of a human monocyte-derived neutrophil chemotactic factor that has peptide sequence similarity to other host defense cytokines. *Proc Natl Acad Sci USA* 1987;**84**:9233–7.

36 Van Damme J, Van Beeumen J, Opdenakker G, Billiau A. A novel, NH_2-terminal sequence-characterized human monokine possessing neutrophil chemotactic, skin-reactive, and granulocytosis-promoting activity. *J Exp Med* 1988;**167**:1364–76.

37 Gregory H, Young J, Schröder J-M, Mrowietz U, Christophers E. Structure determination of a human lymphocyte derived neutrophil activating peptide (LYNAP). *Biochem Biophys Res Commun* 1988;**151**:883–90.

38 Maestrelli P, O'Hehir RE, Lamb JR, Tsai J-J, Cromwell O, Kay AB. Antigen-induced neutrophil chemotactic factor from cloned human T-lymphocytes. *Immunology* 1988;**65**:605–9.

39 Maestrelli P, Tsai J-J, Cromwell O, Kay AB. The identification and partial characterization of a human mononuclear cell-derived neutrophil chemotactic factor apparently distinct from IL-1, IL-2, GM-CSF, TNF and IFN-gamma. *Immunology* 1988;**64**:219–25.

40 Henson PM, Johnston RB Jr. Tissue injury in inflammation; oxidants, proteinases and cationic proteins. *J Clin Invest* 1987;**79**:669–74.

41 Lee L-Y, Bleecker ER, Nadel JA. Effect of ozone on bronchomotor response to inhaled histamine aerosol in dogs. *J Appl Physiol* 1977;**43**:626–31.

42 Chung KF, Becker AB, Lazarus SC, Frick OL, Nadel JA, Gold WM. Antigen-induced airway hyperresponsiveness and pulmonary inflammation in allergic dogs. *J Appl Physiol* 1985;**558**:1347–53.

43 Murphy KR, Wilson MC, Irvin CG *et al.* The requirement for polymorphonuclear leukocytes on the late asthmatic response and heightened airways reactivity in an animal model. *Am Rev Respir Dis* 1986;**134**:62–8.

44 Holtzman MJ, Fabbri LM, O'Byrne PH *et al.* Importance of airway inflammation of hyperresponsiveness induced by ozone in dogs. *Am Rev Respir Dis* 1983;**127**:686–90.

45 O'Byrne PH, Walters EH, Gold BD *et al.* Neutrophil depletion inhibits airway hyperresponsiveness induced by ozone exposure. *Am Rev Respir Dis* 1984;130:214–9.

46 Marsh WR, Irvin CG, Murphy KR, Behrens BL, Larsen GL. Increases in airway reactivity to histamine and inflammatory cells in bronchoalveolar lavage after the late asthmatic response in an animal model. *Am Rev Respir Dis* 1985;131:875–9.

47 Hutchinson AA, Hinson JM Jr, Brigham KL, Snapper JR. Effect of endotoxin on airway responsiveness to aerosol histamine in sheep. *J Appl Physiol* 1983;54:1463–8.

48 Hinson JM Jr, Hutchinson AA, Brigham KL, Meyrick BO, Snapper JR. Effect of granulocyte depletion on pulmonary responsiveness to aerosol histamine. *J Appl Physiol* 1984;56:411–7.

49 Abraham WM, Perruchoud AP, Sielczak MW, Yerger LD, Stevenson JS. Airway inflammation during antigen-induced late bronchial obstruction. *Prof Repiri Res* 1985;19:48–88.

50 Irvin CG, Baltopoulos G, Henson P. Airways hyperreactivity produced by products from phagocytosing neutrophils. *Am Rev Respir Dis* 1985;131:A278.

51 Baltopoulos G, Young SK, Seccombe J, Larsen GL, Henson PM, Irvin CG. Phagocytosing neutrophils release lipid products which increase airways responsiveness. *J Appl Physiol* (submitted).

52 Uchida DA, Kimani GK, Henson PM, Larsen GL, Irvin CG. Effects of products from phagocytosing eosinophils on airways function of the rabbit. *Am Rev Respir Dis* (submitted).

53 Murlas C, Roum JH. Bronchial hyperreactivity occurs in steroid-treated guinea pigs depleted of leukocytes by cyclophosphamide. *J Appl Physiol* 1985;58:1630–7.

54 Hutson PA, Church MK, Clay TP, Miller P, Holgate ST. Early and late phase bronchoconstriction after allergen challenge of nonanesthetised guinea pigs. 1. The association of disordered airway physiology to leucocyte infiltration. *Am Rev Respir Dis* 1988;137:548–57.

55 Church MK, Hutson PA, Holgate ST. Comparison of nedocromil sodium and albuterol against late phase bronchoconstriction and cellular infiltration in guinea pigs. *Am Rev Respir Dis* 1988;137:136.

56 Diaz P, Galleguillos FR, Gonzalez MC, Pantin C, Kay AB. Bronchoalveolar lavage in asthma; the effects of DSCG on leucocyte counts, immunoglobulins and complement. *J Allergy Clin Immunol* 1984;74:41–8.

57 Martin RJ, Cicutto LC, Ballard RD, Szefler SJ. Airway inflammation in nocturnal asthma. *Am Rev Respir Dis* 1988;137:284.

58 Laitinen LA, Heino M, Laitinen A, Kava T, Haahtela T. Damage to the airway epithelium and bronchial reactivity in patients with asthma. *Am Rev Respir Dis* 1985;313:599–606.

59 Salvato G. Some histological changes in chronic bronchitis and asthma. *Thorax* 1968;23:168–72.

60 Durham SR, Kay AB. Eosinophils, bronchial hyperreactivity and late-phase asthmatic reactions. *Clin Allergy* 1985;15:411–8.

61 De Monchy JG, Kauffman HF, Venge P *et al.* Bronchoalveolar eosinophils during allergen-induced late asthmatic reactions. *Am Rev Respir Dis* 1985;131:373–6.

62 Metzger WJ, Zavala D, Richerson HB *et al.* Local allergen challenge and bronchoalveolar lavage of allergic asthmatic lungs. Description of the model and local airway inflammation. *Am Rev Respir Dis* 1987;135:433–40.

63 Filley WV, Holley KE, Kephart GM, Gleich GJ. Identification by immunofluorescence of eosiniphil granule major basic protein in lung tissues of patients with bronchial asthma. *Lancet* 1982;ii:11–16.

64 Gleich GJ, Frigas E, Loegering DA, Wassom DL, Steinmuller D. Cytotoxic properties of the eosinophil major basic protein. *J Immunol* 1979;123:2925–7.

173

65 Jorg A, Henderson WR, Murphy RC, Klebanoff JJ. Leukotriene generation by eosinophils. *J Exp Med* 1982;**155**:390–402.

66 Weller PF, Lee CW, Foster DW, Corey EJ, Austen KF, Lewis RA. Generation and metabolism of 5–lipoxygenase pathway leukotrienes by human eosinophils; predominant production of leukotriene C_4. *Proc Natl Acad Sci USA* 1983;**80**:7626–30.

67 Shaw RJ, Cromwell O, Kay AB. Preferential generation of leukotriene C_4 by human eosinophils. *Clin Exp Immunol* 1984;**56**:716–22.

68 Shaw RJ, Walsh GM, Cromwell O, Moqbel R, Spry CJF, Kay AB. Activated human eosinophils generate SRS-A leukotrienes following physiological (IgG-dependent) stimulation. *Nature* 1985;**316**:150–2.

69 Moqbel R, MacDonald AJ, Kay AB. IgE-dependent release of leukotriene (LT) C_4 from human low density eosinophils. *J Allergy Clin Immunol* 1988;**81**:208.

70 Lam S, Chan H, LeRiche JC, Chan-Yeung M, Salari H. Release of leukotrienes in patients with bronchial asthma. *J Allergy Clin Immunol* 1988;**81**:711–7.

71 Wardlaw AJ, Hay H, Cromwell O, Haslam P, Collins JV, Kay AB. Leukotrienes (LT) B_4 and C_4 in bronchoalveolar lavage fluid in bronchial asthma and other respiratory diseases. *Thorax* 1987;**42**:219.

72 Lee TC, Lenihan DJ, Malone B, Ruddy LL, Wasserman SI. Increased biosynthesis of platelet activating factor in activated human eosinophils. *J Biol Chem* 1984;**259**:5520–30.

73 Champion A, Wardlaw AJ, Moqbel R, Cromwell O, Shepherd D, Kay AB. IgG-dependent generation of platelet-activating factor by normal and 'low density' human eosinophils. *J Allergy Clin Immunol* 1988;**81**:207.

74 Wardlaw AJ, Moqbel R, Cromwell O, Kay AB. Platelet activating factor; a potent chemotactic and chemokinetic factor for human eosinophils. *J Clin Invest* 1986;**78**:1701–6.

75 Kimani G, Tonnesen MG, Henson PM. Stimulation of eosionophil adherence to human vascular endothelial cells *in vitro* by platelet activating factor. *J Immunol* 1988;**140**(9):3161–6.

76 Lopez AF, Sanderson CJ, Gamble JR, Campbell HD, Young IG, Vadas MA. Recombinant human interleukin-5 is a selective activator of human eosinophil function. *J Exp Med* 1988;**167**:219–24.

77 Yamaguchi Y, Hayashi Y, Sugama Y *et al*. Highly purified murine interleukin-5 (IL-5) stimulates eosinophil function and prolongs *in vitro* survival. IL-5 is an eosinophil chemotactic factor. *J Exp Med* 1988;**167**:1737–42.

78 McFadden ER Jr. Corticosteroids and cromolyn sodium as modulators of airway inflammation. *Chest* 1988;**94**:181–4.

79 Howarth PH, Durham SR, Lee TH, Kay AB, Church MK, Holgate ST. Influence of albuterol, cromolyn sodium and ipratropium bromide on the airway and circulating mediator responses to antigen bronchial provocation in asthma. *Am Rev Respir Dis* 1985;**132**:986–92.

80 Holgate ST, Church MK, Cushley MJ, Robinson C, Mann JS, Howarth PH. Pharmacological modulation of airway calibre and mediator release in human models of bronchial asthma. In; Kay AB, Austen KF, Lichtenstein LM, eds. *Asthma, physiology, immunopharmacology and treatment*. London: Academic Press 1984:391–415.

81 Burge PS, Efthimiou J, Turner-Warwick M, Nelmes TJ. Double-blind trials of inhaled beclomethasone dipropionate and fluocortin butyl ester in allergen-induced immediate and late asthmatic reactions. *Clin Allergy* 1982;**12**:523–31.

82 King SJ, Miller HRP, Newlands GFJ, Woodbury RG. Depletion of mucosal mast cell protease by corticosteroids; effect on intestinal anaphylaxis in the rat. *Proc Natl Acad Sci USA* 1985;**82**:1214–8.

83 Otsuka H, Denburg JA, Befus D *et al*. Effect of beclomethasone dipropionate on nasal metachromatic cell subpopulations. *Clin Allergy* 1986;**16**:589–95.

84 Lee TH, Brown MJ, Nagy L, Causon R, Walport MJ, Kay AB. Exercise-induced

release of histamine and neutrophil chemotactic factors in atopic asthmatics. *J Allergy Clin Immunol* 1982;**70**:73–81.

85 Casale TB, Wood D, Richerson HB, Zehr B, Zavala D, Hunninghake GW. Direct evidence of a role for mast cells in the pathogenesis of antigen-induced bronchoconstriction. *J Clin Invest* 1987;**80**:1507–11.

86 Wenzel SE, Fowler AA, Schwartz LB. Activations of pulmonary mast cells by bronchoalveolar allergen challenge. *Am Rev Respir Dis* 1988;**137**:1002–8.

87 De Monchy JG, Keyzer JJ, Kauffman HF, Beaumont F, DeVries K. Histamine in late asthmatic reactions following house dust mite inhalation. *Agents Actions* 1985;**16**:252–5.

88 Metzger WJ, Richerson HB, Warden K, Monick M, Hunninghake GW. Bronchoalveolar lavage of allergic asthmatic patients following allergen provocation. *Chest* 1986;**89**:477–83.

89 Behrens BL, Clark RAF, Marsh W, Larsen GL. Modulation of the late asthmatic response by antigen-specific immunoglobulin G in an animal model. *Am Rev Respir Dis* 1984;**130**:1134–9.

90 Lee TH, Assoufi BK, Kay AB. The link between exercise, respiratory heat exchange, and the mast cell in bronchial asthma. *Lancet* 1983;**i**:520–22.

91 Melewicz FM, Kline NE, Cohen AB, Spiegelberg HL. Characterization of Fc receptor for IgE on human alveolar macrophages. *Clin Exp Immunol* 1982;**49**:364–70.

92 Joseph M, Tonnel AB, Torpier G, Capron A, Arnoux B, Benveniste J. Involvement of IgE in the secretory processes of alveolar macrophages from asthmatic patients. *J Clin Invest* 1983;**71**:221–30.

93 Capron M, Jouault T, Prin C *et al.* Functional study of a monoclonal antibody to IgE-Fc receptor of eosinophils, platelets and macrophages (Fc$_\varepsilon$R$_2$). *J Exp Med* 1986;**164**:72–89.

94 Tonnel AB, Gosset P, Joseph M, Fournier E, Capron A. Stimulation of alveolar macrophages in asthmatic patients after local provocation test. *Lancet* 1983;**i**:1406–8.

95 Kay AB, Diaz P, Carmichael J, Grant IWB. Corticosteroid-resistant chronic asthma and monocyte complement receptors. *Clin Exp Immunol* 1981;**44**:576–80.

96 Grant IWB, Wyllie AH, Poznansky MC, Gordon ACH, Douglas JG. Corticosteroid resistance in chronic asthma. In; Kay AB, Austen KF, Lichtenstein LM, eds. *Asthma. Physiology, immunopharmacology, and treatment.* London: Academic Press 1984:359–74.

97 Haslett C, Henson PM. Resolution of inflammation. In; Clark RAF, Henson PM, eds. *The molecular and cellular biology of wound repair.* New York: Plenum Publishing 1988; 185–211.

98 Mazzoni L, Morley J, Page CP, Sanjar S. Induction of airway hyperreactivity by platelet activating factor in the guinea-pig. *J Physiol* 1985;**365**:107P.

99 Vargaftig BB, Lefort J, Chignard M, Benveniste J. Platelet activating factor induces a platelet-dependent bronchoconstriction unrelated to the formation of prostaglandin derivatives. *Eur J Pharmacol* 1980;**65**:185–92.

100 Stimler NP, O'Flaherty JT. Spasmogenic properties of platelet-activating factor; evidence for a direct mechanism in the contractile response of pulmonary tissue. *Am J Pathol* 1983;**113**:75–84.

101 Lefort J, Rotilio D, Vargaftig BB. The platelet-independent release of thromboxane A2 by PAF-acether from guinea-pig lungs involves mechanisms distinct from those for leukotriene. *Br J Pharmacol* 1984;**82**:565–75.

102 Metzger WJ, Hunninghake GW, Richerson HB. Late asthmatic reactions; inquiry into mechanisms and significance. *Clin Rev Allergy* 1985;**3**:145–65.

103 Lellouch-tubiana A, Lefoit J, Pirotzky E, Vargaftig BB, Pfister A. Ultrastructural evidence for extravascular platelet recruitment in the lung upon intravenous injection of platelet-activating factor (PAF-acether) to guinea pigs. *Br J Exp Pathol* 1985;**66**:345–55.

104 Knauer KA, Lichtenstein LM, Adkinson NF Jr, Fish JE. Platelet activation

during antigen-induced airway reactions in asthmatic subjects. *N Engl J Med* 1981;**304**:1404–7.

105 Durham SR, Dawes J, Kay AB. Platelets in asthma. *Lancet* 1985;ii:36.

106 Joseph M, Auriault C, Capron A, Vorng H, Viens P. A new function for platelets; IgE-dependent killing of schistosomes. *Nature* 1983;**303**:310–2.

107 Maclouf J, Fradin A, Vausbinder L, Henson PM, Murphy RC. Development of an ex vivo model to assess transcellular metabolism of arachidonic acid: towards a reappraisal of the biosynthesis of eicosanoids. In; Fitzgerald, Patrono, eds. *Platelet and vascular occlusion*. Raven Press (in press).

108 Maclouf J, Murphy RC, Henson PM. Transcellular biosynthesis of sulfidopeptide leukotrienes during physiologic stimulation of human neutrophil/platelet mixtures. *J Immunol* (submitted).

109 Leung DYM, Geha RS. Regulation of the human IgE antibody response. *Intern Rev Immunol* 1987;**2**:75–91.

110 Jeffery PK, Nelson FC, Wardlaw AJ, Kay AB. Quantitative analysis of bronchial biopsies in asthma. *Am Rev Respir Dis* 1987;**135**:A316.

111 Jeffery PK, Wardlaw AJ, Nelson FC, Collins JV, Kay AB. Bronchial biopsies in asthma; an ultrastructural quantitative study and correlation with hyper-reactivity. *Am Rev Respir Dis* (in press).

112 Timonen T, Stenius-Aarnala B. Natural killer cell activity in asthma. *Clin Exp Immunol* 1985;**59**:85–90.

113 Poznansky MC, Gordon ACH, Grant IWB, Wyllie AH. A cellular abnormality in glucocorticoid resistant asthma. *Clin Exp Immunol* 1985;**61**:135–42.

114 Poznansky MC, Gordon ACH, Douglas JG, Krajewski AS, Wyllie AH, Grant IWB. Resistance to methylprednisolone in cultures of blood mononuclear cells from glucocorticoid-resistant asthmatic patients. *Clin Sci* 1984;**67**:639–45.

115 Harper TB, Gaumer HR, Waring W, Brannon RB, Salvaggio JE. A comparison of cell-mediated immunity and suppressor T-cell function in asthmatic and normal children. *Clin Allergy* 1980;**10**:555–63.

116 Rola-Pleszczynski M, Blanchard R. Suppressor Cell function in respiratory allergy. *Int Archs Allergy Appl Immun* 1981;**64**:361–70.

117 Rivlin J, Kuperman O, Freier S, Godfrey S. Suppressor T-lymphocyte activity in wheezy children with and without treatment by hyposensitization. *Clin Allergy* 1981;**11**:353–6.

118 Hwang KC, Fikrig SM, Friedman HM, Gupta S. Deficient concanavalin A-induced suppressor-cell activity in patients with bronchial asthma, allergic rhinitis, and atopic dermatitis. *Clin Allergy* 1985;**15**:67–72.

119 Ilfeld D, Kivity S, Feierman E, Topilsky M, Kuperman O. Effects of *in vitro* colchicine and oral theophylline on suppressor cell function of asthmatic patients. *Clin Exp Immunol* 1985;**61**:360–7.

120 Rocklin RE, Sheffer AL, Greineder DR, Melmon KL. Generation of antigen-specific suppressor cells during allergy desensitization. *N Engl J Med* 1980;**302**:1213–9.

121 Gerblich AA, Campbell AE, Schuyler MR. Changes in T-lymphocyte subpopulation in asthmatics. *N Engl J Med* 1984;**310**:1349–52.

122 Gonzalez MC, Diaz P, Gelleguillos FR, Ancic P, Cromwell O, Kay AB. Allergen-induced recruitment of bronchoalveolar (OKT4) and suppressor (OKT8) cells in asthma. Relative increases in OKT8 cells in single early responders compared with those in late-phase responders. *Am Rev Respir Dis* 1987;**136**:600–4.

123 Frew AJ, Kay AB. The relationship between infiltrating CD4 + lymphocytes, activated eosinophils and the magnitude of the allergen-induced late phase cutaneous reaction. *J Immunol* 1988;**141**:4158–64.

124 Corrigan CJ, Hartnell A, Kay AB. T-lymphocyte activation in acute severe asthma. *Lancet* 1988;i:1129–32.

125 Corrigan CJ, Kay AB. Soluble interleukin-2 receptors and gamma-interferon in acute severe asthma ('status asthmaticus'). Relationship to activated

(CD4+) T-lymphocytes with serum concentrations of soluble interleukin-2 receptors, gamma-interferon, and the peak expiratory flow rate. *Am Rev Respir Dis* (in press).

126 Milks LC, Congers GP, Cramer EB. The effect of neutrophil migration on epithelial permeability. *J Cell Biol* 1986;**103**:2729-38.

127 Parsons PE, Sugahara K, Cott GR, Mason RJ, Henson PM. The effect of neutrophil migration and prolonged neutrophil contact on epithelial permeability. *Am J Pathol* 1987;**129**:302-12.

128 Holtzman MJ, Aizawa H, Nadel JA, Goetzl EJ. Selective generation of leukotriene B_4 by tracheal epithelial cells from dogs. *Biochem Biophys Res Commun* 1983;**114**:1071-7.

129 Hunter JA, Finkbeiner WE, Nadel JA, Goetzl EJ, Holtzman MJ. Predominant generation of 15-lipoxygenase metabolites of arachidonic acid by epithelial cells from human trachea. *Proc Natl Acad Sci USA* 1985;**82**:4633-7.

130 Shak S, Perez HD, Goldstein IM. A novel dioxygenation product of arachidonic acid possesses potent chemotactic activity for human polymorphonuclear leukocytes. *J Biol Chem* 1983;**258**:14948-53.

131 Kirsch CM, Sigal E, Djokic TD, Graf PD, Nadel JA. An *in vivo* chemotaxis assay in the dog trachea; evidence for chemotactic activity of 8S, 15S-dihydroxyeicostatetraenoic acid. *J Appl Physiol* 1988;**64**:1792-5.

132 Walsh JJ, Dietlin LF, Low FN, Burch GE, Mogabgab WJ. Bronchotracheal response in human influenza. *Arch Intern Med* 1961;**108**:376-82.

133 Fabbri LM, Aizawa H, Alpert SE, et al. Airway hyperresponsiveness and changes in cell counts in bronchoalveolar lavage after ozone exposure in dogs. *Am Rev Respir Dis* 1984;**129**:288-91.

134 Phillips MJ, Gold WM, Goetzl EJ. IgE-dependent and ionophore-induced generation of leukotrienes by dog mastocytoma cells. *J Immunol* 1983;**131**:906-10.

135 Serhan CN, Hamberg H, Samuelsson B. Lipoxins; novel series of biologically active compounds formed from arachidonic acid in human leukocytes. *Proc Natl Acad Sci USA* 1984;**81**:5335-9.

136 Serhan CN, Nicolaou KC, Webber SE, et al. Lipoxin A stereochemistry and biosynthesis. *J Biol Chem* 1986;**261**:16340-5.

137 Ramstedt U, Serhan CN, Lundberg U, Wignell H, Samuelsson B. Inhibition of human natural killer activity by (14R,15S)-14,15- dihydroxy-5Z,8Z,10E,12E-eicosatetraenoic acid. *Proc Natl Acad Sci USA* 1984;**81**:6914-8.

138 Ramstedt U, Ng J, Wigzell H, Serhan CN, Samuelsson B. Action of novel eicosanoids lipoxin A and B on human natural killer cell cytoxicity; effects on intracellular cAMP and target cell binding. *J Immunol* 1985;**135**:3434-8.

139 Vanderhoek JY, Bryant RW, Bailey JM. Inhibition of leukotriene biosynthesis by the leukocyte product 15-hydroxy-5,8,11,13- eicosatetraenoic acid. *J Biol Chem* 1980;**255**:10064-6.

140 Bruynzeel PLB, Kok PTM, Vretor RJ, Verhagen J. On the optimal conditions of LTC_4 formation by human eosinophils *in vitro*. *Prostaglandins Leukotrienes Med* 1985;**20**:11-22.

141 Sigal E, Grungerger D, Craik CS, Caughey GH, Nadel JA. Arachidonate 15-lipoxygenase (ω-6 lipoxygenase) from human leukocytes; purification and structural homology to other mammalian lipoxygenases. *J Biol Chem* 1988;**263**:5328-32.

142 Sigal E, Craik CS, Highland E et al. Molecular cloning and primary structure of human 15-lipoxygenase. *Biochem Biophys Res Commun*, in press.

143 Maclouf J, Fradin A, Vausbinder L, Henson PM, Murphy RC. Development of an *ex vivo* model to assess transcellular metabolism of arachidonic acid; towards a reappraisal of the biosynthesis of eicosanoids. 1988 (in press).

144 Walters EH, O'Byrne PH, Fabbri LM, Graf PD, Holtzman MJ, Nadel JA. Control of neurotransmission by prostaglandins in canine trachealis smooth muscle. *J Appl Physiol* 1984;**57**:129-34.

145 Leikauf GD, Ueki IF, Nadel JA, Widdicombe JH. Bradykinin stimulates Cl secretion and prostaglandin E_2 release by canine tracheal epithelium. *Am J Physiol* 1985;**248**:F48–F55.

146 Jacoby DB, Ueki IF, Widdicombe JH, Loegering DA, Gleich GJ, Nadel JA. Effect of human eosinophil major basic protein on ion transport in dog tracheal epithelium. *Am Rev Respir Dis* 1988;**137**:13–6.

147 Barnett K, Jacoby DB, Lazarus SC, Nadel JA. Bradykinin stimulates release of an epithelial cell product that inhibits smooth muscle contraction. *Am Rev Respir Dis* 1987;**135**:A274.

148 Flavahan NA, Aarhus LL, Rimele TJ, Vanhoutte PM. Respiratory epithelium inhibits bronchial smooth muscle tone. *J Appl Physiol* 1985;**58**:834–8.

149 Sekiyawa K, Tamaoki J, Nadel JA, Borson DB. Enkephalinase inhibitor potentiates substance P- and electrically induced contraction in ferret trachea. *J Appl Physiol* 1987;**63**:1401–5.

150 Dussen DJ, Nadel JA, Sekiyawa, Graf PD, Borson DB. Neutral endopeptidase and angiotensin converting enzyme inhibitors potentiate kinin-induced contraction of ferret trachea. *J Pharmacol Exp Ther* 1988;**244**:531–6.

151 Nadel JA, Djokic TD, Djokic LT, Borson DB. Neutral endopeptidase inhibitor potentiates neurotensin-induced contraction in guinea pig bronchi. *FASEB J* 1988;**2**:A1383.

152 Varsano S, Basbaum CB, Forsberg LS *et al.* Dog tracheal epithelial cells in culture synthesize sulfated macromolecular glycoconjugate and release them from the cell surface upon exposure to extracellular proteinases. *Exp Lung Res* 1987;**13**:157–83.

153 Varsano S, Rosen SD, Lazarus SC, Gold WM, Nadel JA. Selective adhesion of mast cells to tracheal epithelial cells. *Fed Proc* 1987;**46**:A992.

154 Andersson B, Dahmen J, Frejd T *et al.* Identification of an active disaccharide unit of a glycoconjugate receptor for pneumococci attaching to human pharyngeal epithelial cells. *J Exp Med* 1983;**158**:559–70.

155 Lamb D, Lumsden A. Intra-epithelial mast cells in human airway epithelium; evidence for smoking-induced changes in their frequency. *Thorax* 1982;**37**:334–42.

156 Cutz E, Levison H, Cooper DM. Ultrastructure of airways in children with asthma. *Histopathology* 1978;**2**:407–21.

157 Nadel JA, Widdicombe JH, Peatfield AC. Regulation of airway secretions, ion transport, and water movement. In; Fishman AP, Fisher AB, eds. *Handbook of physiology. The respiratory system.* Volume 1. Bethesda, Maryland: The American Physiological Society 1985:419–45.

158 Olver RE, Davis B, Marin MG, Nadel JA. Active transport of Na$^+$ and Cl$^-$ across the canine tracheal epithelium *in vitro*. *Am Rev Respir Dis* 1975;**112**:811–5.

159 Welsh MJ, Widdicombe JH, Nadel JA. Fluid transport across the canine tracheal epithelium. *J Appl Physiol* 1980;**49**:905–9.

160 Al-Bazzaz FJ, Yadava VP, Westenfelder C. Modification of Na and Cl transport in canine tracheal mucosa by prostaglandins. *Am J Physiol* 1981;**240**:F101–F5.

6: Pharmacology/Treatment

S. T. Holgate, W. M. Abraham, P. J. Barnes & T. H. Lee

INTRODUCTION

Increased responsiveness of the airways to a wide variety of exogenous stimuli is a cardinal feature of asthma and probably underlies much of its symptomatology. Although the pathophysiological mechanisms of increased airway responsiveness are not fully understood in asthma, longitudinal studies have clearly established that it is not a static phenomenon but one that varies from hour to hour, day to day and year by year being dependent upon both exogenous and endogenous influences. Another factor that can modify airways responsiveness is the administration of certain drugs. Indeed the acute and long term effect of anti-asthma drugs in reducing bronchial hyperresponsiveness (BHR) is considered an important factor relating to clinical efficacy. Observation on the effect of anti-asthma drugs on BHR when combined with information obtained from animal studies has greatly increased understanding of the possible mechanisms underlying the abnormality in addition to providing experimental models against which to test novel pharmacological agents.

ANIMAL MODELS OF AIRWAYS HYPERRESPONSIVENESS AND THEIR PHARMACOLOGICAL MODULATION

Animal studies have been important in helping to understand the pathophysiology of BHR as it relates to bronchial asthma in man. Few animal models, however, exhibit the chronic BHR associated with asthma. Therefore, most of our knowledge is derived from studies in which animals are challenged by inhalation with inflammatory agents such as ozone, sulphur dioxide (SO_2), toluene diisocyanate (TDI), cigarette smoke, or a variety of inflammatory mediators including platelet activating factor (PAF), thromboxane-like agents, and leukotriene B_4 (LTB_4), as well as specific antigens, to induce a transient BHR. This transient phenomenon is clearly different from the chronic BHR observed in asthma, but the mechanisms and pathways responsible for these acute and chronic episodes may be the same. One means of identifying these pathways is to use pharmacological probes to prevent or reverse the effects of these inflammatory stimuli. This section will summarise studies in which selective pharmacological intervention has been used to define pathways and mediators that may play a role in the development of BHR in animal models.

Hyperresponsiveness induced by inhaled chemicals

In general, acquired or transient BHR resulting from inhalation challenge with a variety of inflammatory stimuli is mediator dependent. In some[1-6] but not all models[7-9] it is evident that these mediators are released from the inflammatory cells recruited to the airways by the initial insult. There is little or no evidence to suggest that this acquired BHR is a function of increased cholinergic activity because anticholinergic agents have been ineffective in modifying it,[10,11] unlike viral-induced BHR (see below).[12]

Endotoxin produces BHR in sheep[11] and certain inbred strains of rats.[13] Airway inflammation is associated with the increased responsiveness in both species.[13,14] In rats aminophylline treatment has been shown to reduce both the airway inflammatory response and the BHR resulting from endotoxin inhalation, which suggests that airway responsiveness is associated with this inflammatory response.

That mediators released from activated inflammatory cells may be important for the development of BHR has been demonstrated by a sequence of studies which indicated that the increased airway responsiveness to acetylcholine in dogs after exposure to ozone was correlated with the numbers of neutrophils infiltrating the bronchial epithelium.[15] This ozone-induced BHR disappeared after one week as did the neutrophil influx. Furthermore, dogs which did not develop BHR after ozone did not show leucocyte infiltration into the airways. Similar observations have been made using bronchoalveolar lavage (BAL) as an index of airway inflammation.[16] When dogs were made granulocytopenic by hydroxyurea treatment, ozone did not cause BHR and did not increase the numbers of neutrophils in the bronchial epithelium or in BAL.[17] It became clear, however, that it was not the neutrophil recruitment *per se* that was causing the ozone-induced BHR, but that the BHR was dependent on the generation of cyclo-oxygenase metabolites of arachidonic acid by these infiltrating cells.[6] Thus, the cyclo-oxygenase blocker indomethacin prevented the ozone-induced BHR but not the inflammatory response. Similar results have been obtained using the thromboxane synthetase inhibitor OKY-046, indicating that thromboxane might be the active cyclo-oxygenase metabolite in this process. Further studies in dogs showed that aerosol challenge with the thromboxane A_2-mimetic, U-46619, at a dose which did not cause bronchoconstriction, induced neutrophil influx into the airways and increased airways responsiveness.[18] Again, BHR but not neutrophil influx was blocked by OKY-046; these results provided additional support for thromboxane as a mediator in ozone-induced BHR in dogs.[18] Lipoxygenase products of arachidonic acid may also contribute to the ozone-induced BHR in dogs however, because a dual cyclo-oxygenase/lipoxygenase inhibitor, BW755C, blocked this response also.[19]

Although these findings strongly implicate the neutrophil and its products in the development of ozone or endotoxin-induced BHR in dogs, rats and sheep, it is apparent from studies in other species that BHR is not always associated with increased numbers of inflammatory cells in the airways. Guinea-pigs developed BHR after exposure to ozone, but the hyperresponsiveness occurred before a significant accumulation of neutrophils in the airways.[9] It is not surprising, therefore, that guinea-pigs depleted of circulating granulocytes were capable of developing BHR after ozone.[9]

Another example of the independence between BHR and inflammation was offered by studies using TDI. In sensitive patients TDI has been shown to cause early and late phases of bronchoconstriction[20] and BHR.[21] TDI also increases airway responsiveness and caused BHR in guinea-pigs associated with an increased number of neutrophils in the airway wall.[22,23] Treatment of these TDI-exposed guinea-pigs with hydroxyurea inhibited both the neutrophil influx and the BHR.[23] However, treatment with another cytotoxic drug, cyclophosphamide, also inhibited the TDI-induced neutrophil influx but not the BHR.[23] Thus, in guinea-pigs, TDI-induced BHR appears to be granulocyte-independent.

Not only are the cell responses different between dogs and guinea-pigs, but the mediators responsible for the BHR appear to differ as well. Ozone-induced BHR in guinea-pigs was not blocked by indomethacin, but was blocked by BW755C and the leukotriene antagonist FPL-55712.[8] These observations suggest that lipoxygenase metabolites of arachidonic acid might be responsible for the ozone-induced increase in BHR in guinea-pigs. This suggestion is supported further by the finding that U-60,257, a prostaglandin I_1 derivative which is a blocker of leukotriene release[24] also blocked ozone-induced hyperresponsiveness in this model.[25]

The contrasting observations in dogs and guinea-pigs might be explained by different effector cells and mediators causing disordered airway function in the two species. Another possibility, however, is that these species differences could reflect two separate pathways which lead to different hyperrresponsiveness states similar to those observed in human asthma (see following).

Hyperresponsiveness induced by antigens

It is well known that BHR is enhanced on the days following antigen challenge in patients, especially in those who develop late responses.[26-28] It has recently been shown that acquired BHR can occur soon after the resolution of the acute response to allergen or to occupational agents and before the development of the late response.[29,30] How this early BHR relates to that seen in the days following allergen challenge is unclear, but it is conceivable that this early allergen-induced response is mediated by a process similar to that producing BHR in guinea-pigs, while the prolonged allergen-induced BHR could be explained by processes similar to those described in dogs.

Dogs,[1,3] rabbits[4,5,31] and sheep[7,32] have been reported to develop BHR after airway challenge with specific allergen. In dogs, BHR occurs six hours after challenge and persists for up to 96 hours after challenge and is associated with a BAL neutrophilia at six hours.[3] Antigen-induced BHR occurred 72 hours after antigen challenge in rabbits showing late airway responses.[11] Again, this BHR was associated with neutrophil influx at this time. Allergic sheep which develop both immediate and late airway responses to inhaled allergen also develop BHR 24 hours after allergen challenge, whereas sheep which only develop immediate responses to allergen do not.[7] However, BAL 24 hours after allergen challenge recovered similar numbers of neutrophils in both groups. This finding once again points out the independence of airway inflammation and BHR in these animal models.

As with ozone-induced BHR, pharmacological studies on these animal models indicate allergen-induced BHR is mediator dependent. In dogs, the antigen-induced BHR but not the neutrophil influx was blocked by OKY-046, suggesting that thromboxane mediates the increased responsiveness.[1] In sheep, the 24 hour antigen-induced BHR was blocked by treating animals before antigen challenge with either indomethacin,[7] FPL-57231 (a sulphidopeptide leukotriene antagonist),[7] nedocromil sodium (an 'anti-inflammatory' agent)[33] or Sch-37224 (a combined leukotriene-thromboxane synthesis inhibitor).[34] In these studies indomethacin did not block the late allergen-induced response, indicating that different mediators may be responsible for late responses and the 24 hour BHR.[7] Similar findings have been reported in asthma patients.[35] When FPL-57231 was used, both the late allergen-induced response and the BHR were prevented.[7] These findings suggest that peptide leukotrienes may be involved not only in late airway responses but also in BHR that accompanies it. That lipoxygenase products of arachidonic acid metabolism can contribute to transient BHR is supported by studies in guinea-pigs in which leukotrienes have been shown to enhance responsiveness[36] and in which the increase in responsiveness resulting from alveolar hypoxia[37] was blocked by the leukotriene antagonist FPL-57231 but not by indomethacin.[38] It could be argued, however, that the antagonism of leukotriene actions by FPL-57231 inhibited or reduced the generation of cyclo-oxygenase products in the sheep, or that thromboxane receptors were sensitive to this agent.[39]

Nedocromil sodium blocked both the early and late responses in these experiments.[33] It is not surprising, therefore, that nedocromil sodium pretreatment also blocked the 24 hour BHR. By preventing the initial antigen-induced mediator release, this drug presumably inhibited the subsequent inflammatory response and elaboration of mediators by these cells which leads to BHR. Nedocromil sodium was also shown to be effective in blocking the late response and the 24 hour BHR when given three hours after antigen challenge.[33] Again, these findings are consistent with observations in human subjects.[40] Blockade of the 24 hour BHR was also achieved when sheep were treated with glucocorticosteroids one hour before allergen challenge, but not when the glucocorticosteroids were given approximately 20 minutes before allergen challenge.[40] Presumably, the one hour steroid pretreatment acted in a fashion similar to that of nedocromil sodium, whereas the acute pretreatment, although it was effective in blocking the late response, still allowed the initial mediator release to occur. A follow-up treatment with glucocorticosteroids eight hours after antigen challenge in the acutely pretreated group was sufficient to block the subsequent development of the 24 hour BHR.[40]

From studies in both dogs and sheep, it appears that the development of BHR 24 hours after allergen challenge does not necessarily depend on the development of late increases in airflow resistance. Rather, the immediate release of anaphylactic mediators (e.g. LTB_4, PAF) may be more important. These mediators initiate an inflammatory response in the airways and stimulate the release of cyclo-oxygenase metabolites, possibly thromboxane, from the recruited inflammatory cells. Further support for this argument comes from observations that inhaled LTB_4,[41] PAF,[2] and the thromboxane mimetic U-46619[18] caused airway inflammation and BHR in dogs. In all cases the BHR, but not the inflammatory response, was blocked by the thromboxane synthesis inhibitor OKY-046.

That a variety of inflammatory mediators can induce airway inflammation and increased responsiveness suggests that the initial release of anaphylactic mediators provokes a cascade resulting in the release of secondary mediators responsible for the observed physiological effects. In this regard, PAF may be especially important. PAF is a potent pro-inflammatory agent[42] which can induce bronchoconstriction and BHR in both animals[43,44] and man.[45] In rabbits[5] and sheep,[43] inhaled PAF can elicit both early and late bronchial responses, similar to those observed with antigen. In both models, PAF-antagonists have been effective in modifying the late antigen-induced responses.[5,46] In rabbits, the ginkgolide BN52021 reduced the late airway response by 43%, whereas in the sheep the PAF antagonist WEB-2086 reduced the late response by 79%. In the rabbit model, the reduction in the late airway response was accompanied by a reduction in the numbers of neutrophils and eosinophils in BAL. Furthermore, these treated rabbits showed no subsequent increases in airway responsiveness 24 hours after antigen challenge.[5] When taken in conjunction with the observations in dogs, these results indicate that PAF may play an important role in initiating the recruitment of activated inflammatory cells to the airways; these cells, in turn, may be important for generating mediators leading to late responses and BHR.

It has recently been shown that BHR can occur soon after the resolution of the immediate bronchoconstrictor response to antigen or to occupational agents (e.g. TDI or maleic anhydride) but before the onset of the late response.[29,30] The relationship between this acute allergen-induced BHR and the increased responsiveness observed on the days following allergen challenge is unclear. Preliminary findings in allergic patients have shown that acute BHR is blocked by glucocorticosteroid treatment before antigen challenge[47], possibly implicating arachidonic acid metabolites. In allergic sheep, acute antigen-induced BHR (approximately a twofold increase) appears two to three hours after challenge.[48,49] and occurred in all allergic sheep, i.e. those that subsequently developed late responses and those that did not. This suggests that the mechanisms leading to acute BHR[5] differ from those involved in the 24 hour hyperresponsive state. When the sheep were treated before allergen challenge with a thromboxane/endoperoxide antagonist, L-641,953, the acute increase in airways responsivness was markedly reduced. This drug treatment did not affect the immediate antigen-induced bronchoconstriction nor did it affect the subsequent development of the late response.[49] Acute BHR in sheep was also blocked by pretreating them with the anti-inflammatory agent nedocromil sodium.[50] This result was expected because nedocromil sodium also blocked the acute allergen-induced response.

Airway hyperresponsiveness resulting from viral infection

Virus infection has been used to induce hyperresponsiveness in animals[12,51] as well as in man.[52,53] It has been suggested that viral-induced BHR is partially a vagally mediated effect resulting from epithelial damage, and animal studies support this hypothesis.[12] Dogs infected with type C influenza virus, exhibit increased BHR three days after infection, with a peak response occurring between one and three weeks post infection. Unfortunately, no pharmacological studies have been performed to elucidate the mechanisms involved in this process.

Guinea-pigs infected with parainfluenza type 3 (P-3) virus had BHR four days after infection, which was blocked by mid-cervical vagotomy or by administration of the ganglionic blocking agent hexamethonium. Low doses of atropine (1 mg/kg) had no effect, but the hyperresponsiveness was blocked by a higher atropine dose (5 mg/kg).[12] These findings suggested that enhanced reflex activity may be involved in virus provoked BHR in the guinea-pig, although the higher doses of atropine needed to modify this effect indicate that non-cholinergic mechanisms may also be involved.

ANIMAL MODELS OF STABLE AIRWAY HYPERRESPONSIVENESS

Basenji-greyhound dogs are reported to exhibit greater airways responsiveness to inhaled stimuli than do mongrel dogs.[10,54,55] The increased responsiveness in the Basenji-greyhound is not associated with an overt airway inflammation such as is seen in other models following inhalation challenge with antigen or other inflammatory agents.[54] Under basal conditions, these dogs do have more mast cells and lymphocytes and fewer macrophages in BAL than mongrel dogs, and the increased airway responsiveness observed in these dogs could be related to this cellular difference. This hypothesis is supported by studies in asthma patients in which the number of mast cells recovered in BAL correlates with the degree of BHR.[56] Furthermore, mast cells in the airways of asthmatic patients contain less histamine than mast cells of control subjects,[57] suggesting that mast cells from asthma patients are constantly releasing mediators which could contribute to increased responsiveness to inhaled stimuli.

Increased numbers of airway luminal mast cells might also influence airway responsiveness by increasing the frequency of non-immunological and immunological mediator release induced by both immunological and non-immunological mechanisms. In both asthmatic subjects and Basenji-greyhounds, a greater number of these cells in the airways would promote mediator release of a sufficient magnitude to provoke bronchoconstriction, leading to airflow obstruction, sooner than in non-asthmatic patients or normal animals. This mechanism may explain the hyperresponsiveness of the Basenji-greyhound to citric acid challenge.[49] In these dogs, citric acid challenge caused bronchoconstriction which was associated with leukotriene release. The constrictor response to citric acid was blocked by the leukotriene antagonist FPL-55712, and reduced by sodium cromoglycate and isoprenaline.[10] Atropine, however, did not have any protective effect. Mongrel dogs showed no constrictor response or leukotriene release with citric acid. Thus, the mediator-dependent bronchoconstriction induced by this provocation may be the result of the increased numbers, and/or sensitivity, of mediator-containing cells in the airways of the Basenji-greyhound dogs.[58] A similar mechanism could also contribute to the increased bronchial responsiveness to hypotonic aerosols observed in these dogs, since this stimulus also causes mast cell degranulation. These experimental studies provide one explanation for the effectiveness of chronic treatment with anti-inflammatory drugs, such as sodium cromoglycate and nedocromil sodium, in reducing BHR in asthmatic patients.[59]

Other factors which may contribute to the stable BHR observed in asthma include down regulation of specific receptor subtypes and biochemical abnormalities in the phospholipid composition of cell membranes. For example, allergic sheep demonstrate BHR to inhaled histamine when compared to non-allergic animals. This has been suggested to be the result of functional depression of histamine H_2 receptor function of these animals.[60] In guinea-pigs, BHR to histamine was correlated with increased enzyme activities and lysophosphatidyl choline content of tracheal tissues.[61]

MODELS OF BRONCHIAL HYPERRESPONSIVENESS IN HUMANS

The important observation that airway responsiveness to agents such as histamine and methacholine progressively increases after inhalation challenge with an allergen or other sensitising agent, has provided a useful model for observing the effect of anti-asthma drugs.[26-28] Booij-Noord et al.[62] and Pepys and Hutchcroft[63] observed that sodium cromoglycate, when administered prior to allergen provocation of the airways of atopic asthmatics, inhibited both early and late phase bronchoconstriction. This work has recently been extended to show that in both adults and children, this drug, administered prior to challenge, also inhibits the allergen-induced increase in bronchial responsiveness achieved at 7–36 hours.[64,65] However, if the drug is administered after the early response but before the onset of the late response, this latter event is somewhat delayed and foreshortened, but not altered in magnitude.[66] By contrast, sodium cromoglycate inhaled at this later time almost totally inhibits the acquisition of hyperresponsiveness with allergen. This study supports the view that while allergen-provoked late phase bronchoconstriction and hyperresponsiveness develop in parallel, they may have different underlying mechanisms.[67] Other evidence to support this view is the observation of increased responsiveness in patients without late phase reaction, and the persistence of hyperresponsiveness after indices of airway calibre have returned to pre-challenge baseline values.[68]

The role of cholinergic mechanisms in acquired hyperre-sponsiveness is much debated and remains controversial. In contrast to the many animal studies suggesting a role for vagal reflexes in hyperresponsiveness, evidence in asthma is lacking.[68] Part of the reason for this is that sufficiently high doses of muscarinic anticholinergic agents to block most of the functional vagal airway receptors cannot be given to humans because of systemic side effects. One way around this has been to administer high doses of a drug by inhalation. Ipratropium bromide, a methyl congener of atropine, has provided a particularly valuable tool. When inhaled in a dose of up to 1 mg, this drug effectively inhibits bronchoconstriction provoked by such stimuli as SO_2,[69] histamine,[70] prostaglandins,[71] cold air,[72] and osmotic stimuli[73], but it has no overall effect on acquired bronchial responsiveness other than providing an increase in baseline upon which the provocation test is being performed. An anticholinergic agent such as ipratropium, will effectively antagonise any test stimulus for reactivity that depends upon a vagal reflex component, e.g. histamine and prostaglandins. The situation with regard to muscarinic receptors is made more complex by the recent classifi-cation of three subtypes which serve different pre- and post-ganglionic functions. Drugs such as atropine or ipratropium bromide are active against all three receptor substances.[74]

Another group of bronchodilator agents that have been studied for their effects on BHR is the β_2-selective adrenoceptor agonists. By inhalation, and to a much lesser degree by oral administration, these drugs are powerful bronchodilators and functional antagon-ists of bronchoconstrictor mediators. As a consequence, they have found wide use in the symptomatic treatment of airways diseases. Their effect on airway smooth muscle is probably mediated through the second messenger cyclic 3'5'-adenosine monophos-phate, activation of protein kinase A and subsequent phosphory-lation of proteins which are concerned with intracellular Ca^{++} sequestration and Ca^{++} calmodulin activation of myosin light chain kinase.[75] Through this common pathway β_2-adrenoceptor agonists will functionally antagonise any mediator operating through a receptor mechanism to contract airways smooth muscle. Thus, while bio-available to the airways, these drugs will produce a marked reduction in airways responsiveness as defined by a rightward displacement of a stimulus–response curve.[76] There is some evidence to suggest that the ability of a β_2-adrenoceptor agonist to protect against an exogenous constric-tor stimulus has a different dose–response characteristic from that for bronchodilatation.[77] This difference might be explained by the complex action that these drugs exert on other cells in the airways, for example increasing Cl^- ion transport and closing epithelial tight junctions in epithelial cells, increasing mucus secretion in goblet cells, and causing dilatation of the bronchial vascular bed. The recent recognition of pre-synaptic β_2-receptors in ganglia of human airways is an added complication.[78] Functional antagonism of endogenous or exogenous constrictor stimuli produced by a β_2-adrenoceptor agonist will only last as long as the drug is in contact with airway β_2-receptors. With the many inhaled β_2-adrenoceptor agonists now available, this protection lasts from two hours (fenoterol, isoprenaline) to six hours (salbutamol, terbutaline). Clearly, with the availability of longer acting inhaled β_2-stimulant preparations such as salmeterol, functional antagonism may be a realistic target for producing prolonged reduction in responsiveness.

A direct action of β_2-adrenoceptor agonists on airways smooth muscle must be clearly differentiated from any protective effect that they have on the cellular events underlying the pathogenesis of BHR. Cockroft and Murdock have shown that administration of inhaled salbutamol in a single dose prior to allergen challenge abrogated the early asthmatic response but had no significant effect either on the late response or the associated increase in histamine responsiveness measured at seven hours post-challenge.[65] The early bronchoconstrictor response to allergen can largely be accounted for by the IgE-dependent release of both preformed and newly generated bronchoconstrictor mediators such as histamine, PGD_2 and LTC_4 from bronchial mast cells.[79] Since β_2-adrenoceptor agonists are highly effective at inhibiting mediator release from activated mast cells,[80] the lack of any effect of these drugs on the late reaction or increase in responsiveness has been interpreted as these cells playing little or no role in the later airway events.[81] However, studies on mast cells of human lung fragments, dispersed lung cells and BAL have yet to show that β_2-adrenoceptor agonists can completely shut down mediator release. Preliminary studies indicate that macrophages are refractory to the inhibitory action of these drugs when mediator release is measured as thromboxane and LTB_4 release.[82,83] It is suggested that activation of low affinity receptors for IgE ($Fc_\varepsilon R_2$) on these cells released chemoattractants for eosinophils, and that this is responsible for their recruitment into the airways where mediator secretion occurs. These cells are considered to play an important role in the pathogenesis of late phase responses and the associated increase in airways responsiveness.[79]

Xanthines, particularly theophylline, have found wide use in the treatment of asthma as oral bronchodilator agents. In common with β_2-adrenoceptor agonists they are functional antagonists of smooth muscle contraction, but are considerably less potent than β_2-stimulants.[84] Part of their pharmacological action on the airways is to competitively inhibit the hydrolysis of cyclic AMP by phosphodiesterases. The complexity of this system of enzymes is only just being appreciated, but it does appear that the isoenzyme classified as type IV is probably an important target for the inhibitory action of substituted xanthines.[85] Xanthines have other pharmacological actions pertinent to the pathogenesis of asthma such as antagonism of adenosine at its cell surface receptors.[86] When administered as an intravenous infusion throughout an allergen challenge and during the subsequent periods of early and late phase bronchoconstriction, theophylline has a preferential inhibitory effect on the late response.[87] Enprofylline, a xanthine which is free of adenosine antagonistic activity,[88] also exhibits a preferential inhibition of the late, compared with the early, response. However, in the study of Pauwels et al.,[87] theophylline and enprofylline were present at pharmacologically active concentrations in the plasma throughout the period of evaluation of the late phase response. There have been no recorded studies reporting the effect of this treatment regimen on allergen acquired hyperresponsiveness, although it would be anticipated that if an agonist such as histamine or methacholine were used to measure responsiveness, functional antagonism would be found. Cockcroft et al. (personal communication) have recently shown that theophylline administered only during allergen provocation suppressed the immediate response but had no measurable effect on either the late reaction or acquired increase in bronchial responsiveness. These findings are therefore similar to their observations with β_2-adrenoceptor agonists.

Glucocorticosteroids have assumed a central role as modifying agents of BHR. Soon after the initial description of late phase bronchoconstriction, the inhibitory action of single dose oral prednisolone on the late but not the early reaction was described.[62] Subsequent studies have shown that inhaled corticosteroids such as beclomethasone dipropionate[89] and budesonide,[90] shared with sodium cromoglycate the property of inhibiting both late phase bronchoconstriction and increased responsiveness following allergen challenge. Similar results have been observed with this class of drugs against TDI challenge.[91] The inhibitory effects of glucocorticosteroids on eosinophil,[92] T-lymphocyte,[93] and macrophage[94] function, together with their indirect suppressive effect on phospholipase A_2 activity, are likely to contribute to the pharmacology of corticosteroids in inhibiting the induction of BHR or reducing its baseline level. The recent demonstration that inhaled beclomethasone dipropionate was far more effective than oral prednisolone in reducing basal BHR is evidence for their local action on the bronchial mucosa.[95] Although Laitinen *et al.* have reported that oral prednisolone promotes repair of the epithelium in asthma,[96] activity of this class of drugs on infiltrating inflammatory cells at this site has yet to be shown. While sodium cromoglycate and corticosteroids are highly effective in inhibiting allergen-induced airways responsiveness,[64,65] their effect on basal hyperresponsiveness in asthma is less impressive. Although when administered regularly to asthmatics these drugs produce measurable reductions in histamine, methacholine and exercise responsiveness, the magnitude of this change is small.[97-102] This has led some investigators to view BHR at two different levels, possibly with different mechanisms—one accessible to reversal with prophylactic drugs and the other not.[103] Until more is known of the cellular events underlying the mechanism of this measure of disordered airway function, mechanistic interpretations of any effects of drugs remain speculative.

THE ROLE OF MEDIATORS IN BRONCHIAL HYPERRESPONSIVENESS AND THEIR PHARMACOLOGICAL MODULATION

Although animal studies have strongly suggested a role for individual mediators in the pathogenesis of BHR, evidence implicating any single chemical substance in hyperresponsiveness associated with asthma is deficient. Based on animal studies and the limited information on the contribution of various mediators to human asthma, attention has been focused on the newly formed lipid derived products as potential candidates against which drug development has been targeted.

The leukotrienes

The structural identification of slow reacting substance of anaphylaxis (SRS-A) as the three sulphidopeptide leukotrienes LTC_4, LTD_4 and LTE_4, and the potent activity that these mediators had on human airways smooth muscle, led to the suggestion that they may be important mediators of acquired BHR. The demonstration that asthmatic, compared to non-asthmatic, subjects appeared to be less responsive to both LTC_4 and LTD_4 relative to their airways response to histamine or methacholine, has added strength to the idea that these mediators contribute towards the basic abnormality of 'non-specific BHR'.[104-106] It is suggested that the relative lack of leukotriene responsiveness is due to the endogenous release of these substances and the presence of some tachyphy-

has been shown to enhance airways responsiveness to histamine,
methacholine and $PGF_{2\alpha}$.[107–109] After a single inhalation of LTD_4
or LTE_4, asthmatic patients may exhibit increased methacholine
responsiveness of their airways for up to one week which[108]
compares with similar changes reported for PAF (see below).

A number of LTD_4 antagonists which have been modelled on
the acetophenone FPL 55712 have been shown to be active in
animal studies and subsequently developed as potential therapeutic agents for asthma. However while both LY-171883 and
L-649,923 were shown to produce a three to fivefold protection of
normal airways against the constrictor effects of inhaled
LTD_4,[110–113] and produce a small inhibition of the later time
points of an allergen provoked early reaction,[114,115] no significant
effect has been detected on the late reaction. Unfortunately, in
both of these studies bronchial responsiveness was not measured
in relation to the allergen challenge. Only with the development of
more potent antagonists will it be possible to determine with any
confidence a role for this class of mediator in the pathogenesis of
BHR.

Another leukotriene of potential importance in asthma is LTB_4.
Single inhalations of this dihydroxy derivative of arachidonic acid
increase bronchial responsiveness and neutrophil influx into the
airways of dogs,[41] but in normal and asthmatic humans a similar
effect has not been seen. Since LTB_4 is a potent chemotactic factor
for neutrophils and, to a lesser extent, eosinophils, antagonists of
its receptor mediator effects would be worthy of study.

An alternative approach to this problem has been the development of inhibitors of the 5-lipoxygenase pathway which, theoretically, inhibit both the generation of LTB_4 and the sulphidopeptide
leukotrienes.[116] Although several of these compounds have
reached the stage of clinical study,[117,118] none have shown any
effect on either allergen provoked late reactions or increased
airways responsiveness. Again, the development of more potent
compounds which are selective and of proven bio-availability will
be the only way of testing whether this is a promising approach
for developing a drug active against this component of disordered
airway function.

Dietary manipulation of lipid derived mediators

A novel approach found to influence the generation and release of
lipid derived mediators is the manipulation of the dietary intake of
polyunsaturated fatty acids. The two major types of polyunsaturated fatty acids prominent in marine fish oils are eicosapentaenoic
acid (EPA) (20:5, n-3) and docosahexaenoic acid (DCHA) (22:6,

n-3) (Figure 6.1). EPA and DCHA competitively inhibit the conversion of arachidonic acid by the cyclo-oxygenase pathway to prostanoid metabolites.[119,120] To the extent they are formed, the endoperoxide and thromboxane A_3 derived from EPA are substantially less active than the arachidonic acid-derived counterparts in eliciting aggregation of human platelets.[121,122] DCHA is not metabolised to any cyclo-oxygenase product. With respect to the metabolism of EPA and DCHA by the 5-lipoxygenase

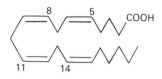

Arachidonic acid (AA)

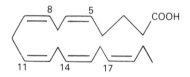

Eicosapentaenoic acid (EPA)

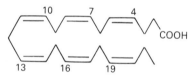

Docosahexaenoic acid (DCHA)

Fig. 6.1 Chemical structure of arachidonic, eicosapentaenoic and docosahexaenoic acids.

cascade, EPA is converted to LTB_5, LTC_5 and LTE_5 (Figure 6.2). DCHA is metabolised only to the 7- and 4-hydroperoxy DCHA and their reduction products, 7- and 4-hydroxy DCHA, respectively. LTB_5 is substantially less active than LTB_4 in a number of pre-inflammatory functions,[122–126] but LTC_5, LTD_5 and LTE_5 are equiactive as LTC_4, LTD_4 and LTE_4 in constricting non-vascular smooth muscle.[127,128] Thus EPA is capable of inhibiting the elaboration of inflammatory mediators by the cyclo-oxygenase pathway and is metabolised to LTB_5 with attenuated biological activity.

Non-esterified EPA and DCHA did not alter the release of arachidonic acid from ionophore-activated polymorphonuclear leucocytes (PMN).[129] LTB_4 production was diminished throughout the EPA dose–response, beginning at 5 µg/ml EPA and reaching 50% suppression at 10 µg/ml and 85% suppression at 40 µg/ml. DCHA did not stimulate the metabolism of membrane-derived arachidonic acid, did not inhibit LTB_4 generation and was

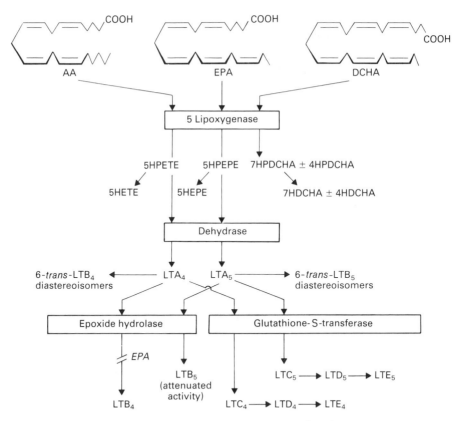

Fig. 6.2 Pathways for the oxidative metabolism of arachidonic acid (AA), eicosapentaenoic (EPA) and docosahexaenoic acids (DCHA).

not a substrate for leukotriene formation. Thus, in contrast to DCHA, EPA attenuated the generation of LTB_4 and was converted to LTB_5.

Human leucocytes also generate PAF from membrane alkyl phospholipids through the release of arachidonic acid or other fatty acids from the 2-position and subsequent acetylation.[130] Non-esterified arachidonic acid of 1 µg/ml resulted in a 64% increase of calcium ionophore-induced PAF generation from 7.75 ± 0.78 ng/10^6 cells for untreated monolayers to 12.70 ± 1.21 ng/10^6 cells (mean $\pm$ SE). Treatment of monolayers with EPA at the optimal concentration of 1 µg/ml decreased PAF generation by 28%.[131] Treatment of monocyte monolayers with DCHA did not appreciably affect PAF generation. The changes in PAF release with each fatty acid added *in vitro* paralleled those in total PAF generation; the percentage PAF release remained unaffected.

The effects of supplementing the diet with fatty acids derived from fish oil on the 5-lipoxygenase pathway activity of PMN and monocytes have recently been studied in seven normal human subjects, who supplemented their usual diets for six weeks with daily doses of Maxepa containing 3.2 g of EPA and 2.2 g of DCHA. The diet increased the EPA content in PMN and monocytes more than sevenfold without changing the quantities of arachidonic acid and DCHA.[132] When the PMN were activated *in vitro* with the ionophore A23187, the release of arachidonic acid and its metabolites was reduced by a mean of 37% and the maximum generation of the major 5–lipoxygenase metabolites, including LTB_4, was reduced by a mean of 48%. When monocyte monolayers were activated with the ionophore A23187, the release of arachidonic acid and its metabolites was reduced by a mean of 39% and the generation of LTB_4 was suppressed by 58%. In addition, the generation of PAF was inhibited by approximately 50%. The adherence of PMN to endothelial cell monolayers which had been pretreated with LTB_4 was inhibited completely and their average chemotactic response to LTB_4 was inhibited by 70% as compared with values determined before the diet was started.[132] The margination of leucocytes to endothelial surfaces is the initial step in the recruitment of cells by a chemotactic stimulus to an inflammatory focus. Thus, the impairment of leucocyte function caused by the dietary incorporation of fish oil fatty acids into membrane phospholipids would be expected to be anti-inflammatory. This effect would be amplified by the substantial suppression of the biosynthesis of arachidonic acid-derived metabolites and PAF. The leucocyte biochemical and functional suppression had recovered by six weeks after the diet was discontinued.

Since airway inflammation may be important in the pathophysiology of bronchial asthma, the effects of a fish oil enriched diet on the disease have been investigated.[133] Subjects received either 18 capsules a day of fish oil (3.2 g EPA and 2.2 g DCHA) or identical placebo capsules containing olive oil in a double-blind fashion. Aspects of neutrophil function, airways response to both specific and non-specific stimuli, and severity of disease were assessed before and after the treatment period. There was incorporation of EPA into PMN phospholipids from barely detectable amounts prior to treatment to comprising 2.6% of total PMN fatty acids following dietary supplementation with fish oil. In addition PMN from subjects who had received fish oil demonstrated a 50% reduction in the generation of LTB (LTB_4 and LTB_5) in response to calcium ionophore, and a substantial attenutation of their chemotactic responses to FMLP and LTB_4. In subjects who had received placebo, the phospholipid content of EPA, LTB_4 generation and chemotactic responses to PMN were unchanged. The change in neutrophil function in subjects who had ingested EPA was not accompanied by any change in airways non-specific responsiveness, or severity of asthma.

Payan *et al.* have studied the effects of EPA in subjects with

Two groups of six subjects received either 0.1 or 4.0 g of purified EPA a day in a double-blind fashion for eight weeks. Both doses of EPA led to a small but significant generation of LTB_5 by PMN and mixed mononuclear leucocytes in response to calcium ionophore A23187. Only high dose EPA suppressed ionophore induced LTB_4 generation by PMN and mononuclear leucocytes. High dose EPA also abolished neutrophil, but not mononuclear leucocyte, chemotaxis to C5a, the chemotactic peptide F-mlp and LTB_4. Neither dose of EPA attenuated ionophore induced PAF generation by mixed mononuclear cells. In addition both low dose and high dose EPA led to an enhanced T-lymphocyte proliferation in response to mitogen, although whether this is restricted to either helper-inducer or suppressor-cytotoxic lymphocytes has not been defined. Moreover, changes in leucocyte function were not accompanied by changes in severity of asthma as assessed by history, clinical examination or a panel of pulmonary function tests.[135]

The effect of a six week fish oil enriched diet containing 3 g EPA has been studied in 10 patients with aspirin-sensitive asthma.[136] Peak flow rates were lower, and bronchodilator use greater, during the fifth and sixth week of the fish oil diet than during the control diet. This suggests that a fish oil diet may have a deleterious effect on asthmatic patients with aspirin sensitivity. Arm *et al.* have recently studied the effect of a fish oil enriched diet on both early and late asthmatic responses to allergen challenge.[137] Whilst there were no changes in the acute airways response to allergen, there was a significant (approximately 35%) attenuation of the late asthmatic response in subjects who had received fish oil. There were no changes in immediate cutaneous responses to antigen, total serum IgE, or airway responses to histamine in the same subjects. Insofar as airways inflammation is believed to be central to the pathophysiology of the allergen-induced late asthmatic response, the attenuation of the late phase reaction by fish oil is consistent with an anti-inflammatory effect.

These studies extend previous observations in normal subjects and demonstrate that a fish oil enriched diet attenuated PMN and mononuclear cell functions in subjects with asthma. The associated attenuation of the allergen-provoked late asthmatic response suggests that these alterations in leucocyte function were sufficient to reduce the induction of airways inflammation. The lack of any clinical benefit in subjects with either mild disease[133] or severe persistent asthma[135] who ingested fish oil, may have been due to insufficient time for resolution of the chronic inflammatory response and regeneration of airways epithelium to effect a change in clinical variables. In addition, the ingestion of fish oil may lead to a deterioration of asthma in patients with aspirin sensitivity.

Platelet activating factor

One mediator that has attracted most attention in relation to hyperresponsiveness in asthma is PAF. PAF is generated from membrane phospholipids by phospholipase A_2, and is synthesised and released (usually in small quantities) from several inflammatory cells, including macrophages, eosinophils (the richest known source), neutrophils, platelets and possibly some mast cells.[130,138] Macrophages and eosinophils from asthmatics generate more PAF than those from normal subjects.[139,140] PAF has several effects which are relevant to asthma.[141,142]

Inhaled PAF causes bronchoconstriction, in both normal and asthmatic subjects, by an indirect mechanism since it has no direct contractile action on human airways *in vitro*.[143] Of particular interest however, is its reported effect in causing a prolonged increase in non-specific bronchial responsiveness.[45] The mechanism for this increased responsiveness is not certain. In the skin of atopic subjects,[144] injection of PAF causes eosinophil infiltration and may therefore recruit eosinophils into the airways (Figure 6.3). A similar effect does not occur in the skin of non-atopic subjects where the eosinophil is replaced by the neutrophil as the dominant leucocyte. PAF has been shown to 'prime' and activate eosinophils for mediator secretion induced by other stimuli and is a potent stimulant of basic protein release from the granules of these cells.[145] There is some evidence to suggest that eosinophils of asthmatics are activated to a greater extent than those of atopic non-asthmatic individuals.[146] Interestingly, PAF antagonists reduce allergen-induced eosinophil infiltration into animal airways. Other properties of PAF relevant to asthma are its capacity to increase microvascular leakage,[147] stimulate mucus secretion,[148] and impair mucociliary transport.[149]

The role of PAF in the pathogenesis of asthma, and particularly in eosinophil recruitment and activation and in BHR must now be determined. The imminent availability of specific PAF antagonists should make this feasible. The ginkgolide PAF antagonist (BN52063) has already been shown to reduce skin and platelet responses to PAF after oral administration,[150] and to reduce the late (cell infiltration) response to allergen in the skin.[151] The effect of this and more potent receptor antagonists on allergen-induced responses in human airways and in clinical asthma must now be determined. The ginkgolide mixture is only weakly effective in blocking airway responses to PAF, but not allergen.[152] More potent antagonists given by inhalation may be necessary.[153] It is also possible that there might be an abnormality in production or degradation of PAF in asthmatics—such as an increase in the rate-limiting enzyme PAF acetyltransferase, or a defect in PAF

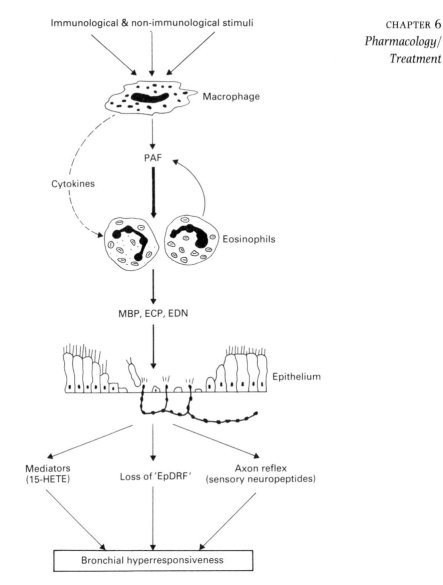

Fig. 6.3 Schematic representation for the involvement of platelet activating factor in the pathogenesis of bronchial hyperresponsiveness in asthma (ECP, eosinophil cationic protein; EDN, eosinophil derived neurotoxin; EpDRF, epithelial derived relaxant factor; MBP, major basic protein).

acetyl hydrolase. At present no drugs are available that selectively inhibit these enzymes.

Other chemical mediators of bronchial hyperresponsiveness

It is highly likely that more than one mediator is involved in the pathogenesis of BHR. Between individuals or in the same individual but at different times, hyperresponsiveness may comprise different functional and structural changes within the airways (Figure 6.4).[154] Thus a drug which inhibits the effects of any single mediator will only have a major impact on BHR in asthma if that mediator is situated in a key position in the cascade of inflammatory events. Histamine, prostaglandins, thromboxane, bradykinin and adenosine are additional mediators generated within human airways whose combined effect may contribute to their increased responsiveness in asthma. Thromboxane A_2 is of particular interest since the thromboxane synthetase inhibitor OKY-046 has been shown to reduce airways responsiveness to inhaled methacholine when administered continuously for two weeks.[155] Further evidence of at least some contribution by

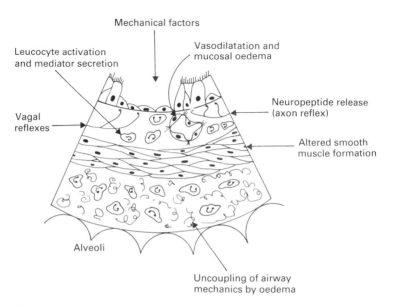

Fig. 6.4 Possible contributing factors to the pathogenesis of bronchial hyper-responsiveness.

prostanoids to hyperresponsiveness is the observation that flurbi-profen, the cyclo-oxygenase inhibitor, reduces histamine respon-siveness when administered for five days.[156] However, the com-plexity of action of non-steroidal anti-inflammatory drugs is highlighted by the observation that in approximately 10% of all asthmatics, these drugs can provoke bronchoconstriction.[157] A number of mechanisms have been suggested including increased synthesis of the endoperoxide PGH_2 and division of oxidative arachidonic acid metabolism to lipoxygenase products such as the leukotrienes.[158] The recent availability of receptor agonists for the thromboxane TP_1 receptor GR 32191,[159] and the recognition that a common receptor exists for most of the contractile effect of prostanoids should enable a more definitive dissection of the role of this mediator class in BHR and other aspects of asthma.

Histamine, which is known to play an important role in the immediate airways response to allergen, may also be released during late phase bronchoconstriction. Increased plasma concentrations of histamine have been reported in association with late phase bronchoconstriction,[160] but whether it plays a role in disordered airway function, as it does in the nose[161], is not known. The recognition that T-lymphocytes, macrophages and other leucocytes are capable of releasing cytokines which stimulate histamine release, and that these contribute to histamine release in the nasal late phase response to allergen is of considerable interest[162] particularly since mast cell numbers both in lavage,[56,57,163] and biopsies[164] of airways have been shown to be increased in asthma. The clinical efficacy of some of the newer and more potent H_1-anti-histamines such as terfenadine,[165] azelastine,[166] and citirizine[167] in asthma might indicate a greater role for histamine than has been appreciated previously. It is unlikely, however, that this mediator alone contributes much towards BHR in asthma. Several studies have shown that different mediators acting in combination may have greater functional effects on the airways than either mediator alone. For example, low concentrations of PGD_2 or sulphidopeptide leukotriene, enhance airways responsiveness to histamine.[109,168] Experiments designed to study mediator interactions are difficult to interpret when agonists alone are used and probably more information will be obtained with combinations of receptor antagonists.

NEURAL MECHANISMS OF BRONCHIAL HYPERRESPONSIVENESS

Neural control of human airways is complex and the contribution of neurogenic mechanisms to the pathogenesis of asthma and BHR is not certain.[169-171] Because changes in bronchomotor tone in asthma occur rapidly, it was suggested many years ago that there may be an abnormality in autonomic neural control with an imbalance between excitatory and inhibitory pathways, resulting in excessively twitchy airways. Over the years, several types of autonomic defect have been proposed in asthma, including enhanced cholinergic, α-adrenergic and non-adrenergic non-cholinergic excitatory mechanisms or reduced β-adrenergic and non-adrenergic inhibitor mechanisms. Various abnormalities in airway control have been described in asthma, although it has always been difficult to determine whether these are primary defects, or secondary to the disease and its treatment. There is even evidence for autonomic abnormalities outside the airways,[172] although the magnitude of these defects is small and their significance is dubious. Nevertheless, it is likely that neural mechanisms contribute to the features of asthma, and may be particularly important in producing the symptoms of asthma.

The recognition that inflammation plays a key role in asthma has suggested that there may be some interaction between neural

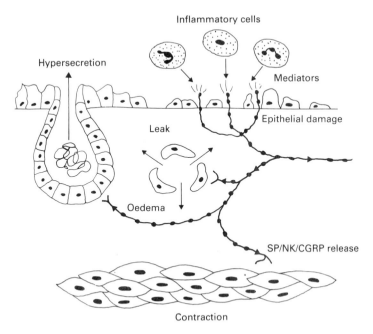

Fig. 6.5 Neurogenic inflammation in asthma.

and inflammatory mechanisms (Figure 6.5).[173] Several inflammatory mediators may have effects on the release of neurotransmitters from airway nerves, or may act on autonomic receptors. Similarly, neural mechanisms may contribute to the inflammatory reaction in the airway wall, and the concept of neurogenic inflammation, which is well established in skin, may also apply to the airways.[174]

Cholinergic mechanisms

Cholinergic nerves are the dominant neural bronchoconstrictor pathway in human airways and there has been considerable interest in whether cholinergic mechanisms are exaggerated in asthma. This view is supported by the observation that many stimuli which produce bronchospasm (such as SO_2, prostaglandins, histamine and cold air) also stimulate afferent receptors and may therefore lead to reflex cholinergic bronchoconstriction.[68,175,176] There are several mechanisms which might lead to increased cholinergic activity in asthma.

There may be an increase in central vagal drive, although there is no direct evidence for this in asthma. Indirect evidence which may suggest such an increase in vagal tone is the enhanced vagal cardiac tone (as determined by the Valsalva manoeuvre and sinus arrhythmia) which has been demonstrated in asthma subjects.[177]

Reflex bronchoconstriction

There may be increased reflex bronchoconstriction due to stimulation of sensory receptors in the airway (irritant receptors and C-fibre endings) by inflammatory mediators. Several mediators, such as histamine, prostaglandins and bradykinin, have been shown to stimulate sensory receptors, and it is possible that these receptors may be more easily triggered in asthma, since airway epithelium may be damaged.

Increased acetylcholine release

There may be enhanced neurotransmission in cholinergic ganglia, perhaps because of release of other neurotransmitters or mediators, or facilitation of acetylcholine release from post-ganglionic nerve terminals. Thus, both serotonin and thromboxane analogues facilitate acetylcholine release in dog airways,[178,179] whereas tachykinins have a similar action in guinea-pig and rabbit airways.[180,181] Since adrenergic nerves may inhibit acetylcholinergic release, either via β-receptors[78,182] or via α_2-receptors,[183] it is possible that a defect in adrenergic nerves or receptors may be reflected by an increase in cholinergic tone.

Muscarinic receptor effects

Enhanced muscarinic cholinergic effects on airway smooth muscle may occur through an increase in receptor density or affinity, or an increase in the efficiency of receptor activation-contraction coupling. Asthmatic patients show an exaggerated bronchoconstrictor response to cholinergic agonists,[184] but a similar increased responsiveness is observed with other spasmogens, such as histamine, leukotrienes or prostaglandins, suggesting that an isolated defect in muscarinic receptors is unlikely. There are conflicting reports about the response of asthmatic airways *in vitro* to cholinergic agonists and other spasmogens, as discussed above, and an exaggerated response to cholinergic agonists has not consistently been demonstrated. In guinea-pigs which become hyperresponsive to acetylcholine after intravenous or inhaled PAF, there is no increase in response of airways *in vitro* to acetylcholine, no change in muscarinic receptors, as determined by direct receptor binding, and no change in coupling or biochemical consequences of receptor activation, as measured by cholinergic stimulation of phosphoinositide turnover.[185]

Although there are several reasons why cholinergic mechanisms might be enhanced in asthma, the evidence for this is not convincing, since cholinergic antagonists are generally less effective as bronchodilators irrespective of the contractile stimulus. This implies that airway smooth muscle is contracted by mechanisms other than vagal tone, and, presumably, several mediators may act directly on airway smooth muscle, against which cholinergic antagonists would not be effective. Thus, histamine bronchoconstriction is weakly affected by anticholinergic treatment in human subjects, whereas in the dog histamine bronchoconstriction is largely abolished by vagal nerve section or by atropine.

Recent studies have demonstrated the presence of inhibitory muscarinic receptors (autoreceptors) on cholinergic nerves of airways in animals *in vivo*,[186,187] and in human airways *in vitro*.[74] These receptors inhibit acetylcholine release and therefore limit vagal bronchoconstriction. Drugs such as atropine, which block with equal affinity both pre-junctional receptors and those on smooth muscle, increase acetylcholine release to overcome the post-junctional blockade. This means that such drugs will not be as effective against vagal bronchoconstriction as against cholinergic agonists, so it may be necessary to re-evaluate the contribution of cholinergic nerves, when drugs which are selective for the muscarinic receptors on airway smooth muscle are developed. Recently, the presence of muscarinic autoreceptors has been demonstrated in human subjects *in vivo*. A cholinergic agonist, which selectively activates these receptors, inhibits cholinergic reflex bronchoconstriction in normal subjects. This inhibitory mechanism does not appear to operate in asthmatic subjects, suggesting that there may be some impaired function of these autoreceptors.[188] Such a defect in muscarinic autoreceptors may then result in exaggerated cholinergic reflexes in asthma, since the normal feedback inhibition of acetylcholine release may be lost. This might also explain the sometimes catastrophic bronchoconstriction which occurs with β-blockers in asthma, since antagonism of inhibitory β-receptors on cholinergic nerves would result in an increased release of acetylcholine which could not switch itself off.

M1–receptors, which are excitatory, are present in airway ganglia of animals and may be inhibited by pirenzepine.[189] Similar receptors are also present in human airways, since pirenzepine inhibits reflex bronchoconstriction at doses which do not inhibit the direct effect of cholinergic agonists in airway tone.[190]

Adrenergic mechanisms

Since adrenergic agonists have a dramatic effect in relieving asthmatic bronchoconstriction, it was logical to suggest that there may be some defect in adrenergic mechanisms in asthma. Adrenergic mechanisms involve sympathetic nerves, circulating catecholamines and α- and β-adrenoceptors, and there are several possible defects which could be present in asthma.[191]

Adrenergic innervation

Adrenergic nerves do not control airway smooth muscle directly,[170] but could influence cholinergic neurotransmission, as discussed above. There is no evidence to suggest that sympathetic neurotransmission may be abnormal in asthma, but it is possible that inflammatory mediators, such as histamine, might impair the release of noradrenaline from adrenergic nerves. Adrenergic neural control of the bronchial vasculature may also be important in asthma.

Circulating catecholamines

Since adrenergic nerves do not directly control airway smooth muscle, it seems probable that circulating catecholamines may play a more important role in regulation of bronchomotor tone.[192] Although the catecholamines noradrenaline, adrenaline and dopamine, are present in the circulation, only adrenaline has physiological effects and is secreted by the adrenal medulla.[193] Since β-blockers cause bronchoconstriction in asthmatic patients, but not normal subjects, this suggests that there is an increase in adrenergic drive to the airways and in the absence of adrenergic innervation this might be provided by circulating adrenaline. However, plasma adrenaline concentrations are not elevated in asthmatic patients, even in those who bronchoconstrict with intravenous propranolol.[192] Even during acute exacerbations of asthma there is no elevation of plasma adrenaline,[194] suggesting that severe bronchoconstriction is not a stimulus to adrenaline release. Furthermore, plasma adrenaline is not elevated during bronchoconstriction induced by inhaled histamine allergen or by hyperventilation. Exercise of a sufficient magnitude to precipitate exercise-induced asthma fails to elevate plasma adrenaline, although such a rise is seen in normal subjects who perform the same degree of exercise.[192] This suggests that there may be a problem in mobilisation of adrenaline in asthma, but this is unlikely to be due to a defect in adrenal medullary secretion, since hypoglycaemia stimulates a large rise in plasma adrenaline, as in normal subjects.

β-adrenoceptors

The possibility that β-receptors are abnormal in asthma has been extensively investigated. The original suggestion that there was a primary defect in β-receptor function in asthma[195] has not been substantiated, and any defect in β-receptors is likely to be secondary to the disease, perhaps as a result of inflammation or adrenergic therapy. Two recent studies have demonstrated that airways from asthmatic patients fail to relax normally in response to isoprenaline, suggesting a possible defect in β-receptor function in airway smooth muscle.[196,197] Whether this is due to a reduction in β-receptors, a defect in receptor coupling or some abnormality in the biochemical pathways leading to relaxation is not yet known.

It is possible that inflammation might lead to such abnormalities in β-receptor function. In guinea-pig trachea oxygen radicals released from activated macrophages may cause a reduction in β-receptors.[198] However, airways from guinea-pig which are hyperresponsive after PAF exposure relax normally to isoprenaline *in vitro* and there is no reduction in β-receptor density or affinity.[199] Recent studies have suggested that stimulation of phosphoinositide hydrolysis may lead to down regulation and uncoupling of β-receptors in airway smooth muscle, probably via the activation of protein kinase C which occurs in response to diacylglycerol generated by phosphatidyl inositol hydrolysis.[200] Since many inflammatory mediators and spasmogens may stimulate phosphatidylinositol hydrolysis it is possible that this provides a mechanism for impaired β-receptor function in asthma.

α-adrenoceptors

Alpha-receptors which mediate bronchoconstriction have been demonstrated in airways of several species, including humans, but α-adrenoceptor mediated contraction may only be demonstrated under certain conditions. In canine trachea, histamine and serotonin facilitate α-adrenergic bronchoconstriction *in vitro* and *in vivo*,[201-203] an effect which is not due to any change in α-receptor density or affinity.[204] Such facilitation has not been demonstrated in human airways *in vitro*. If α-adrenergic facilitation were important in asthma, then α-blocking drugs should be beneficial. However, specific α-blockers have little or no effect in asthma.[205,206] It is difficult to understand how α-receptors on airway smooth muscle would be activated in the absence of direct adrenergic innervation, and in any case, noradrenaline causes bronchodilatation rather than bronchoconstriction in asthmatic patients.[207] The situation is complicated by the demonstration of inhibitory $α_2$-receptors on airway smooth muscle,[183] and the demonstration that α-agonists reduce microvascular leakiness in airways.[208]

Non-adrenergic non-cholinergic neural mechanisms

The role of non-adrenergic non-cholinergic nerves in asthma remains uncertain, since the neurotransmitters involved have been conclusively identified and no specific blockers are available. There is increasing evidence that neuropeptides may act as neurotransmitters of non-adrenergic non-cholinergic nerves, and many neuropeptides, which have potent effect on airway function, have now been identified in human airways.[209,210]

Defective non-adrenergic non-cholinergic nerves

A defect in non-adrenergic inhibitory nerves has been proposed, since this is the only neural bronchodilator pathway in human airways. This could arise from an intrinsic defect in these nerves (which seems unlikely), or be due to a secondary abnormality such as increased breakdown of the neurotransmitter (which may be vasoactive intestinal polypeptide (VIP)) or a defect in the non-adrenergic non-cholinergic inhibitory receptors. Inflammatory cells release a variety of peptidases which may lead to more rapid breakdown of VIP in asthmatic airways.[211] Since VIP may normally act as a braking mechanism to cholinergic nerves in airways this may lead to exaggerated bronchoconstriction. Non-adrenergic non-cholinergic bronchodilatation has now been demonstrated in human airways *in vivo*,[212] but does not appear to be defective in mild asthma.

Increased non-adrenergic non-cholinergic excitatory nerves

Perhaps a more likely abnormality is an increase in activity of non-adrenergic non-cholinergic excitatory nerves. Evidence from animal studies suggests that non-adrenergic non-cholinergic bronchoconstriction is due to release of neuropeptides such as substance P and neurokinin A from C-fibre sensory nerve endings.[213] If these sensory endings are activated in asthma by exposure of epithelial nerve endings and release of mediators such as bradykinin and prostaglandins, then an axon reflex may be triggered. Release of sensory neuropeptides would then lead to bronchoconstriction, hyperaemia, microvascular leakage and mucus hypersecretion. These local reflexes may, therefore, amplify and spread airway inflammation. In addition, sensory nerves may provide an input to cholinergic ganglia in the airways leading to a local reflex bronchoconstriction. There are no suitable antagonists of tachykinin receptors, so it is difficult to be certain of the role of axon reflexes in asthma. However, sensory neuropeptide release may be modulated by opioid receptors *in vitro* and *in vivo*.[214,215] Since the relevant nerves are present, and sensory neuropeptides have potent effects on human airways,[216] it seems likely that neurogenic inflammation may play an important role in amplifying inflammation in asthmatic airways, as occurs in the skin (Figure 6.6).

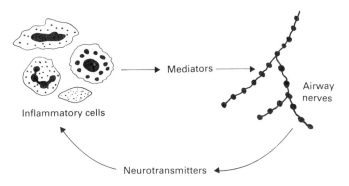

Fig. 6.6 Interrelationship between leucocytes and sensory nerves in the pathogenesis of airway inflammation in asthma.

EXERCISE-INDUCED ASTHMA AS AN ENVIRONMENTAL MANIFESTATION OF PHARMACOLOGICAL BRONCHIAL HYPERRESPONSIVENESS

With current methods used to quantify airways responsiveness, to refer to an abnormal response as 'non-specific' is probably incorrect. As discussed in Chapter 1, stimuli that provoke bronchoconstriction indirectly, i.e. by release of constrictor mediators, are probably of more relevance to natural factors that provoke day to day asthma. One such stimulus that deserves specific attention as a common inciting stimulus is exercise. Exercise-induced asthma is reversed rapidly in most patients by the administration of a β_2-sympathomimetic aerosol. Since brief exercise induces bronchodilatation, recovery from exercise-induced asthma can be aided by a further minute of exercise prior to aerosol therapy.[217] As the airways obstruction is reversed, the hyperinflation and hypoxaemia also recovers. In about 10% of patients, the exercise-induced asthma is much more severe and a β_2-sympathomimetic aerosol may not be effective. In these individuals, it may be necessary to administer aerosol via a nebuliser. The failure of the metered dose aerosol to reverse airflow obstruction in these cases may be due to the inability of the patient to take a deep inspiration.

It is not always convenient to administer medication during exercise. Therefore, it is preferable to use prophylactic therapy. A drug is most effective in the prevention of exercise-induced asthma when delivered as an aerosol. A β-adrenoceptor agonist, sodium cromoglycate, anti-histamine and anti-cholinergic agents have all been shown to inhibit exercise-induced asthma when given by aerosol.[218,219] The failure to inhibit exercise-induced asthma when these same drugs are given orally in higher doses is now well described.

The duration of action of drugs in preventing exercise-induced asthma is less than the effective duration for broncho-dilatation.[220,221] This suggests that the concentration of the drug in the airways is an important determinant of its efficacy. This concept is supported by the fact that the β_2-sympathomimetic agents or theophylline when given as elixirs or tablets, are less effective in preventing exercise-induced asthma, even though they induce significant bronchodilatation at rest.[222] These findings indicate that the efficacy of β_2-sympathomimetic agents in preventing exercise-induced asthma is more likely to be due to its effect on the initiating event such as mast cell mediator release, rather than on the smooth muscle.

Zielinski and Chodosowska have reported a significant reduction in exercise-induced asthma following the intramuscular administration of thiazinamium, 30 minutes prior to exercise.[223] Clemastine, delivered as an aerosol prior to exercise, may also be useful in preventing exercise-induced asthma in some patients.[224] Many of the studies with anti-histamines, however, have been limited by the sedative effects of these drugs. More recently, using potent and selective H_1 histamine antagonists without sedative effects such as terfenadine, there is a clear partial inhibition of exercise-induced asthma and hyperventilation-induced asthma,[225,226] supporting the view that histamine released from airway mast cells contributes to the pathogenesis of these responses.

The finding that sodium cromoglycate and calcium antagonists inhibit exercise-induced asthma without bronchoconstriction indicates that a drug does not have to be a bronchodilator to prevent exercise-induced asthma. This is supported by the finding that exercise-induced asthma can be prevented by inhaling water given as a vapour at $37°C$; an action which is independent of bronchodilator activity and may relate to the inhibition of water and possibly heat loss during exercise. In contrast, ipratropium bromide may exert its protective effect on exercise-induced asthma by its effect on resting lung function.[227] Thompson *et al.* have demonstrated that sodium cromoglycate, ipratropium bromide, and ipratropium bromide plus sodium cromoglycate all significantly inhibited the percentage fall in FEV_1 after exercise in patients whose site of airflow obstruction was in the large airways.[228] Ipratropium bromide had no preventive action in subjects whose site of airflow obstruction was in the small airways, unlike sodium cromoglycate and ipratropium bromide plus sodium cromoglycate. They postulated that mediator release may be an important factor in the development of exercise-induced asthma in most asthmatics, whereas cholinergic mechanisms are relevant only in those patients in whom the main site of airflow obstruction is in the large central airways (Figure 6.7).

An advance in the treatment of severe exercise-induced asthma was the demonstration by Henriksen and Dahl that budesonide, an aerosol corticosteroid, reduced the severity of exercise-induced asthma when given in a daily dose of 400 µg over four weeks.[229] Oral steroids do not usually protect asthmatic individuals from the bronchospastic effects of exercise. Studies investigating the effects of aerosolised corticosteroids, given immediately prior to exercise, have reported no inhibition of exercise-induced asthma.[230]

Bianco *et al.* reported that an α-blocking agent, indoramin, was shown to be effective in preventing exercise-induced asthma.[231]

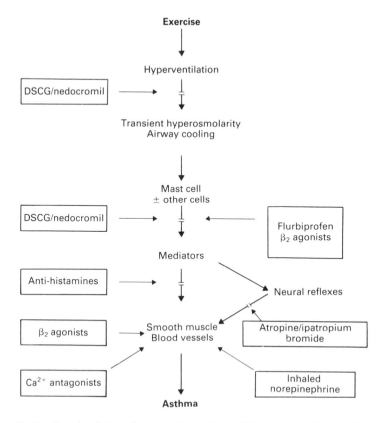

Fig. 6.7 Postulated sites of action of drugs that inhibit exercise-induced asthma (DSCG, cromolym).

However, other studies do not confirm this finding.[232] The failure of the drug may have been due to its oral route of administration since thymoxamine, another α-blocking agent, when delivered as an aerosol, was shown to be effective in inhibiting exercise-induced asthma.[233]

Other agents, such as aspirin, indomethacin, dextropropoxyphene and ketotifen have all been shown to have no significant effect on exercise-induced asthma and, in some cases, exercise-induced asthma has been worse following therapy.[218,234–236] Diethylcarbamazine pamoate, an anti-filarial agent which inhibits the release of slow reacting substance of anaphylaxis, inhibited exercise-induced asthma when given as an aerosol prior to exercise.[237] This drug is an irritant for the airways and has not been studied extensively. Indeed, as with allergen responses, it is most unlikely that any single mediator or mechanism can account for airway obstruction following exercise in asthma.

CONCLUDING COMMENTS

Hyperresponsiveness is a key abnormality in asthma and deserves recognition both in the clinical presentation of asthma and its pathogenesis. Available evidence strongly suggests that inflammatory processes are important in producing this aspect of disordered airway physiology. Pharmacological studies have greatly increased our knowledge of mechanisms involved in hyperresponsiveness but fall short of a complete explanation of the phenomenon. It is most likely that hyperresponsiveness, as measured in the laboratory, has many different components and that any single mechanism will be an insufficient explanation.

REFERENCES

1 Chung KF, Aizawa H, Becker AB, Frick O, Gold WM, Nadel JA. Inhibition of antigen-induced airway hyperresponsiveness by a thromboxane synthetase inhibitor (OKY-046) in allergic dogs. *Am Rev Respir Dis* 1986;**134**:258–61.

2 Chung KF, Aizawa H, Leikauf GD, Ueki IF, Evans TW, Nadel JA. Airway hyperresponsiveness induced by platelet-activating factor; role of thromboxane generation. *J Pharmacol Exp Ther* 1986;**236**;580–4.

3 Chung KF, Becker AB, Lazarus SC, Frick OL, Nadel JA, Gold WM. Antigen-induced airway hyperresponsiveness and pulmonary inflammation in allergic dogs. *J Appl Physiol* 1985;**58**:1347–53.

4 Marsh WR, Irvin CG, Murphy KR, Behrens BL, Larsen GL. Increases in airway reactivity to histamine and inflammatory cells in bronchoalveolar lavage after the late asthmatic response in an animal model. *Am Rev Respir Dis* 1985;**131**:875–9.

5 Metzger WJ, Sjoerdsma K, Brown L, Coyle T, Page C, Touvay C. The late phase asthmatic response in the allergic rabbit; a role for platelet-activating factor (PAF) and modification by PAF antagonist, ginkgolide BN 52021. *Am Rev Respir Dis* (in press).

6 O'Byrne PM, Walters EH, Gold BD *et al.* Indomethacin inhibits the airway hyperresponsiveness but not the neutrophil influx induced by ozone in dogs. *Am Rev Respir Dis* 1984;**130**:220–4.

7 Lanes S, Stevenson JS, Codias E *et al.* Indomethacin and FPL-57231 inhibit antigen-induced airway hyperresponsiveness in sheep. *J Appl Physiol* 1986;**61**:864–72.

8 Lee HK, Murlas C. Ozone-induced bronchial hyperreactivity in guinea pigs is abolished by BW 755C and FPL 55712 but not indomethacin. *Am Rev Respir Dis* 1985;**132**:1005–9.

9 Murlas C, Roum JH. Sequence of pathologic changes in the airway mucosa of guinea pigs during ozone-induced bronchial hyperreactivity. *Am Rev Respir Dis* 1985;**131**:314–20.

10 Hirshman CA, Peters J, Butler J, Hanifin JM, Downes H. Role of mediators in allergic and non-allergic asthma in dogs with hyperreactive airways. *J Appl Physiol* 1983;**54**:1108–14.

11 Hutchison AA, Hinson JM, Brigham KL, Snapper JR. Effect of endotoxin on airway responsiveness to aerosol histamine in sheep. *J Appl Physiol* 1983;**54**:1463–8.

12 Buckner CK, Songsiridej V, Dick EC, Busse WW. *In vivo* and *in vitro* studies on the use of the guinea pig as a model for virus-provoked airway hyperreactivity. *Am Rev Respir Dis* 1985;**132**:305–10.

13 Pauwels R. The effects of theophylline on airway inflammation. *Chest* 1987;**92**:32S–37S.

14 Hinson JM Jr, Hutchison AA, Brigham KL, Meyrick BO, Snapper JR. Effects of granulocyte depletion on pulmonar responsiveness to aerosol histamine. *J Appl Physiol* 1984;**56**:411–7.

15 Holtzman MN, Fabbri LM, O'Byrne PM. Importance of airway inflammation for hyperresponsiveness induced by ozone. *Am Rev Respir Dis* 1983;**127**:686–90.

16 Fabbri LM, Aizawa H, Alpert SE *et al.* Airway hyperresponsiveness and changes in cell counts in bronchoalveolar lavage after ozone exposure in dogs. *Am Rev Respir Dis* 1984;**129**:288–91.

17 O'Byrne PM, Walters EH, Gold BD *et al.* Neutrophil depletion inhibits airway hyperresponsiveness induced by ozone exposure. *Am Rev Respir Dis* 1984;**130**:214–9.

18 Aizawa H, Chung KF, Leikauf GD *et al.* Significance of thromboxane generation in ozone-induced airway hyperresponsiveness in dogs. *J Appl Physiol* 1985;**59**:1918–23.

19 Fabbri LM, Aizawa H, O'Byrne PM *et al.* An anti-inflammatory drug (BW755C) inhibits airway hyperresponsiveness induced by ozone in dogs. *J Allergy Clin Immunol* 1985;**76**:162–6.

20 Fabbri LM, Boschetto P, Zocca E *et al.* Bronchoalveolar neutrophilia during late asthmatic reactions induced by toluene diisocyanate. *Am Rev Respir Dis* 1987;**136**:36–42.

21 Fabbri LM, Chiesura-Corona P, dal Vecchio L *et al.* Prednisone inhibits late asthmatic reactions and the associated increase in airway responsiveness induced by toluene-diisocyanate in sensitized subjects. *Am Rev Respir Dis* 1985;**132**:1010–4.

22 Cibulas W Jr, Murlas CG, Miller ML *et al.* Toluene-diisocyanate-induced airway hyperreactivity and pathology in the guinea pig. *J Allergy Clin Immunol* 1986;**77**:828–34.

23 Thompson JE, Scypinski LA, Gordon T, Sheppard D. Hydroxyurea inhibits airway hyperresponsiveness in guinea pigs by granulocyte-independent mechanism. *Am Rev Respir Dis* 1986;**134**:1213–6.

24 Bach MK, Braschler JR, Smith HW, Fitzpatrick FA, McGuire JC. 6,9-deepoxy-6,9-(phenylimino-$\Delta^{6,8}$-prostaglandin I$_1$, (U-60,257), a new inhibitor of leukotriene C and D synthesis; *In vitro* studies. *Prostaglandins* 1982;**23**:759–71.

25 Murlas C, Lee HK. U-60,257 inhibits O_3-induced bronchial hyperreactivity in the guinea pig. *Prostaglandins* 1985;**30**:563-72.

26 Cartier A, Thomson NC, Frith PA, Roberts R, Hargreave FE. Allergen-induced increase in bronchial responsiveness to histamine; relationship to the late asthmatic response and change in airway caliber. *J Allergy Clin Immunol* 1982;**70**:170-7.

27 Cockcroft DW, Ruffin RE, Dolovich J, Hargreave FE. Allergen-induced increase in non-allergic bronchial reactivity. *Clin Allergy* 1977;**7**:503-13.

28 Cockcroft DW, Murdoch KY. Changes in bronchial responsiveness to histamine at intervals after allergen challenge. *Thorax* 1987;**42**:302-8.

29 Durham SR, Graneek BJ, Hawkins R, Taylor AJN. The temporal relationship between increases in airway responsiveness to histamine and late asthmatic responses induced by occupational agents. *J Allergy Clin Immunol* 1987;**79**:398-406.

30 Thorpe JE, Steinberg D, Bernstein IL, Murlas CG. Bronchial reactivity increases soon after the immediate response in dual responding asthmatic subjects. *Chest* 1987;**91**:15-21.

31 Murphy KR, Wilson MC, Irvin CG. The requirement for polymorphonuclear leukocytes in the asthmatic response and heightened airway reactivity in an asthmatic model. *Am Rev Respir Dis* 1986;**134**:62-8.

32 Abraham WM, Lanes S, Stevenson JS, Yerger LD. Effect of an inhaled glucocorticosteroid (budesonide) on post-antigen induced increases in airway responsiveness. *Clin Respir Physiol* 1986;**22**:387-92.

33 Abraham WM, Stevenson JS, Eldridge M, Garrido R, Nieves L. Nedocromil sodium in allergen-induced bronchial responses and airway hyperresponsiveness in allergic sheep. *J Appl Physiol* 1988;**65**:1062-8.

34 Abraham WM, Stevenson JS, Garrido R. A leukotriene and thromboxane inhibitor (Sch 37224) blocks antigen-induced immediate and late responses and airway hyperresponsiveness in allergic sheep. *J Pharm Exper Ther* 1988;**247**:1004-11.

35 Kirby JG, Hargreave FE, O'Byrne PM. Indomethacin inhibits allergen-induced airway hyperresponsiveness but not allergen-induced asthmatic responses (abstract). *Am Rev Respir Dis* 1987;**135**:A312.

36 Stewart AG, Thompson DC, Fennessy MR. Leukotriene D_4 potentiates histamine-induced bronchoconstriction in guinea pigs. *Agents Actions* 1984;**15**:146-52.

37 Ahmed TA, Marchette B. Hypoxia enhances non-specific bronchial reactivity. *Am Rev Respir Dis* 1985;**132**:839-44.

38 D'Brot J, Ahmed T. Hypoxia-induced enhancement of non-specific bronchial reactivity; role of leukotrienes. *Am Rev Respir Dis* 1987;**135**(4):A88.

39 Weichman BM, Wasserman MA, Cleason JG. SK&F 88046; a unique pharmacologic antagonist of bronchoconstriction induced by leukotriene D_4, thromboxane and prostaglandins F_2 and D_2 *in vitro*. *J Pharmacol Exp Ther* 1984;**228**:128-32.

40 Mattoli SA, Foresi A, Corbo GM, Polidori G, Ciappi G. Protective effect of disodium cromoglycate on allergen-induced bronchoconstriction and increased hyperresponsiveness; a double-blind placebo-controlled study. *Ann Allergy* 1986;**57**:295-300.

41 O'Byrne OM, Leikauf GD, Aizawa H *et al*. Leukotriene B_4-induced airway hyperresponsiveness in dogs. *J Appl Physiol* 1985;**59**:1941-6.

42 McManus LM. Pathophysiology of platelet-activating factor. *Path Immunopathol Res* 1986;**5**:104-17.

43 Abraham WM, Stevenson JS, Garrido R. A possible role for platelet activating factor in allergen-induced late responses. Modification by a selective antagonist. *J Appl Physiol* (in press).

44 Morley J. Platelet activating factor and the search for prophylactic antiasthma drugs. In: Jenne JW, Murphy S eds. *Asthma drugs: theory and practice. Lung biology series*. New York: Marcel Dekker 1987: 997-1020.

45 Cuss FM, Dixon CMS, Barnes PJ. Effects of inhaled platelet activating factor on pulmonary function and bronchoresponsiveness in man. *Lancet* 1986;ii:189–92.

46 Stevenson JS, Tallent M, Blinder L, Abraham WM. Modification of antigen-induced late responses with an antagonist of platelet activating factor (WEB 2086) (abstract). *Fed Proc* 1987;**46**:6683.

47 Murlas C, Bernstein DI, Bernstein IL, Steinberg DR. Prednisone inhibits the early increase in bronchial reactivity that occurs soon after the immediate response in dual responding asthmatics (abstract). *Am Rev Respir Dis* 1987;**135**:A321.

48 Abraham WM, Blinder L, Wanner A, Stevenson JS, Tallent M. Inhibition of antigen-induced airway hyperresponsiveness in allergic sheep with a thromboxane antagonist (L641,953) (abstract). *Fed Proc* 1987;**46**:349.

49 Abraham WM, Blinder L, Wanner A, Stevenson JS, Tallent MW. Antigen-induced airway hyperresponsiveness does not contribute to airway late responses (abstract). *Am Rev Respir Dis* 1987;**135**:A97.

50 Abraham WM, Stevenson JS, Tallent M. Effect of nedocromil sodium on antigen-induced airway responsiveness in allergic sheep (abstract). *Am Rev Respir Dis* 1987:**135**:A318.

51 Inoue H, Horio S, Ichinose M *et al.* Changes in bronchial reactivity to acetylcholine with type C influenza virus infection in dogs. *Am Rev Respir Dis* 1986;**133**:367–71.

52 Empey DW, Laitinen LA, Jacobs L, Gold WM, Nadel JA. Mechanisms of bronchial hyperreactivity in normal subjects after upper respiratory tract infection. *Am Rev Respir Dis* 1976;**113**:131–9.

53 Little JW, Hall WJ, Douglas RG Jr, Mudholkar GS, Speers DM, Patel K. Airway hyperreactivity and peripheral airway dysfunction in Influenza A infection. *Am Rev Respir Dis* 1978;**118**:295–303.

54 Hirshman CA, Austin DR, Klein W, Hanifin JM, Hulbert W. Increased metachromatic cells and lymphocytes in bronchoalveolar lavage fluid of dogs with airway hyperreactivity. *Am Rev Respir Dis* 1986;**133**:482–7.

55 Hirshman CA, Peters J, Downes H, Leon D, Lynn RK, Butler J, Hanifin JM. Citric acid airway constriction in dogs with hyperreactive airways. *J Appl Physiol* 1983;**54**:1101–7.

56 Kirby J, Hargreave FE, Gleich GJ, O'Byrne PM. Bronchoalveolar cell profiles of asthmatic and non-asthmatic subjects. *Am Rev Respir Dis* 1987;**136**:379–83.

57 Tomioka M, Ida S, Shindoh Y, Ishihara T, Takishima T. Mast cells in bronchoalveolar lumen of patients with bronchial asthma. *Am Rev Respir Dis* 1984;**129**:1000–5.

58 Osborne ML, Evens TW, Sommerhoff CP *et al.* Hypotonic and isotonic aerosols increase bronchial reactivity in Basenji-greyhound dogs. *Am Rev Respir Dis* 1987;**135**:345–9.

59 Lowhagen O, Rak I. Modification of bronchial hyperreactivity after treatment with sodium cromoglycate during pollen season. *J Allergy Clin Immunol* 1985;**75**:460–7.

60 Ahmed T, Krainson JP, Yerger LD. Functional depression of H_2 histamine receptors in sheep with experimental allergic asthma. *J Allergy Clin Immunol* 1983;**72**:310–20.

61 Nath P, Joshi AP, Agrawal KP. Biochemical correlates of airway hyperreactivity in guinea pigs: role of lysophosphatidyl choline. *J Allergy Clin Immunol* 1983;**72**:351–8.

62 Booij-Noord H, Orie NGM, DeVries K. Immediate and late bronchial obstructive reactions to inhalation of house dust and protective effects of disodium cromoglycate and prednisolone. *J Allergy Clin Immunol* 1971;**48**:344–54.

63 Pepys J, Hutchcroft BJ. Bronchial provocation tests on the etiologic diagnosis and analysis of asthma. *Am Rev Respir Dis* 1975;**112**:829–59.

64 Mattoli S, Foresi A, Corbo GM, Polidori G, Ciappi G. Protective effect of disodium cromoglycate on allergen-induced bronchoconstriction and increased hyperresponsiveness. *Ann Allergy* 1986;**57**:295–300.

65 Cockcroft DW, Murdock KY. Comparative effects of inhaled salbutamol, sodium cromoglycate and beclomethasone dipropionate on allergen-induced early asthmatic responses, late asthmatic responses and increased bronchial responsiveness to histamine. *J Allergy Clin Immunol* 1987;**79**:734–40.

66 Mattoli S, Foresi A, Corbo GM, Valente S, Ciappi G. Effect of two doses of cromolyn on allergen-induced late asthmatic response and increased responsiveness. *J Allergy Clin Immunol* 1987;**79**:747–54.

67 Boushey HA, Holtzman J, Sheller JR, Nadel JA. Bronchial hyperreactivity, state of the art. *Am Rev Respir Dis* 1980;**121**:389–413.

68 Barnes PJ. Neural control of human airways in health and disease. *Am Rev Respir Dis* 1986;**134**:1289–314.

69 Nadel JA, Salem H, Tamplin B, Tokiwa G. Mechanism of bronchoconstriction during inhalation of sulphur dioxide. *J Appl Physiol* 1965;**20**:164–7.

70 White J, Eiser NM. The role of histamine and its receptors in the pathogenesis of asthma. *Br J Dis Chest* 1983;**77**:215–26.

71 Beasley R, Varley J, Robinson C, Holgate ST. Direct and reflex bronchoconstrictor actions of prostaglandins (PG) D$_2$, its initial metabolite 9α,11β-PGF$_{2α}$ in asthma. *Am Rev Respir Dis* 1987;**136**:1140–4.

72 Sheppard D, Epstein J, Holtzman MJ, Nadel JA, Boushey HA. Dose-dependent inhibition of cold air-induced bronchoconstriction by atropine. *J Appl Physiol* 1982;**53**:169–74.

73 Anderson SD, Smith CM. Heat and water loss from the airways as a provoking stimulus for asthma. *Prog Clin Biol Res* 1988;**163**:283–99.

74 Minette PA, Barnes PJ. Prejunctional inhibitory muscarinic receptors on cholinergic nerves in human and guinea pig airways. *J Appl Physiol* 1988;**64**:2532–7.

75 Krall JF. Receptor-mediated regulation of tension in smooth muscle cells. In: Jenne JW, Murphy J eds. *Asthma drugs: theory and practice. Lung biology series.* 1987;**31**:97–128.

76 Bendouvakis J, Cartier A, Roberts R, Ryan G, Hargreave FE. The effect of ipratropium and fenoterol on methacholine- and histamine-induced bronchoconstriction. *Br J Dis Chest* 1981;**75**:295–305.

77 Salome CM, Shcoeffel RE, Yan K, Woolcock AJ. Effect of aerosol fenoterol on the severity of bronchial hyperreactivity in patients with asthma. *Thorax* 1983;**38**:854–8.

78 Rhoden RJ, Meldrum LA, Barnes PJ. Beta-adrenergic modulation of cholinergic neurotransmission in human airways (abstract). *Am Rev Respir Dis* 1987;**135**:A91.

79 Holgate ST, Finnerty JP. Recent advances in understanding the pathogenesis of asthma and its clinical implications. *Q J Med* 1988;**249**:5–19.

80 Church MK, Hiroi J. Inhibition of IgE-dependent histamine release from human dispersed lung mast cells by anti-allergic drugs and salbutamol. *Br J Pharmacol* 1987;**90**:421–9.

81 Barnes PJ. The changing face of asthma. *Q J Med* 1987;**63**:359–65.

82 O'Malley G, Baker AJ, MacDermot J, Fuller RW. β-receptor stimulation does not inhibit human alveolar macrophage activation (abstract). *Thorax* 1987;**42**:747.

83 Tonnel AB, Joseph M, Capron A. Alveolar macrophage and allergic asthma. In: Kay Ab ed. *Allergy and inflammation.* Academic Press: London 1987: 139–50.

84 Bergstrand H. Phosphodiesterase inhibition and theophylline. *Eur J Respir Dis* 1980;**61**(Suppl.109):37–44.

85 Reeves ML, Leigh BK, England PJ. The identification of a new cyclic nucleotide phosphodiesterase activity in human and guinea pig cardiac ventricle. *Biochem J* 1987;**241**:535–41.

86 Holgate ST. Mechanisms and significance of adenosine-induced bronchoconstriction in asthma. *Allergy* 1987;**42**:727–30.

87 Pauwels R, Vanrenterghem D, Van der Straeten M, Johannesson N, Persson CGA. The effect of theophylline and enprofylline on allergen-induced bronchoconstriction. *J Allergy Clin Immunol* 1985;**76**:583–90.

88 Persson CGA, Ekman M, Kjellin G. Enprofylline, a principally new antiasthmatic xanthine. *Acta Pharmacol Toxicol* 1981;**49**:313–16.

89 Pepys J, Davies RJ, Breslin AB, Hendricks DJ, Hutchcroft BJ. The effect of inhaled beclomethasone dipropionate (Becotide) and sodium cromoglycate on asthmatic reactions to provocation tests. *Clin Allergy* 1974;**4**:13–24.

90 Dahl R, Johansson S-A. Importance of duration of treatment with inhaled budesonide on the immediate and late bronchial reaction. *Eur J Respir Dis* 1982;**122**(Suppl.):167–75.

91 Mapp CE, Boschetto P, Zocca E *et al.* Pathogenesis of late asthmatic reactions induced by exposure to isocyanates. *Clin Respir Physiol* 1987;**23**:583–6.

92 Altman LC, Hill JS, Harfield WM *et al.* Effect of corticosteroids on eosinophil chemotaxis and adherence. *J Clin Invest* 1981;**67**:28–36.

93 Gerblich MA, Urda G, Schugler M. Atopic asthma; T-cell response to corticosteroids. *Chest* 1985;**87**:44–50.

94 Poznansky MC, Gordon ACH, Grant IWB, Wyllie AH. A cellular abnormality in glucocorticoid resistant asthma. *Clin Exp Immunol* 1985;**61**:135–42.

95 Jenkins CR, Woolcock AJ. Effect of prednisolone and beclomethasone dipropionate on airway responsiveness in asthma; a comparative study. *Thorax* 1988;**43**:378–84.

96 Laitinen LA, Heino M, Karjolainen J, Ylikoski J, Laitinen A. Inflammation of bronchial epithelium and oral steroid treatment of patients with asthma at early stages of their disease (abstract). *Am Rev Respir Dis* 1987;**135**:A474.

97 Rocchiccioli K, Pickering CAC, Cole M, Horsfield N. Effect of regular treatment with sodium cromoglycate on non-specific bronchial hyperreactivity. *Thorax* 1984;**33**:706.

98 Lowhagen O, Rak S. Modification of bronchial hyperreactivity after treatment with sodium cromoglycate during pollen season. *J Allergy Clin Immunol* 1985;**75**:460–7.

99 Israel RH, Poe RH, Wicks CM, Greenblatt DW, Kallay MC. The protective effect of methyl prednisolone on carbachol-induced bronchospasm. *Am Rev Respir Dis* 1984;**130**:1019–22.

100 Bhagat RG, Grunstein MM. Effect of corticosteroids on bronchial responsiveness to methacholine in asthmatic children. *Am Rev Respir Dis* 1985;**131**:902–6.

101 Ryan G, Latimer KM, Juniper EF, Roberts RS, Hargreave FE. Effect of beclomethasone dipropionate on bronchial responsiveness to histamine in controlled non-steriod dependent asthma. *J Allergy Clin Immunol* 1985;**75**:25–30.

102 Kraan J, Koeter GH, Mark TN, Sluiter HJ, de Vries K. Change in bronchial hyperreactivity induced by four weeks of treatment with antiasthmatic drugs in patients with allergic asthma; a comparison between budesonide and terbutaline. *J Allergy Clin Immunol* 1985;**76**:628–36.

103 Lowhagen O, Rak S. Bronchial hyperreactivity after treatment with sodium cromoglycate in atopic asthmatic patients not exposed to relevant allergens. *J Allergy Clin Immunol* 1985;**75**:343–7.

104 Griffin M, Weiss JW, Leitch AG *et al.* Effects of leukotriene D on human airways in asthma. *N Engl J Med* 1983;**308**:436–9.

105 Adelroth E, Morris MM, Hargreave FE, O'Byrne PM. Airway responsiveness to leukotrienes C_4 and D_4 and to methacholine in patients with asthma and normal controls. *N Engl J Med* 1986;**315**:480–4.

106 Drazen JM, Austen KF. Leukotrienes and airway responses. *Am Rev Respir Dis* 1987;**136**:985–98.

107 Barnes NC, Piper PJ, Costello JF. Action of inhaled leukotrienes and their

interactions with other allergic mediators. *Prostaglandins* 1984;**28**:629–31.

108 Arm JP, Spur BW, Lee TH. The effects of inhaled leukotriene E$_4$ (LTE$_4$) on the airway responsiveness to histamine in subjects with asthma and normal subjects. *J Allergy Clin Immunol* 1988;**82**:654–60.

109 Phillips GD, Holgate ST. The interaction of inhaled leukotriene C$_4$ with histamine and prostaglandin D$_2$ on airway calibre in asthma. *J Appl Physiol* (in press).

110 Jones TR, Young R, Champion E *et al.* L-649,923, sodium (beta S*, gamma R*)-4-(3-(4-acetyl-3-hydroxy-2-propylphenoxy)-propylthio)-gamma-hydroxy-beta-methyl benzenebutanoate, a selective, orally active leukotriene receptor antagonist. *Can J Physiol Pharmacol* 1986;**64**:1068–75.

111 Fleisch JH, Rinkema LE, Haisch KD *et al.* LY-171883, 1-⟨2hydroxy-3-propyl-4-⟨4-(1H-tetrazol-5-yl) butoxy⟩phenyl⟩ethanone, an orally active leukotriene D$_4$ antagonist. *J Pharmacol Exp Ther* 1985;**233**:148–57.

112 Barnes J, Piper PJ, Costello J. The effect of an oral leukotriene antagonist L-649,923 on histamine and leukotriene D$_4$-induced bronchoconstriction in normal man. *J Allergy Clin Immunol* 1987;**79**:816–21.

113 Phillips GD, Rafferty P, Robinson C, Holgate ST. Dose-related antagonism of LTD$_4$-induced bronchoconstriction by oral administration of LY-171883 in non-asthmatic subjects. *J Pharmacol Exp Ther* (in press).

114 Britton JR, Hanley SP, Tattersfield AE. The effect of an oral leukotriene D$_4$ antagonist L-649,923 on the response to inhaled antigen in asthma. *J Allergy Clin Immunol* 1987;**79**:811–6.

115 Fuller RW, Black PN, Dollery CT. Effect of oral LY-171883 on inhaled and intradermal antigen and LTD$_4$ in atopic subjects (abstract). *Br J Clin Pharmacol* 1988;**25**:626P.

116 Bach MK. Prospects for the inhibition of leukotriene synthesis. *Biochem Pharmacol* 1984;**33**:515–21.

117 Mann JS, Holgate ST. Effect of piriprost (U-60,257) a novel leukotriene inhibitor on allergen- and exercise-induced asthma. *Thorax* 1986;**41**:741–52.

118 Fuller RW, Maltby N, Richmond R *et al.* Oral nafazatrom in man; effect of inhaled antigen challenge. *Br J Clin Pharmacol* 1987;**23**:677–81.

119 Needleman P, Raz A, Minkes NS, Ferendelli A, Sprecher H. Triene prostacyclin and thromboxane biosynthesis and unique biological properties. *Proc Natl Acad Sci USA* 1979;**76**:944–8.

120 Corey EJ, Shih C, Cashman JR. Docosahexaenoic acid is a strong inhibitor of prostaglandin but not leukotriene biosynthesis. *Proc Natl Acad Sci USA* 1983;**80**:3581–4.

121 Dyerberg J, Bang HO, Stofferson E, Moncada S, Vane JR. Eicosapentaenoic acid and prevention of thrombosis and atherosclerosis. *Lancet* 1978;**ii**:117–9.

122 Whitaker MO, Wyche A, Fitzpatrick F, Sprecher H, Needleman P. Triene prostaglandins; Prostaglandin D$_3$ and eicosapentaenoic acid as potential antithrombotic substances. *Proc Natl Acad Sci USA* 1979;**76**:5919–23.

123 Goldman DW, Pickett WC, Goetzl EJ. Human neutrophil chemotactic and degranulating activities of leukotriene B$_5$ (LTB$_5$) derived from eicosapentaenoic acid. *Biochem Biophys Res Commun* 1983;**117**:282–8.

124 Lee TH, Mencia-Huerta JM, Shih C, Corey EJ, Lewis RA, Austen KF. Characterisation and biological properties of 5,12-dihydroxy derivatives of eicosapentaenoic acid including leukotriene B$_5$ and the double lipoxygenase product. *J Biol Chem* 1984;**259**:2383–9.

125 Terano T, Salmon JS, Moncada S. Biosynthesis and biological activity of leukotriene B$_5$. *Prostaglandins* 1984;**27**:217–32.

126 Lee TH, Sethi T, Crea AET *et al.* Characterisation of leukotriene B$_3$. Comparison of its biological activities with leukotriene B$_4$ and leukotriene B$_5$ in complement receptor enhancement, lysozyme release and chemotaxis of human neutrophils. *Clin Sci* 1988;**74**:467–75.

127 Dahlen SE, Hedqvist P, Hammarstrom S. Contractile activities of several cystein-containing leukotrienes in the guinea pig lung strip. *Eur J Pharmacol* 1982;**86**:207–15.

128 Leitch AG, Lee TH, Ringel EW *et al.* Immunologically-induced generation of tetraene and pentaene leukotrienes in the peritoneal cavities of menhaden-fed rats. *J Immunol* 1984;**132**:2559–64.

129 Lee TH, Mencia Huerta JM, Shih C, Corey EJ, Lewis RA, Austen KF. Effects of exogenous arachidonic, eicosapentaenoic, and docosahexaenoic acids on the generation of 5-lipoxygenase pathway products by ionophore-activated human neutrophils. *J Clin Invest* 1984;**74**:1922–33.

130 Benveniste J, Tence M, Varenne P, Bidault J, Boullet C, Polansky J. Semi-synthese et structure proposé du facteur activant les plaquettes (PAF); paf-acether, un alkyl ether analogue de la lysophosphatidylcholine. *CR Acad Sci Paris* 1979;**289**D:1037–40.

131 Sperling RI, Robin JL, Kylander KA, Lee TH, Lewis RA, Austen KF. The effects of N-3 polyunsaturated fatty acids on the generation of platelet-activating factor-acether by human monocytes. *J Immunol* 1987;**139**:4126–91.

132 Lee TH, Hoover RL, Williams JD *et al.* Effect of dietary enrichment with eicosapentaenoic and docosahexaenoic acids on *in vitro* neutrophil and monocyte leukotriene generation and neutrophil function. *N Engl J Med* 1985;**312**:1217–24.

133 Arm JP, Horton CE, Mencia-Huerta JM *et al.* Effect of dietary supplementation with fish oil lipids on mild asthma. *Thorax* 1988;**43**:84–92.

134 Payan DG, Wong YS, Chernov-Rogan T. Alterations in human leukocyte function induced by ingestion of eicosapentaenoic acid. *J Clin Immunol* 1986;**78**:937–42.

135 Kirsch CM, Payan DM, Wong MYS *et al.* The effect of eicosapentaenoic acid in asthma. *Clin Allergy* 1988;**18**:177–87.

136 Picado C, Castillo JA, Schinca N *et al.* Effects of a fish oil enriched diet on aspirin intolerant asthmatic patients; a pilot study. *Thorax* 1988;**43**:93–7.

137 Arm JP, Horton CE, Eiser NM, Clark TJH, Lee TH. The effects of dietary supplementation with fish oil on asthmatic responses to antigen. *Am Rev Respir Dis* (in press).

138 Braquet P, Shen TY, Touqui L, Vargaftig BB. Perspectives in platelet-activating factor research. *Pharmacol Rev* 1987;**39**:97–145.

139 Godard P, Chaintreuil J, Damon M *et al.* Functional assessment of alveolar macrophages; comparison of cells from asthmatics and normal subjects. *J Allergy Clin Immunol* 1982;**70**:88–93.

140 Lee TC, Lenihan DJ, Malone B, Roddy LL, Wasserman SI. Increased biosynthesis of platelet activating factor in activated human eosinophils. *J Biol Chem* 1984;**259**:5526–30.

141 Barnes PJ, Chung KF. PAF closely mimics pathology of asthma. *Trends Pharmacol Sci* 1987;**8**:285–7.

142 Barnes PJ, Chung KF, Page CP. Platelet-activating factor as a mediator of allergic disease. *J Allergy Clin Immunol* 1988;**81**:919–34.

143 Schellenberg RR, Walker B, Snyder F. Platelet-dependent contraction of human bronchus by platelet activating factor (abstract). *J Allergy Clin Immunol* 1983;**71**:145.

144 Henocq E, Vargaftig BB. Accumulation of eosinophils in response to intracutaneous PAF-acether and allergens in man. *Lancet* 1986;**i**:1378–9.

145 Kroegel C, Yukawa T, Dent G, Chanwz P, Chung KF, Barnes PJ. Platelet activating factor induces eosinophil peroxidase release from purified human eosinophils. *Immunology* 1988;**64**:559–62.

146 Chanez P, Dent G, Yukawa T, Chung KF, Barnes PJ. Increased eosinophil responsiveness to platelet-activating factor in asthma (abstract). *Clin Sci* 1988;**74**:5P.

147 Evans TW, Chung K, Rogers DF, Barnes PJ. Effect of platelet-activating factor

on airway vascular permeability; possible mechanisms. *J Appl Physiol* 1987;**63**:479–84.

148 Goswami SK, Ohashi M, Panagiotis S, Marom Z. Platelet activating factor enhances mucous glycoprotein release from human airways *in vitro* (abstract). *Am Rev Respir Dis* 1987;**135**:A159.

149 Aursudkij B, Rogers DF, Evans TW, Alton EWFW, Chung KF, Barnes PJ. Reduced tracheal mucus velocity in guinea pig *in vivo* by platelet activating factor (abstract). *Am Rev Respir Dis* 1987;**35**:A160.

150 Chung KF, Dent G, McCusker M, Guinot Ph, Page CP, Barnes PJ. Effect of a ginkgolide mixture (BN 52063) in antagonising skin and platelet responses to platelet activating factor in man. *Lancet* 1987;**i**:248–51.

151 Roberts NM, Page CP, Chung KF, Barnes PJ. The effect of a specific PAF antagonist, BN 52063, on antigen-induced cutaneous responses in man. *J Allergy Clin Immunol* 1988;**82**:236–41.

152 Roberts NM, McCusker M, Chung KF, Barnes PJ. Effect of a PAF antagonist, BN 52063, on PAF-induced bronchoconstriction in human subjects. *Br J Clin Pharmacol* 1988;**26**:65–72.

153 Chung KF, Barnes PJ. PAF antagonists; their therapeutic potential in asthma. *Drugs* 1988;**35**:93–103.

154 Holgate ST, Beasley R, Twentyman RO. The pathogenesis and significance of bronchial hyperresponsiveness in airways disease. *Clin Sci* 1987;**73**:561–72.

155 Fujimara M, Sasaki F, Nakatsumi Y *et al*. Effects of thromboxane synthetase (AA-861) on bronchial responsiveness to acetylcholine in asthmatic subjects. *Thorax* 1986;**41**:955–9.

156 Curzen N, Rafferty P, Holgate ST. Cyclooxygenase inhibition and H_1-histamine receptor antagonism alone and in combination on allergen-induced bronchoconstriction in man. *Thorax* 1987;**42**:946–52.

157 Samter M, Beers RF. Intolerance to aspirin. Clinical studies and consideration of its pathogenesis. *Ann Intern Med* 1986;**68**:975–83.

158 Ferreri NR, Howland WC, Stevenson DD, Spiegelberg HL. Release of leukotrienes, prostaglandins and histamine into nasal secretions of aspirin sensitive asthmatics during reaction to aspirin. *Am Rev Respir Dis* 1988;**137**:847–54.

159 Beasley CRW, Featherstone RL, Church MK *et al*. The effect of a thromboxane receptor antagonist GR32191 on PGD_2- and allergen-induced bronchoconstriction. *J Appl Physiol* 1989 (in press).

160 Durham SR, Lee TH, Cromwell O *et al*. Immunologic studies in allergen-induced late-phase asthmatic reactions. *J Allergy Clin Immunol* 1984;**74**:41–60.

161 Naclerio RM, Proud D, Togias AG *et al*. Inflammatory mediators in late antigen-induced rhinitis. *N Engl J Med* 1985;**313**:65–70.

162 Lichtenstein LM. Histamine releasing factors and IgE-heterogeneity. *J Allergy Clin Immunol* 1988;**81**:821–8.

163 Flint KF, Leung KBP, Hudspith BN, Brostoff J, Pearce FL, Johnson NMcI. Bronchoalveolar mast cells in extrinsic asthma; a mechanism for the initiation of antigen-specific bronchoconstriction. *Br Med J* 1985;**291**:923–6.

164 Lozewicz S, Gomez E, Ferguson H, Davies RJ. Mast cells and eosinophils in the bronchial mucous membrane in asthma (abstract). *Thorax* 1988;**43**:238P.

165 Taytard A, Beaumont D, Pajet JC, Sapere M, Lewis PS. Treatment of bronchial asthma with terfenadine in a randomized controlled trial. *Br J Clin Pharmacol* 1987;**24**:743–6.

166 Spector SL, Perhach JL, Rohr AS, Rachelefsky GS, Katz RM, Siegel SC. Pharmacodynamic evaluation of azelastine in subjects with asthma. *J Allergy Clin Immunol* 1987;**80**:75–80.

167 Storms W, Middleton E, Dvorin D *et al*. Azelastine (azel) in the treatment of asthma (abstract). *J Allergy Clin Immunol* 1985;**75**:167.

168 Fuller RW, Dixon CMS, Dollery CT, Barnes PJ. Prostaglandin D_2 potentiates

airway responsiveness to histamine and methacholine. *Am Rev Respir Dis* 1986;133:252–4.

169 Nadel JA, Barnes PJ, Holtzman MJ. Autonomic factors in the hyperreactivity of airway smooth muscle. In: Fishman AP ed. *Handbook of physiology: the respiratory system III.* American Physiological Society 1986:693–702.

170 Nadel JA, Barnes PJ. Autonomic regulation of airways. *An Rev Med* 1984;35:451–67.

171 Kaliner MA, Barnes PJ *The airways; neural control in health and disease.* New York: Marcel Dekker 1987.

172 Kaliner M, Shelhamer J, Davis PB, Smith LJ, Venter JC. Autonomic nervous system abnormalities and allergy. *Ann Intern Med* 1982;96:349–57.

173 Barnes PJ. Airway inflammation and autonomic control. *Eur J Respir Dis* 1986;69(Suppl.147):80–7.

174 Barnes PJ. Asthma as an axon reflex. *Lancet* 1986;1:242–45.

175 Nadel JA. Autonomic regulation of airway smooth muscle. In: Nadel JA ed. *Physiology and pharmacology of the airways.* New York: Marcel Dekker 1980:217–57.

176 Barnes PJ. Cholinergic control of airway smooth muscle. *Am Rev Respir Dis* 1987;136:S42–S54.

177 Kallenbach JM, Webster T, Dowdeswell R, Reinach SG, Millar Scott RN, Swi S. Reflex heart rate control in asthma. *Chest* 1985;87:644–8.

178 Sheller JR, Holtzman MJ, Skoogh B-E, Nadel JA. Interaction of serotinin with vagal and acetylcholine-induced bronchoconstriction in canine lungs. *J Appl Physiol* 1982;52:964–6.

179 Chung KF, Evans TW, Graf PD, Nadel JA. Modulation of cholinergic neurotransmission in canine airways by thromboxane-mimetic U 46619. *Eur J Pharmacol* 1985;117:373–5.

180 Hall AK, Barnes PJ, Meldrum LA, MacLagan J. Facilitation by tachykinins of neurotransmission in guinea pig pulmonary parasympathetic nerves. *Br J Pharmacol* (in press).

181 Tanaka DT, Grunstein MM. Mechanisms of substance P-induced contraction of rabbit airway smooth muscle. *J Appl Physiol* 1984;57:1551–7.

182 Danser AHJ, van den Ende R, Lorenz RR, Flavahan NA, Vanhoutte PM. Prejunctional β_1-adrenoceptors inhibit cholinergic neurotransmission in canine bronchi. *J Appl Physiol* 1987;62:785–90.

183 Andersson RGG, Fugner A, Lundgren BR, Maucevic G. Inhibitory effects of clonidine on bronchospasm induced in guinea pigs by vagal stimulation of antigen challenge. *Eur J Pharmacol* 1986;123:181–5.

184 Boushey HA, Holtzman MJ, Sheller JR, Nadel JA. Bronchial hyperreactivity. *Am Rev Respir Dis* 1980;121:389–413.

185 Robertson DM, Rhoden KJ, Grandordy B, Page CP, Barnes PJ. The effects of platelet activating factor on histamine and muscarinic receptor function in guinea pig airways. *Am Rev Respir Dis* 1988;137:1317–22.

186 Fryer AD, MacLagen J. Muscarinic inhibitory receptors in pulmonary parsympathetic nerves in the guinea pig. *Br J Pharmacol* 1984;83:973–8.

187 Blaber LC, Fryer AD, MacLagen J. Neuronal muscarinic receptors attenuate vagally-induced contraction of feline bronchial smooth muscle. *Br J Pharmacol* 1985;36:723–8.

188 Minette P, Lammers J-W, Barnes PJ. Inhibitory muscarinic receptors on airway cholinergic nerves in man; evidence for a defect in asthma. *J Appl Physiol* (in press).

189 Bloom JW, Yamamura HI, Baumgartner C, Halonen M. A muscarinic receptor with high affinity for pirenzepine vagally induced bronchoconstriction. *Eur J Pharmacol* 1987;133:21–7.

190 Lammers J-W, Minette P, McCusker M, Barnes PJ. The role of pirenzepine-sensitive (M_1) muscarinic receptors in vagally mediated bronchoconstriction in humans. *Am Rev Respir Dis* 1989 (in press).

191 Barnes PJ. Adrenoceptors in bronchial asthma. In: Szbadi E, Bradshw CM,

Nahorski SR eds. *Pharmacology of adrenoceptors.* London: Macmillan 1985;205–14.

192 Barnes PJ. Endogenous catecholamines and asthma. *J Allergy Clin Immunol* 1986;**77**:791–6.

193 Cryer PE. Physiology and pathophysiology of the human sympathoadrenal neuroendocrine system. *N Engl J Med* 1980;**303**:436–44.

194 Ind PW, Causon RC, Brown MJ, Barnes PJ. Circulating catecholamines in acute asthma. *Br Med J* 1985;**290**:267–9.

195 Szentivanyi A. The β-adrenergic theory of the atopic abnormality in bronchial asthma. *J Allergy Clin Immunol* 1968;**42**:203–32.

196 Cerrina J, Ladurie ML, Labat C, Raffestin B, Bayol A, Brink C. Comparison of human bronchial muscle responses to histamine *in vivo* with histamine and isoprotenerol agonists *in vitro*. *Am Rev Respir Dis* 1986;**134**:57–61.

197 Goldie RG, Spina D, Henry PJ, Lulich KM, Paterson JW. *In vitro* responsiveness of human asthmatic blockers to carbachol, histamine, α-receptor agonists and theophylline. *Br J Clin Pharmacol* 1986;**22**:669–76.

198 Engels F, Oosting RS, Nijkamp FP. Pulmonary macrophages induce deterioration of guinea pig tracheal β-adrenergic function through release of oxygen radicals. *Eur J Pharmacol* 1985;**111**:143–4.

199 Barnes PJ, Grandordy B, Page CP, Rhoden KJ, Robertson DN. The effect of platelet-activating factor on pulmonary β-adrenoceptors. *Br J Pharmacol* 1987;**90**:709–15.

200 Grandordy B, Rhoden K, Barnes PJ. Effects of protein kinase C activation on adrenoceptors in airway smooth muscle. *Biochem Biophys Res Commun* 1989 (in press).

201 Kneussl MP, Richardson BJ. α-adrenergic receptors in human and canine tracheal and bronchial smooth muscle. *J Appl Physiol* 1978;**45**:307–11.

202 Barnes PJ, Skoogh B-E, Brown JK, Nadel JA. Activation of α-adrenergic responses in tracheal smooth muscle; a post-receptor mechanism. *J Appl Physiol* 1983;**54**:1469–76.

203 Brown JK, Shields R, Jones C, Gold WM. Augmentation of α-adrenergic responsiveness in trachealis muscle of living dogs. *J Appl Physiol* 1983;**54**:1558–66.

204 Barnes PJ, Skoogh B-E, Nadel JA, Roberts JM. Postsynaptic α$_2$-adrenoceptors predominate over α$_1$-adrenoceptors in canine tracheal smooth muscle and mediate neuronal and humoral α-adrenergic contraction. *Mol Pharmacol* 1983;**23**:570–5.

205 Barnes PJ, Ind PW, Dollery CT. Inhaled prazosin in asthma. *Thorax* 1981;**36**:378–81.

206 Barnes PJ, Wilson NM, Vickers H. Prazosin, an α$_1$ adrenoceptor antagonist partially inhibits exercise-induced asthma. *J Allergy Clin Immunol* 1981;**68**:411–5.

207 Larsson K, Martinsson A, Hjemdahl P. Influence of circulating α-adrenoceptor agonists on pulmonary function and cardiovascular variables in patients with exercise induced asthma and healthy subjects. *Thorax* 1986;**41**:552–7.

208 Boschetto P, Roberts NM, Rogers DF, Barnes PJ. The effect of antiasthma drugs on microvascular leakage in guinea pig airways. *Am Rev Respir Dis* 1988 (in press).

209 Barnes PJ. Non-adrenergic non-cholinergic neural control of human airways. *Arch Int Pharmacodyn* 1986;**230**(Suppl.):208–28.

210 Barnes PJ. Neuropeptides in the lung; Localization, function and pathophysiologic implications. *J Allergy Clin Immunol* 1987;**79**:285–95.

211 Barnes PJ. Airway neuropeptides and asthma. *Trends Pharm Sci* 1987;**8**:24–7.

212 Lammers J-W, Minette P, McCuster MT, Chung KF, Barnes PJ. Non-adrenergic bronchodilator mechanisms in normal human subjects *in vivo*. *J Appl Physiol* 1988;**64**:1817–22.

213 Lundberg HM, Saria A, Lundblad L *et al.* Bioactive peptides in capsaicin-sensitive C-fiber afferents of the airways; functional and pathophysiological implications. In: Kaliner MA, Barnes PJ eds. *The airways; neural control in health and disease.* New York: Marcel Dekker 1987:417–45.

214 Lammers J-W, Minette P, McCusker M, Chung KF, Barnes PJ. Non-adrenergic non-cholinergic bronchodilatation stimulated by capsaicin inhalation in normal and asthmatic subjects (abstract). *Am Rev Respir Dis* 1988;**137**:A240.

215 Frossard N, Barnes PJ. u-Opioid receptors modulate non-cholinergic constrictor nerves in guinea pig airways. *Eur J Pharmacol* 1987;**141**:519–21.

216 Belvisi MG, Chung MF, Jackson DM, Barnes PJ. Opioid control of non-cholinergic bronchoconstriction in the guinea pig *in vivo*. *Br J Pharmacol* 1988;**95**:413–8.

217 Joseph J, Bandler L, Anderson SD. Exercise as a bronchodilator. *Aust J Physiother* 1976;**12**:47–50.

218 Anderson SD, Seale JP, Ferris L, Schoeffel RE, Lindsay DA. An evaluation of pharmacotherapy for exercise-induced asthma. *J Allergy Clin Immunol* 1979;**64**:612–24.

219 Anderson SD. Current concepts of exercise-induced asthma. *Allergy* 1983;**36**:289–302.

220 Anderson SD, Silverman M, Konig P, Godfrey S. Exercise-induced asthma; a review. *Br J Dis Chest* 1975;**69**:1–39.

221 Schoeffel RE, Anderson SD, Seale JP. The protective effect and duration of action of metaproterenol on exercise-induced asthma. *Ann Allergy* 1981;**46**:273–5.

222 Anderson SD, Seale JP, Rozea P, Bandler L, Theobald G, Lindsay DA. Inhaled and oral salbutamol in exercise-induced asthma. *Am Rev Respir Dis* 1976;**114**:493–500.

223 Zielinski J, Chodosowska E. Exercise-induced bronchoconstriction in patients with bronchial asthma. Its prevention with an anti-histaminic agent. *Respiration* 1977;**34**:31–5.

224 Hartley JPR, Nogrady SG. Effect of an anti-histamine on exercise-induced asthma. *Thorax* 1980;**35**:675–9.

225 Patel KR. Terfenadine in exercise induced asthma. *Br Med J* 1984;**288**:1496–7.

226 Badier M, Beaumone and Orehek J. Attenuation of hyperventilation-induced bronchospasm by terfenadine; a new antihistamine. *J Allergy Clin Immunol* 1988;**81**:437–40.

227 Anderson SD. Exercise-induced asthma. The state of the art. *Chest* 1985;**875**:191-5.

228 Thomson NC, Patel KR, Kerr JW. Sodium cromoglycate and ipratropium bromide in exercise-induced asthma. *Thorax* 1978;**33**:694–9.

229 Henriksen JM, Dahl R. Effects of inhaled Budesonide alone and in combination with low-dose terbutaline in children with exercise-induced asthma. *Am Rev Respir Dis* 1983;**128**:993–7.

230 Konig P, Jaffe P, Godfrey S. Effects of corticosteroids on exercise-induced asthma. *J Allergy Clin Immunol* 1974;**54**:14–9.

231 Bianco S, Griffin JP, Kamburoff PL, Prime FJ. Prevention of exercise-induced asthma by indoramin. *Br Med J* 1974;**4**:18–20.

232 Seale JP, Anderson SD, Lindsay DA. A trial of an α-adrenoceptor blocking drug (indoramin) in exercise-induced bronchoconstriction. *Scand J Respir Dis* 1976;**57**:261–6.

233 Patel KR, Kerr JW, MacDonald EB, McKenzie AM. The effect of thymoxamine and cromolyn on post-exercise bronchoconstriction in asthma. *J Allergy Clin Immunol* 1976;**57**:285–92.

234 Rudolf M, Grant BJ, Saunders KB, Brostoff J, Salt PJ, Walker DI. Letter; aspirin in exercise-induced asthma. *Lancet* 1975;i:450.

235 Smith AP, Dunlop L. Prostaglandins and asthma. *Lancet* 1975;i:39.

236 Wallace D, Grieco MH. Double-blind, cross-over study of exercise-induced bronchospasm in adults. *Ann Allergy* 1976;37:153–63.
237 Sly RM, Matzen K. Effect of diethylcarbamazine pamoate upon exercise-induced obstruction in asthmatic children. *Ann Allergy* 1974;33:138–44.

7: Epidemiology

P. G. J. Burney, H. R. Anderson, B. Burrows,
M. Chan-Yeung, N. B. Pride & F. E. Speizer

Disease arises either from genetic variation or from an environmental exposure. Inflammatory and other pathophysiological explanations of disease represent intermediate events which may link gene products and environmental exposures to the disease process, but are not themselves sufficient explanations of disease. It is the principal task of epidemiology to define and quantify these genetic and environmental risks.

The experimental and morphological evidence linking inflammation and bronchial hyperresponsiveness (BHR) therefore raises two important epidemiological questions. What genetic and environmental origins might there be for such an inflammatory response, and how much of the variation in the prevalence of BHR could be explained by such risk factors? Mechanisms which can induce pathological changes under experimental conditions are only of epidemiological interest if they also help to explain the observed variation in disease prevalence. The effect of any agent is determined not only by its potential for doing harm, but also by levels of exposure and often by other exposures that may modify its effect. For this reason, the question of whether a potential risk factor, identified from experimental data, causes an important amount of clinical disease cannot receive a definitive answer that will apply for all places and at all times. Even so, mechanisms that seem to explain the distribution of disease must remain more interesting than those that do not.

There is, unfortunately, relatively little epidemiological information on the origins and distribution of BHR, and much of what follows will necessarily address the question of the origins of 'asthma' instead. This raises a further important issue. Dolovich and Hargreave have made a useful distinction between 'inducers' and 'inciters' of asthma. Inducers make subjects hyperresponsive to stimuli to which they would not have previously responded. Inciters, by contrast, simply stimulate bronchoconstriction in those who are already hyperresponsive.[1] Induction is clearly the more important process in the causation of asthma as it is normally understood. However, exposure to inciters will also increase the prevalence of symptoms and, if BHR itself has not been measured, it will be difficult to distinguish between the two processes. A range of irritant and potentially inflammatory agents are known or would be expected to be powerful inciters of asthma, and will therefore be associated with increased prevalence of asthmatic symptoms. It cannot be assumed that this is evidence for the induction of BHR without further evidence from studies that have measured BHR.

Epidemiological studies with direct evidence of airway inflammation are even rarer than epidemiological studies of BHR. This chapter will, therefore, review those environmental risk factors which have a clear association with inflammation and which have also been related to the origins of asthma. The central questions are whether there is good evidence that these risk factors cause BHR and, if so, whether this hyperresponsiveness is a marker of asthma as it is commonly understood, and to what extent these risk factors can explain the known distribution of asthma. The first risk factor, atopy, is the least controversial. The other risk factors that will be discussed are infection, pollution, occupation, and smoking.

ATOPY

Atopy is a poorly defined term referring to conditions which, as a group, tend to cluster in families, though each individual condition appears more sporadically. The conditions include hay fever (allergic rhinitis), eczema and other specific and non-specific allergic states, as well as asthma. Because atopy is defined as a clinical syndrome of which asthma is one component, there is an inevitable circularity in associating asthma with atopy. Atopy is, therefore, often inferred from immunological changes associated with this group of conditions including a positive response to allergen challenge in the skin and high concentrations of circulating IgE. In this chapter the term atopy will be used in this sense.

The idea that asthma might be associated with an abnormal response to allergens pre-dates any direct measurements of BHR. It has seemed for almost as long, however, that there are subjects who have asthma but who are not obviously atopic, and the condition was therefore divided into 'extrinsic' (apparently allergic) and 'intrinsic' (apparently non-allergic) disease. The question whether this was correct is an interesting one to which we shall return. The point here is that although the new classification may have provided some temporary solution to the discrepancy, it pre-empted once again any attempt to test the hypothesis that asthma was associated with, let alone caused by, atopy.

The advent of tests for BHR raised the question whether atopy is a risk factor for BHR and, if so, whether atopy causes BHR. A further question, and one that is central to the subject of this book, is whether any effect of atopy on BHR is mediated through some process which can be described under the general heading of 'inflammation'.

The findings of many studies now suggest that there is an association between BHR and atopy.[2–9] One study has suggested, however, that the association between positive skin tests and BHR depends on age. In the young, positive skin tests are very strong predictors of BHR, but this effect becomes progressively less pronounced with age.[7] This weakening association in older subjects is not entirely explained either by smaller skin weal responses or by the increasing proportion of subjects who have BHR associated with smoking and reduced baseline lung function (see below).

The causative nature of such a relation is supported by the effect on BHR of both avoidance of allergens and allergen challenge. Platts-Mills *et al.* have shown that avoidance of allergen leads to a lower BHR.[10] On the other hand, allergen challenge leads to an increased response to inhaled histamine and methacholine in some subjects;[11] this increase seems to follow only where subjects have had some evidence of a late response to the allergen challenge. The change does not seem to depend on a reduction in initial airway calibre.[12] Similar changes in BHR have been observed during the pollen season[13,14] and the ability to prevent the increase in BHR with corticosteroids suggests that the increase in reactivity may be mediated by an inflammatory mechanism.[14] Subjects with allergic rhinitis have also been shown to develop BHR during the pollen season.[15]

Atopy as an explanation of BHR

Several studies have raised important questions about the association between atopy and BHR. There are those studies which have failed to show an association[16–19] and not all of these findings can be explained by the age of the subjects studied or by the confounding effects of cigarette smoking and age. A body of research strongly suggests that BHR and atopy are, to a considerable extent, independent of each other. It has even been suggested that they are independently inherited characteristics.[20] This hypothesis that they are independent is supported by the observation that non-specific BHR and atopy are independent predictors of the bronchial response to allergens.[21] If atopy were the cause of non-specific BHR this would not be the case.

In any event, atopy does not explain the distribution of BHR and asthma observed in epidemiological studies. For example, current data do not suggest that those areas with the lowest prevalence of allergy are also those with the lowest prevalence of BHR. The evidence on this is poor, not least because of the difficulties that arise from the selection of allergens for a survey. The sensitivity to individual allergens may vary widely between areas; where a large enough battery of allergens is used, these areas may still be shown to have the same prevalence of positive skin tests.[22] The selection of appropriate areas to study in this respect is also difficult, and the common practice of selecting just two areas for comparison may lead to very substantial selection biases and seriously flawed conclusions. There are, however, some interesting data to be obtained from the National Health and Nutrition Examination Survey II (NHANES II) study. In this study on a stratified representative sample from the United States not only were answers recorded to questions about asthma and wheeze[23] but also the results of allergen skin tests were recorded.[24] Although the results have not yet been presented fully, an initial assessment of the published data shows that the distributions of the two sets of results are different. Asthma among children is most prevalent in the western and southern States. By contrast, the skin sensitivity tests showed a lower prevalence of atopy in the South than in any of the other regions. This is true not only for regional allergens such as ragweed, but also for indoor allergens such as house dust mites, which would be expected to thrive in the warm humid climate of the South. Possible confounding factors, such as the migration of asthmatics and asthmatic families to certain areas in the United States, will have to be controlled before further conclusions can be drawn from these data.

Atopy and asthma

Non-specific BHR is almost always present in any case of diagnosed asthma, and diagnosed asthma has been shown to be closely correlated with both skin test reactivity to common allergens[25] and to total serum IgE concentrations[26] in studies of general populations. Even the very persistent form of the disease characterised by chronic airflow obstruction (CAO)—a condition almost certainly closely associated with chronic airway inflammation—is related to evidence of allergy.[27] Recent observations strongly suggest that some type of IgE mediated process has a role in almost all asthmatic conditions, even when skin test reactivity to common allergens cannot be shown.[28] This seems to be true regardless of smoking history or age.

Atopy is undoubtedly associated with increased bronchial reactivity, and it seems likely that this is a causal association. Atopy in one form or another may be a necessary condition for true BHR that is not associated with a reduced baseline lung function. It seems most unlikely, however, that atopy is a sufficient cause for BHR. In so far as the secondary increase in BHR after exposure to an allergen seems to depend on a late phase response and is prevented by steroids, it is unlikely to be mediated through an inflammatory response. The inflammatory response induced by allergic mechanisms is relatively distinctive, and even if it is essential for the development of BHR in asthma, one cannot infer that other types of inflammation in the airways would have a similar effect.

It is because atopy is not a wholly satisfactory explanation for asthma that further causes or risk factors have been sought. The hypothesis that asthma might be induced through some common inflammatory mechanism has led to the exploration of other risk factors that are associated with an inflammatory response.

INFECTION

Measures of infection

The term 'infection' has no standard definition in epidemiological studies. Most studies rely on a report, often by the subject or parent, of a diagnosis which implies inflammation of a part of the respiratory tract, with infection being implied to a greater or lesser extent depending on the actual label (pneumonia, bronchitis, wheezy bronchitis). The reporting bias and failure of recall associated with such recollections make the data unreliable. Criteria based on clinical symptoms such as fever, malaise, headache, running nose, sore throat, cough, rash, response to antibiotics, are not universally agreed. The respiratory tract responds in a limited number of ways and these responses tend not to be specific for particular pathological processes. In many studies only illness has been assessed and it is uncertain how many of these illnesses represent infections. Nevertheless, there are some data based on well defined and specific infections which are associated with respiratory syncytial virus in infants and other viruses in older children.

Some epidemiological evidence, particularly that of a descriptive type, relies on routine statistics—mortality, notifications, surveillance systems—and all these present the usual problems of completeness, diagnostic variability, and peculiarities of the information system, particularly in relation to coding rules. Data from hospitals, clinics, and GPs vary for non-epidemiological reasons such as shifts in diagnosis and in the balance of care.

The short-term effects of clinical infections may be particularly difficult to distinguish among asthmatics. Tarlo *et al.* studied 19 married couples who were discordant for a diagnosis of asthma.[29] The same number in each group reported that they had had a 'cold' during the year, but the asthmatics had a greater number of 'colds', particularly in the spring and summer. Of 21 'colds' fully investigated among the asthmatics, however, only three were confirmed as being associated with a viral infection; six of the 10 'colds' fully investigated among the non-asthmatic spouses were confirmed as being associated with viral infections.

Infection and short-term increases in BHR/asthma

It has long been held that bacteria, by acting as allergens, may be asthmogenic, and this idea was the basis for the use of hyposensitisation treatment with bacterial allergens. The efficacy of this was never established, and it is no longer in vogue.[30] The belief that bacterial infection may precipitate or secondarily infect asthma remains strong and is supported by studies which have identified bacteria in the respiratory secretions of asthmatics. This is the rationale of antibiotic regimens though where trials have been carried out no effect on the natural history of the attack has been shown.[31,32] In the United Kingdom at least, there is evidence that this type of treatment is becoming less popular.[33] An increased prevalence of specific IgE against bacterial antigens in smokers has raised the possibility of a role for bacteria in the pathogenesis of chronic airway disease in this group.[34]

Many studies have identified viruses in patients who have asthmatic or wheezy episodes.[2,35-42] Wheezy children seem more likely to get wheezy if infected with some viruses, particularly rhinoviruses. The evidence about whether subjects prone to wheeze have an increased susceptibility to infection is conflicting.

The presence of clinical upper respiratory tract infection (URTI) in otherwise normal subjects has been associated with increased BHR[43] and increases in BHR have been observed following influenza A infection in college students.[44] A recent population survey found increased BHR with concomitant URTI but these findings were not significant.[7] No association has been found between clinical URTI and increased BHR in another large cross-sectional survey,[8] or in a smaller prospective survey.[45] An association between acute bronchitis and an increased BHR has been shown and was thought to be most likely due to a tendency for subjects with increased BHR to develop acute bronchitis.[46]

Hudgel *et al.* followed up 19 asthmatics by taking regular virological samples both at routine follow-up and whenever there was an exacerbation of the asthma.[47] They found evidence of viral infection in subjects during eight of 84 (9.5%) exacerbations compared with eight of 243 (3.3%) routine visits. It may be inferred from this that about 6% of all exacerbations were attributable to viral infection. Studies in children show rather larger risks for wheezing attributable to infection. Horn *et al.* showed viral infections in 26% of children with wheezy bronchitis, but in only 3.2% of the same children after recovery.[48] Viruses are less often isolated from atopic children than non-atopic children during wheezy episodes.[49]

The findings of studies on vaccines and their effects on BHR have reached varying conclusions. Ouellette and Reed,[50] Anand et al.,[51] and Banks et al.[52] all showed increased reactivity after killed influenza vaccine had been given to asthmatics. Sly and Schumbrecht,[53] Kiviloog[54] and de Jongste et al.[55] all failed to show such a change. Laitinen et al.,[56] de Jongste et al.[55] and Kava[57] have shown an effect of live attenuated influenza vaccine on BHR in asthmatics; de Jongste et al.,[55] Lowenberg et al.[58] and Kava[57] have all failed to show an effect of this vaccine on normal subjects and subjects with CAO. Kumar has shown an increase in BHR in children after they had been given live measles vaccine.[59]

We conclude that there is little evidence to associate bacterial infections with precipitation of asthma attacks. There is more evidence to associate viral infections with the precipitation of attacks in subjects who are already asthmatic. The association of clinical evidence of BHR with viral infections may be stronger among children. There is no evidence to suggest that infections are the only, or even a particularly common, cause of attack. Viral infections of both upper and lower respiratory tracts do seem to be associated with increased BHR.

The mechanisms that have been proposed to explain these changes include damage to the epithelium which exposes nerve endings to stimulation by inhaled agents,[43] the sensitisation of nerve endings by mediators,[60] changes in adrenergic responses and by viruses,[61] and the enhanced release of specific IgE from basophils by virus infections[62]

Do infections cause asthma/BHR?

Ecological considerations

The prevalence of respiratory infections tends to be similar between developed and underdeveloped countries, though the latter experience more variability in mortality.[63,64] Yet almost without exception, asthma tends to be less common in developing countries and varies between developed countries.[65] Population studies have confirmed that in underdeveloped countries a low prevalence of asthma and BHR coexist with high levels of upper and lower respiratory tract infections and levels of atopy which are similar to those in developed societies.[18,66]

In the United Kingdom the indicators of infection derived from data on mortality and prevalence do not correspond closely to those of asthma. Pneumonia and bronchitis tend to be more common in the North rather than the South, in urban rather than in rural areas, in manual rather than non-manual classes, and in relatively more crowded households, and where there is passive smoking.[67,68] By contrast, asthma and wheezing is more prevalent in the South, if anything, and is not usually found to be associated with the other factors, with the variable exception of passive smoking in early life.[69,70] Evidence based on a diagnosis of asthma shows an even greater disparity that is explained by social influences on labelling rather than on differences in morbidity. The above comments refer to children, the only group for whom adequate data on prevalence are available.

On the other hand, the high incidence of infections in early childhood and infancy corresponds to the relatively high incidence of wheezing illness at this time. Thereafter, however, asthma/BHR continue throughout childhood affecting 10% of the population while acute respiratory infections of the lower respiratory tract diminish. The associations with gender are also similar with a preponderance in boys until middle childhood.

Trends over time are difficult to describe, and it is probably futile to conjecture whether those for infections have corresponded to asthma (there are no data on trends in BHR). It is possible only to say that mortality from infections in childhood has declined noticeably over this century, including recent years, while the prevalence of asthma and wheezing illness has remained fairly steady since the 1950s.[71] Mortality from asthma increased in the mid-1960s but this did not correspond to any known infective epidemic. The same goes for the more recent rise in deaths from asthma in the United Kingdom.[72]

The demonstration of a seasonal association would be useful but again the evidence does not fit nicely with a precipitating infective agent. Most deaths from asthma in children and young people occur in the July–September quarter and most hospital admissions in the autumn.[73] The reasons for this are not clear but there are other possibilities apart from infection. Epidemics of respiratory syncytial virus tend to occur in the winter.[74] Most epidemics of asthma seem to be related to non-infective factors.[75] In older adults deaths and hospital admissions for asthma increase in the winter which corresponds to the time when infections are most common. The impossibility of distinguishing asthma from an exacerbation of chronic bronchitis and emphysema in routine statistical data makes this association difficult to interpret.

If infections were important for the induction of asthma in early life, and if this was more likely in those who are more vulnerable immunologically, one might expect asthma to be associated with births in certain seasons; there is such an association but studies are not consistent as to which season.[76]

Analytical studies

These general considerations can be compared with the results of studies on individuals. These studies have not all been designed to test assumptions as to whether infection may lead to the induction of asthma, but prevalence, case control, and cohort studies all provide some information that may be relevant to the question.

Prevalence studies in both children and adults tend to show an association between current or past asthma or wheezing and past infections such as bronchitis and pneumonia or 'chest trouble'.[70,77-79] Whether this is a real association is a difficult and often unanswerable question because of recall bias and lack of specificity and uniformity in the way past diseases have been described. An even more serious defect is the lack of evidence about the relative timing of onset of these illnesses.

Studies of specific infections identified from records or notifications and confirmed by microbiology and serology overcome some of these problems. Most have compared a cohort of cases with contemporary controls some years later. Bronchiolitis associated with respiratory syncytial virus has been linked to subsequent attacks of asthma and wheezing[80-83] and with increased BHR.[80-84] Children who had had whooping cough did not show increased BHR some years later, in spite of reporting more current wheezing at the time of follow up.[85] Two large studies of the sequelae of whooping cough have also found associations with subsequent wheezing.[86,87] This was also found in two cohort studies where whooping cough was assessed by parental interview alone.[70,77] The study of Johnston *et al.* was unable to show increased BHR in cases of whooping cough.[86] This study also showed that the higher tendency of these patients to wheeze existed before the date at which the whooping cough occurred; this suggests that the whooping cough did not cause the subsequent asthma.

The question of which comes first is best answered by cohort studies in which the relevant events are measured prospectively. In the National Childhood Development Study reports of pneumonia and whooping cough obtained from children at the age of seven were found to be predictive of the subsequent onset of asthma/wheeze.[70] Thus there is evidence that infections are associated with asthma/wheeze, and that either may precede the other. The evidence relating to BHR specifically is consistent for bronchiolitis caused by respiratory syncytial virus but not for other infections.

Given that these associations are statistically sound—which is a large assumption in view of the methodological difficulties—one can go on to consider the possible causal relations. These are: (i) that infection may cause BHR and asthma; (ii) that BHR and asthma predispose to infections or make them more severe, or recognisable, or symptomatically different; and (iii) that both are related to some other factor. There is little evidence to distinguish between the first two factors but what there is suggests that it is just as likely that BHR comes first. This is not to say that it may not also be exacerbated by infection. The third model is a plausible explanation for most of the associations that exist between early infections and later asthma. Atopy could be a common link by increasing the chance both of being susceptible to infection and of wheezing once infected. The evidence on this is conflicting.[81,84,88,89] As far as the connection between asthma and infection is concerned, BHR could be the common link.

Conclusion

Infections can precipitate asthma/wheezing and cause or exacerbate BHR in the short-term, but the extent to which infections are responsible for natural variations in BHR may have been exaggerated.

On a global basis the distribution of infections does not correspond at all to that of asthma.

In the United Kingdom the epidemiology of infection does not correspond to that of asthma in terms of geography, social class, crowding, environment or trends over time or by season. Analytical studies show an association between infection and the induction of asthma and in some instances BHR, but this may not be causal.

ENVIRONMENTAL POLLUTION

Exposure to a wide variety of stimuli will incite a response in subjects with non-specific BHR. Some common air pollutants such as sulphur dioxide (SO_2), ozone, nitrous oxide and particulates are irritant and can be included among these stimuli. Two questions arise from these observations:

1 Does exposure to these air pollutants account for a significant part of the variation in the observed prevalence of BHR and its symptoms?

2 Does exposure to these air pollutants cause BHR, as distinct from inciting a response in those who already have BHR?

Air pollution and exacerbations of clinical asthma

The heavy smog that occurred at Donora, Pennsylvania, in October 1948 was accompanied by an increase in symptoms in the population, particularly cough. The most severely affected people were those who identified themselves as having a history of asthma; though those with chronic bronchitis and heart disease were also affected.[90] This pattern of disease was also noted in the episode of air pollution reported in the Meuse Valley in 1930.[91] In most other similar episodes, however, elderly subjects with chronic bronchitis have primarily been affected.

The London smog of December 1952 was accompanied by a significant increase in mortality, particularly in the older age groups. There was at that time little evidence for an increase in mortality, or even of morbidity among non-smoking asthmatics. Fry noted in 1953 that in his general practice population the asthmatic children had not been affected by this very serious episode.[92]

The reports of a severe asthma-like illness among American servicemen and their dependants in the Tokyo-Yokahama plain of Japan in the mid-1950s were associated with high levels of air pollution.[93] The worst symptoms again seem to have been most commonly associated with heavy smokers,[94] while about 10% of asthmatics developed severe dyspnoea.[95] Oshima *et al.* were, however, unable to find any cases of 'Tokyo-Yokohama' asthma in a sample of Japanese workers living in the same highly polluted area.[96]

Outbreaks of asthma potentially associated with air pollution have also been studied in several places including, most notably, New Orleans and Barcelona. In New Orleans those affected were typical atopic asthmatics, subjects with chronic bronchitis were not affected. One would have expected these patients to be also affected if the cause of these epidemics was simple chemical air pollution, but there was no correlation between measures of chemical air pollutants and the timing of the outbreaks. In Barcelona there was one outbreak of asthma at the time of a temperature inversion and high levels of chemical air pollution, but subsequent studies have shown no association between symptoms and increased concentrations of nitrous oxide or SO_2.[97]

Goldstein and Weinstein studied the number of patients admitted to the emergency room and air pollution data (SO_2) for selected areas of New York in the period 1969–72.[98] They could find no association between the two, nor did they find a decrease in the number of patients with asthma visiting emergency rooms as the air pollution levels fell during this period. Unfortunately, a single monitoring station was taken to be representative of exposure in these studies. More recent studies by Bates and Sizto in Canada have shown a correlation between admissions of patients with asthma to hospital and seasonally adjusted exposures to higher levels of pollution from the products of combustion.[99] However, out of 21 regressions run for seven measures of pollution and three time lags, only three were significant at the 1% level. Two of the three associations were stronger for respiratory disease other than asthma and none were significant for asthma in 0–14 year olds. It is at least plausible that the associations noted are due to increased admissions of subjects with other chronic obstructive pulmonary disease.

Wittemore and Korn showed some effect of high concentrations of oxidant and particulate pollution on the likelihood of an attack in a panel of asthmatic volunteers.[100] Asthmatics in this study experienced about 20% more attacks on days when the levels of pollution were at the upper limit of the National Air Quality Standards for oxidants and particulates. Charpin *et al.* showed an association between wheeze and cough in children and daily mean SO_2 levels in areas with high pollution levels, but no such association in the less polluted areas.[101] In a sample of school children stratified by their responses to a respiratory symptom questionnaire, Vedal *et al.* failed to show any association between increased symptoms and higher concentrations of SO_2, though all these levels were consistently lower than the current air quality standards.[102] Kagamimori *et al.* have shown changes in respiratory symptoms associated with pollution by concentrations of SO_2 that are well within the current World Health Organisation standards.[103] Much of their evidence, however, is based on correlations between time trends and may be misleading. Hunt and Holman were unable to show an association between mean annual pollution level and admission to hospital in Kwinana, Western Australia, with very similar mean annual SO_2 concentrations.[104] Schenker *et al.* found no association between persistent wheeze and SO_2 concentrations at a range of levels of annual exposure that were all below the current ambient standards.[105] Although there was no association between wheeze and pollution level among children in the six city study, children with wheeze had a higher prevalence of cough and bronchitis than non-wheezy children and a steeper gradient of symptoms across increasing levels of pollution.

The epidemiological evidence as it stands provides little support for the view that the onset of asthma is affected to any major extent by levels of ambient chemical air pollution. There is some evidence that high levels of pollution may cause asthmatics to have some symptoms.

Air pollution as a cause of BHR/asthma

With such slight evidence for an association between air pollution and asthma/BHR, it seems unlikely that one could be an important risk factor for the other. This conclusion is further supported by Anderson's study of a population with very high exposure to air pollutants and virtually no asthma. Anderson studied 112 children from the highlands of New Guinea who were exposed to levels of particulate air pollution between 0.57 and 1.98 mg/m³ between the hours of 6.00 p.m. and 4.00 a.m.[106] These are very high levels, yet there was a virtual absence of asthma in these children. The failure of Oshima *et al.* to find asthma in Japanese workers in the highly polluted Tokyo-Yokohama plain is a further example of a highly exposed population with apparently little adverse effect.[96] If air pollution causes asthma it must be a very specific form of air pollution, or else it can only cause asthma under very specific circumstances. Until a more sophisticated hypothesis can be elaborated which will explain exceptions such as these, the evidence is only very tenuous that asthma can result from exposure to general air pollution.

OCCUPATION

Many agents in the working environment can cause asthma. The mechanism responsible for bronchoconstriction in many instances of occupational asthma is unknown. By far the largest number of occupational agents causing asthma have known or suspected allergenic properties. They cause asthma through sensitisation.

Almost all patients with symptomatic occupational asthma have evidence of BHR. When challenged with the offending agent by inhalation, most of these patients develop an immediate asthmatic reaction, or a biphasic reaction (immediate phase followed by a late phase).[107] The development of the late phase asthmatic reaction is associated with an increase in BHR.[108] Several studies have shown that removal of patients with occupational asthma from further exposure led to complete recovery in only about 40%; this recovery was associated with a decrease in, or a loss of BHR.[109] These findings suggest that BHR is the result of occupational exposure and that it is not the predisposing factor.

In patients with occupational asthma caused by exposure to western red cedar, toluene diisocyanate (TDI), bronchoalveolar lavage (BAL) studies showed an increase in neutrophils and eosinophils and an increase in protein and albumin in the bronchial fluid during the late asthmatic reaction induced by the offending agent. This suggests that airway inflammation is associated with an increase in BHR in these patients.[110,111]

When exposed to high concentrations of TDI (2 ppm), guinea-pigs developed BHR; depletion of leucocytes by hydroxyurea abolished this, suggesting that an inflammatory process is associated with BHR.[112] There are no cross-sectional or longitudinal studies, however, to show that exposure to high doses of irritant gases or fumes leads to an increase in BHR or asthma.

234

Evidence from the above clinical and experimental studies shows that airway inflammation is associated with BHR induced by occupational agents. It is, however, not possible to provide direct epidemiological evidence that airway inflammation is responsible for BHR. One can only provide epidemiological evidence that exposure to some occupational agents is associated with a higher prevalence of asthma or BHR, or both. Studies of 652 workers in red cedar sawmills showed that 4.1% had occupational asthma, and 19.4% had BHR (methacholine $PC_{20} <$ 8 mg/ml). The corresponding figures for the control group (440 office workers) were 1.6%, and 11.6%, respectively.[113] The differences between the groups were statistically significant. Similarly, 19.7% of workers exposed to dimethylphenyl diisocyanate in an iron and steel foundry had evidence of BHR.[114] To assess whether exposure to the above occupational agents is associated with an increase in BHR in the absence of asthma (or sensitisation) workers with current or past asthma from the analysis were excluded. After adjusting for initial FEV_1, cigarette smoking, age and atopy, there was no effect of exposure on the prevalence of BHR (methacholine $PC_{20} < 8$ mg/ml) to suggest that the above occupational agents cause BHR other than by causing asthma.[115]

'Reactive airways dysfunction syndrome' was described in 13 workers who developed asthma associated with BHR after one single exposure to a very high concentration of irritants, such as smoke, ammonia, chlorine, or welding fumes.[116] These patients did not have any existing respiratory symptoms. Evidence of airway inflammation was found in the bronchial biopsy specimens of two such patients which showed bronchial-bronchiolar epithelial desquamation and infiltration of the bronchial wall by plasma cells and lymphocytes.

An increased sensitivity to occupational allergens has been noted among smokers in some groups of workers.[117,118] The resulting allergies were specific to agents encountered in the workplace; there was no increase in sensitivity to common inhaled allergens. This is consistent with other studies which have failed to show greater sensitivity to inhaled allergens in smokers. Zetterstrom *et al.* showed that when rats were exposed to cigarette smoke they were more easily sensitised to inhaled allergens, but not to allergens injected subcutaneously.[119] They argued that this supported the view that cigarette smoking disrupted the airway epithelium and increased access of the allergen to deeper structures. Holt has suggested that the enhanced IgE and reduced IgG response seen in cigarette smokers is similar to that seen in conditions which are known to be associated with a specific defect in T-suppressor cell function.[120] His argument that this may be the mechanism in cigarette smokers is also supported by the observation that children born to mothers who are smokers have high cord IgE[121] and reduced T-suppressor cell function.[122] This supports the view that enhanced IgE production is a specific toxic effect of cigarettes rather than a non-specific inflammatory effect.

There is no good epidemiological evidence to suggest that exposure to occupational agents causes BHR other than by inducing asthma. Clinical and experimental studies have shown that occupational asthma is associated with BHR and airway inflammation.

SMOKING

Association between smoking, airway inflammation and BHR

A consistent feature of cross-sectional studies in non-asthmatic smokers is that the lower the baseline function, the more common and intense the BHR.[123-128] This relationship between BHR and baseline function appears to be much stronger in smokers than in asthmatic subjects.[127] Whether smokers whose lung function is within conventional normal limits show increased BHR is more controversial. Most early studies were based on small groups of smokers who were not drawn from any defined population. The results were highly variable with different studies claiming that smokers were less reactive than non-smokers,[129] more re-active than non-smokers,[130,131] and similarly reactive to non-smokers.[126,132-136] Interpretation of these studies is confounded by differences in the concentrations of bronchoconstric-tor agents used, whether a cut-off was used to divide 'responders' from 'non-responders', the exclusion of subjects with atopy, and differing assessment methods. However, a longer smoking history appears important in the two studies which showed increased reactivity.[130,131]

Community-based studies also have given varied results, but three studies conducted in the Netherlands which showed no, or only a very small, effect of smoking were biased towards younger individuals and may not have contained many heavy smokers.[137-139] Studies of BHR in the United Kingdom,[140] Australia,[141] and Italy,[142] have all found smoking an important factor, at least in older subjects,[140] while studies biased towards middle-aged or older men in Sweden[143] and the United States[144] have also shown an effect of smoking after controlling for baseline lung function.

Because considerable disease can be present in the periphery of the lung while total lung function remains normal, the finding of BHR in the presence of normal lung function does not necessarily imply that the BHR precedes, rather than follows, significant lung damage. Overall, the cross-sectional data support the idea that, at least in men, the BHR of non-asthmatic smokers is commonly acquired many years after the onset of smoking.

The development of chronic airway obstruction (CAO), conventionally due to varying combinations of obliteration and narrowing of small bronchi and bronchioles and of alveolar destruction, is itself the result of a current or previous inflammatory process. Even in the stable state between clinically evident episodes of bronchopulmonary infections, there is often evidence of CAO, with an increase in polymorphonuclear cells in sputum[145] and BAL fluid,[146] and a chronic increase in the number of neutrophils and total white cells in the venous blood.[147-150] Some large studies have found a positive correlation between total white cell count in the peripheral blood and daily consumption of cigarettes, and a negative correlation between white cell count and baseline FEV_1.[147,149]

Because of the coexistence of BHR, reduced lung function and airway inflammation in many smokers, there is considerable difficulty in elucidating whether airway inflammation has a direct role in inducing BHR over and beyond its role in causing structural damage to the lungs. The only study that has directly correlated non-specific responsiveness with airway pathology in smokers was based on lobectomy specimens and found that inflammation in membranous bronchioles (but not in larger airways) was related to the intensity of bronchial responsiveness.[128] This relationship appeared to be independent of the correlation also present between BHR and baseline lung function.

Nevertheless, so far it has not been possible to show that two interventions expected to reduce airway inflammation without greatly altering baseline lung function in smokers—quitting smoking and treatment with inhaled corticosteroids—attenuate bronchial responsiveness in smokers. Three months' treatment with a daily dose of 800 or 1200 μg of an inhaled corticosteroid which attenuates BHR in subjects with asthma[145,151,152] has failed to attenuate BHR in smokers in two separate studies, so far only published as abstracts.[153,154] Although sequential studies of the effects of quitting smoking on BHR are not very satisfactory, they do fail to show consistent changes in BHR.[131,155] The National Heart Lung Blood Institute Study now in progress should provide definitive data on this point. In a study in which 17 ex-smokers with BHR were restudied after an interval of 4 years, BHR was on average unchanged, although FEV_1 showed only the expected 'normal' age-related change. Indeed, for a given impairment of FEV_1, BHR was on average actually greater in ex-smokers than continuing smokers.[156] Although it is conceivable that smokers with BHR are more likely to quit, and there is evidence that ex-smokers do show more allergic features (positive skin tests and raised IgE) than expected, smoking would nevertheless be expected to be interactive with atopy[140] (see Figure 7.1), and the failure of BHR to attenuate in subsequent years after giving up smoking emphasises the importance of baseline dimensions in determining BHR in smokers and ex-smokers. A weakness in this argument is that ex-smokers have not been shown to have increased bronchial responsiveness in several cross-sectional

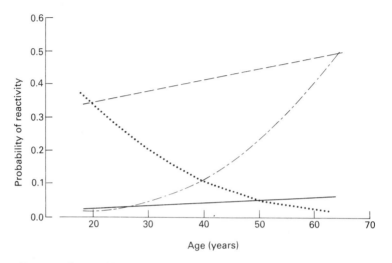

Fig. 7.1 Relation of bronchial hyperresponsiveness to age, skin sensitivity and smoking history. Estimated proportion of reactive subjects according to age among (i) non-smoking, non-atopic subjects (——); (ii) non-smoking subjects with 4 mm mean skin weal diameters (.....); (iii) non-atopic smokers (– · – · –); and (iv) current smokers with 4 mm mean skin weal diameter (– – – –).

studies;[138,143,144] but the length of smoking history in these individuals is not clear, nor whether they had increased responsiveness when they were smoking. Another possible objection can be found in the results from a morphological study which suggested that inflammation in the peripheral airways was as severe in ex-smokers as in current smokers;[157] but most other evidence suggests that inflammation is reduced in ex-smokers and that there is also a decreased sputum volume,[158] fewer neutrophils in BAL fluid,[159] lower blood total WBC count,[150] and slower annual decline in FEV_1[126,156,158] than in continuing smokers.

Differences between BHR in asthmatic subjects and smokers

In asthma the dominant current hypothesis for the development of BHR proposes that sensitisation to inhaled antigen leads to airway inflammation which, in turn, induces BHR. In the original Dutch hypothesis, smoking was regarded as amplifying an endogenous, allergic constitution and recent interest in the role of allergic factors in smokers has been revived by the observations of greater sensitisation to certain occupational allergens,[117,118] raised levels of total serum IgE,[150,160] and increased blood eosinophil counts[150,161] in non-asthmatic smokers. However, Taylor *et al.*[126] were unable to show any relationship between blood eosinophil count or total IgE levels and BHR in non-asthmatic smokers. Also, Burrows *et al.*[162] have recently found that once subjects in whom asthma has been diagnosed are excluded, these allergic markers are no longer related to ventilatory impairment in the community. Bronchial wall biopsies show that eosinophil involvement is more important in asthma than in smokers with chronic bronchitis.[163] There are probably other differences in the nature of the inflammatory process in the two conditions which may account for the observation that inhaled corticosteroids and quitting smoking are apparently effective in attenuating BHR in asthmatic subjects[151,152,164] than in non-asthmatic smokers.[131,153–155] Other differences between the BHR of asthma and of smokers, such as the closeness of the relation to baseline lung function and to diurnal variation in lung function, the presence of limits to bronchial narrowing, the response to isocapnic hyperventilation, or to inhaled β-adrenoceptor blocking drugs have been described (see Chapter 1) but at present these are descriptive and do not allow further speculation on the pathogenesis of BHR in the two conditions.

Effects of smoking on bronchial responsiveness in subjects with asthma

The BHR of asthma would be expected to be worsened by active smoking. This is a very difficult area to study without selection bias because asthmatic children are particularly discouraged from taking up smoking and some who experiment with smoking presumably quit rapidly because of acute worsening of symptoms. Any adverse effect of smoking is not so strong and universal as to make smoking a rarity among asthma subjects[165] while the onset of asthma in middle-age has been stated to be no more common in smokers than non-smokers.[166] Indeed, there is a contrary strand of reports of asthma first emerging after quitting smoking.[167] Direct evidence on changes in BHR is sparse, but recently large decreases in BHR have been reported in asthmatic smokers within 1–7 days of quitting smoking[164] which is presumably well before inflammatory changes in the airways would be expected to settle. Further studies are obviously needed.

The transient bronchoconstrictor effects of inhaling cigarette smoke have been extensively studied.[168,169] These effects presumably occur in asthmatic as well as normal subjects and could account for the frequent complaint that asthma is worsened by passive exposure to cigarette smoke. A more sustained effect on non-specific bronchial responsiveness has also been proposed. In young adults with asthma, one study has shown a reduction in intensity of BHR shortly after passive exposure to cigarette smoke for one hour,[170] while another study showed worsening of BHR four hours after similar exposure.[171] Several studies have shown a relation between passive smoking and decreased levels of pulmonary function in children, and passive smoking may enhance bronchial responsiveness in asthmatic children,[172,173] but it is uncertain whether it actually induces BHR or increases the risk of development of asthma.[173,174]

CONCLUSION

The hypothesis that asthma or BHR might be caused by airway inflammation raises two important epidemiological questions. What are the important environmental or genetic origins of this inflammation, and what proportion of BHR can be attributed to them? Answering these questions at the present time, however, raises a number of difficulties.

Firstly, there is the problem that relatively little epidemiological work has yet been done on the distribution of BHR, and the data that do exist are largely related to clinical symptoms or diagnosed illness. This poses a major problem for studies of the origin of BHR, as symptoms may be provoked by agents that do not necessarily induce hyperresponsiveness and yet this will lead to an increase in the prevalence of symptoms and even of diagnosed cases. It is not possible, therefore, to draw a simple conclusion concerning the origins of BHR from the association of agents with the presence of symptoms.

Secondly, there are very few epidemiological studies that look directly at airway inflammation. The only question that can be tackled by epidemiologists at the moment, therefore, is the rather less direct question of whether those agents that are thought to be likely causes of airway inflammation, are also causes of BHR.

There is some evidence that common inflammatory agents are associated with exacerbations of asthma and an increase in symptoms in asthmatic individuals. This evidence is not, however, consistent, and it is hard to implicate the common causes of airway inflammation in more than a small proportion of episodes of worsening asthma. There is evidence that viral infections exacerbate asthma particularly among children, but there is little evidence that viral infections are responsible for more than a small number of exacerbations in adults, even in known asthmatics. Similarly, there is some evidence for increasing symptoms with increasing levels of air pollution, but this effect has only been shown at relatively high levels of air pollution, and some major episodes of pollution have appeared to have little effect even on known asthmatics.

Evidence for the stronger hypothesis, that BHR is itself induced by inflammation, is even more difficult to find. The broad distribution of asthma, in any case, runs contrary to such a hypothesis. Asthma seems to be, if anything, less common in those groups that would be expected to have the greatest exposure to agents that are thought to cause inflammation in the airway. Areas in the developing world where asthma has, at least in the past, been extremely rare, are areas where there is as much respiratory tract infection, and a great deal more serious respiratory tract infection than in the West. In the West, poorer areas do not seem to have more asthma, nor has the prevalence of asthma shown any marked decline to parallel the decline in serious chest infections in children. There are also counter-instances that make it unlikely that air pollution can, by itself, induce BHR.

Other evidence from cigarette smokers strongly suggests that inflammation itself cannot induce hyperresponsiveness. There is little doubt that smokers do have inflammation of the airway and an increased response to inhaled histamine and methacholine, but current evidence favours the hypothesis that this is due to the long term decline in airway calibre seen in this group. The failure of this hyperresponsiveness to diminish on stopping smoking and the failure to attenuate it with anti-inflammatory agents strongly suggest that current inflammation does not adequately explain the BHR seen in non-atopic smokers.

It is, perhaps, too simple to expect that there would be a straightforward association between inflammation and hyper-responsiveness, as both of these terms encompass a range of heterogeneous conditions. If inflammation in general does not cause BHR, it is of interest to know the type of inflammation that may do so, or under what particular circumstances. It is not clear that the idea that 'atopy is an inflammatory condition' adds much to the general proposition that 'atopy is a risk factor for BHR' unless some more specific meaning can be attached to the term 'inflammation'. The question naturally arises whether some more specific formulation of the hypothesis might be more successful, but this question can only be answered empirically when a more specific formulation has been proposed, and it would appear that this is still a long way off. Until such a new formulation has been proposed, conjectures that inflammation 'causes' BHR are probably either wrong or not very meaningful.

From the point of view of the epidemiologist trying to explain the distribution of asthma, the 'inflammatory process' does not look promising. Until some more precise and convincing version of the hypothesis can be provided, it would appear that other clues are more likely to repay investigation. These would include the observation of a very strong link between serum IgE levels and the clinical 'asthma' of all kinds and the relation between dietary sodium and BHR. These are more precisely formulated hypotheses that can be explored further, both in the direction of their environmental and genetic determinants, and in the direction of pathogenic mechanisms.

REFERENCES

1 Dolovich J, Hargreave FE. The asthma syndrome; inciters, inducers and host characteristics. *Thorax* 1981;**36**:641–4.

2 Kreukiet J, Pijper MM. Response to inhaled histamine and to inhaled allergens in atopic patients. *Respiration* 1973;**30**:345.

3 Muranaka M, Suzuki S, Miyamoto T, Takeda K, Okumura H, Makino S. Bronchial reactivities to acetylcholine and IgE levels in asthmatic subjects after long term remission. *J Allergy Clin Immunol* 1974;**54**:32.

4 Stevens WJ, Lins RL, Vermeire PA. Comparative study of bronchial reactivity and atopic status in asthma and rhinitis. *Thorax* 1978;**33**:533–4.

5 Cockcroft D, Murdock K, Berscheid B. Relationship between atopy and bronchial responsiveness to histamine in a random population. *Ann Allergy* 1984;**53**:26–9.

6 Coockson WOCM, Musk AW, Ryan G. Associations between asthma history, atopy, and non-specific bronchial responsiveness in young adults. *Clin Allergy* 1986;**16**:425–32.

7 Burney PGJ, Britton JR, Chinn S *et al*. Descriptive epidemiology of bronchial reactivity in an adult population; results from a community study. *Thorax* 1987;**42**:38–44.

8 Woolcock AJ, Peat JK, Salome CM *et al*. Prevalence of bronchial hyperresponsiveness and asthma in a rural adult population. *Thorax* 1987;**42**:361–8.

9 Kennedy S, Burrows B, Enerson D, Chan-Yeung M. Bronchial hyperresponsiveness, once adjusted for FEV_1 level, is not increased in non-atopic smokers. *Am Rev Respir Dis* 1988;**137**:A31.

10 Platts-Mills T, Mitchell E, Nock P, Tovey E, Maszoro H, Wilkins SR. Reduction of bronchial hyperreactivity during prolonged allergen avoidance. *Lancet* 1972;**ii**:675–8.

11 Cockcroft DW, Killian DN, Mellor JJA, Hargreave FE. Bronchial reactivity to inhaled histamine; a method and clinical survey. *Clin Allergy* 1977;**7**:235–43.

12 Cartier A, Thomson NC, Frith PA, Roberts R, Hargreave FE. Allergen-induced increase in bronchial responsiveness to histamine; relationship to the late asthmatic response and change in airway caliber. *J Allergy Clin Immunol* 1982;**70**:170–7.

13 Boulet LP, Cartier A, Thomson NC, Roberts RS, Dolovich J, Hargreave FE. Asthma and increases in non-allergic bronchial responsiveness from seasonal pollen exposure. *J Allergy Clin Immunol* 1983;**71**:399–406.

14 Sotomayor H, Badier M, Vervloet D, Orehek J. Seasonal increase of carbachol airway responsiveness in patients allergic to grass pollen. Reversal by corticosteroids. *Am Rev Respir Dis* 1984;**130**:56–8.

15 Madonini E, Briatico-Vangosa G, Pappacoda A, Maccagni G, Cardani A, Saporiti F. Seasonal increase of bronchial reactivity in allergic rhinitis. *J Allergy Clin Immunol* 1987;**79**:358–63.

16 van der Lende R, Visser BF, Wever-Hess J, de Vries K, Orie NGM. Distribution of histamine threshold values in a random population. *Rev Inst Hyg Mines* (Hasselt) 1973;**28**:186–90.

17 Bryant DH, Burns MW. The relationship between bronchial histamine reactivity and atopic status. *Clin Allergy* 1976;**6**:373–81.

18 Woolcock AJ, Colman MH, Jones MW. Atopy and bronchial reactivity in Australian and Melanesian populations. *Clin Allergy* 1978;8:155–64.

19 Welty C, Weiss ST, Tager IB *et al.* The relationship of airway responsiveness to cold air, cigarette smoking, and atopy to respiratory symptoms and pulmonary function in adults. *Am Rev Respir Dis* 1984;130:198–203.

20 Sibbald B, Horn MEC, Brain EA, Gregg I. Genetic factors in childhood asthma. *Thorax* 1980;35:671–4.

21 Cockcroft D, Ruffin RE, Frith PA *et al.* Determinants of allergen induced asthma; dose of allergen, circulating IgE antibody concentration and bronchial responsiveness to inhaled histamine. *Am Rev Respir Dis* 1979;120:1053–8.

22 Britton WJ, Woolcock AJ, Peat JK, Sedgwick CJ, Lloyd DM, Leeder SR. Prevalence of bronchial hyperresponsiveness in children; the relationship between asthma and skin reactivity to allergens in two communities. *Int J Epidemiol* 1986;15:202–9.

23 Gergen PJ, Mullally DI, Evans R. National survey of prevalence of asthma among children in the United States 1976 to 1980. *Pediatrics* 1988;81:1–7.

24 Gergen PJ, Turkeltaub PC. Percutaneous immediate hypersensitivity to eight allergens. In: *United States 1976–80. Vital and health statistics*, Series 11, no. 235. Washington: Public Health Service 1986.

25 Burrows B, Lebowitz MD, Barbee RA. Respiratory disorders and allergy skin-test reactions. *Ann Intern Med* 1976;84:134–9.

26 Burrows B, Halonen M, Lebowitz MD, Knudson RJ, Barbee RA. The relationship of serum immunoglobulin E, allergy skin tests, and smoking to respiratory disorders. *J Allergy Clin Immunol* 1982;70:199–204.

27 Burrows B, Bloom JW, Traver GA, Cline MG. The course and prognosis of different forms of chronic airways obstruction in a sample from the general population. *N Engl J Med* 1987;317:1309–14.

28 Burrows B, Martinez FD, Halonen M, Barbee RA, Cline MG. Association of asthma with serum IgE levels and skin-test reactivity to allergens. *New Engl J Med* 1989;320:271–7.

29 Tarlo S, Broder I, Spence L. A prospective study of respiratory infection in adult asthmatics and their normal spouses. *Clin Allergy* 1979;9:293–301.

30 Stenius-Aarniala B. The role of infection in asthma. *Chest* 1987;91:157S–60S.

31 Graham VAL, Knowles GK, Milton AF, Davies RJ. Routine antibiotics in hospital management of acute asthma. *Lancet* 1982;i:418–20.

32 Berman SZ, Mathison DA, Stevenson DD, Tan EM, Vaughan JH. Transtracheal aspiration studies in asthmatic subjects in relapse with 'infective' asthma and in subjects without respiratory disease. *J Allergy Clin Immunol* 1975;56:206–14.

33 Anderson HR, Bailey P, West S. Trends in the hospital care of acute childhood asthma 1970–8; a regional study. *Br Med J* 1980;281:1191.

34 Bloom JW, Halonen M, Dunn AM, Pinnas JL, Burrows B. Pneumococcus-specific immunoglobuline in cigarette smokers. *Clin Allergy* 1986;16:25–32.

35 Stempel DA, Boucher RC. Respiratory infection and airway reactivity. *Med Clin North Am* 1981;65:1045–53.

36 Horn MEC, Brain E, Gregg I, Yealland SJ, Inglis JM. Respiratory viral infection in childhood. A survey in general practice, Roehampton 1967–1972. *J Hyg Camb* 1975;74:157–68.

37 Horn MEC, Brain EA, Gregg I, Inglis JM, Yealland SJ, Taylor P. Respiratory viral infection and wheezy bronchitis in childhood. *Thorax* 1979;34:23–8.

38 Mitchell I, Inglis H, Simpson H. Viral infections in wheezy bronchitis and asthma in children. *Arch Dis Child* 1976;51:707–11.

39 Minor TE, Dick EC, Baker JW, Ouellette JJ, Cohen M, Reed CE. Rhinoviruses and influenza type A infections as precipitants of asthma. *Am Rev Respir Dis* 1976;113:149–53.

40 Minor TE, Baker JW, Dick EC *et al*. Greater frequency of viral respiratory infections in asthmatic children as compared with their nonasthmatic siblings. *J Pediatrics* 1974;**85**:472–7.

41 Minor TE, Dick EC, De Meo AN, Ouellette JJ, Cohen M, Reed CE. Viruses as precipitants of asthmatic attacks in children. *JAMA* 1974;**227**:292–8.

42 Lambert HP, Stern H. Infective factors in exacerbations of bronchitis and asthma. *Br Med J* 1972;**3**:323–7.

43 Empey DW, Laitinen LA, Jacobs L, Gold WM, Nadel JA. Mechanisms of bronchial hyperreactivity in normal subjects after upper respiratory tract infection. *Am Rev Respir Dis* 1976;**113**:131–9.

44 Little JA, Hall WJ, Douglas RG, Mudholker GS, Speers DM, Patel K. Airway hyperreactivity and peripheral airway dysfunction in influenza A infection. *Am Rev Respir Dis* 1978;**118**:295–303.

45 Jenkins CR, Breslin ABX. Upper respiratory tract infections and airway reactivity in normal and asthmatic subjects. *Am Rev Respir Dis* 1984;**130**:879–83.

46 Boldy DAR, Ayres JG. Acute bronchitis and bronchial hyperreactivity to histamine; a descriptive study in the community. *Thorax* 1988;**43**:247P.

47 Hudgel DW, Langston L, Selner JC, McKintosh K. Viral and bacterial infections in adults with chronic asthma. *Am Rev Respir Dis* 1979;**120**:393–7.

48 Horn MEC, Brain EA, Gregg I, Inglis JM, Yealland SJ, Taylor P. Respiratory viral infection and wheezy bronchitis in childhood. *Thorax* 1979;**34**:23–8.

49 Horn MEC, Reed SE, Taylor P. Role of viruses and bacteria in acute wheezy bronchitis in childhood; a study of sputum. *Arch Dis Child* 1979;**54**:587–92.

50 Ouellette JJ, Reed CE. Increased response of asthmatic subjects to methacholine after influenza vaccine. *J Allergy* 1965;**36**:558–63.

51 Anand SC, Itkin IH, Kind LS. Effect of influenza vaccine on methacholine (Mecholyl) sensitivity in patients with asthma of known and unknown origin. *J Allergy* 1968;**42**:187–92.

52 Banks J, Bevan C, Fennerty A, Ebden P, Walters EH, Smith AP. Association between rise in antibodies and increase in airway sensitivity after intramuscular injection of killed influenza virus in asthmatic patients. *Eur J Respir Dis* 1985;**66**:268–72.

53 Sly RH, Schumbrecht L. Effect of influenza vaccine upon susceptibility to the induction of bronchospasm by exercise. *J Allergy* 1968;**42**:182–6.

54 Kiviloog J. Variability of bronchial reactivity to exercise and methacholine in bronchial asthma. *Scan J Respir Dis* 1973;**54**:359–68.

55 de Jongste JC, Degenherdt HJ, Neijens HJ, Duiverman EJ, Raatgeep HC, Kerrebijn FK. Bronchial responsiveness and leucocyte reactivity after influenza vaccine in asthmatic patients. *Eur J Respir Dis* 1984;**65**:196–200.

56 Laitinen LA, Elkin RB, Empey DW *et al*. Changes in bronchial reactivity after administration of live attenuated influenza virus. *Am Rev Respir Dis* 1976;**113**:194.

57 Kava T. Acute respiratory infection, influenza vaccination and airway reactivity in asthma. *Eur J Respir Dis* 1987;**70**:(Suppl.150).

58 Lowenberg A, Orie NGM, Sluiter HJ, Vries K. Bronchial hyperreactivity and bronchial obstruction in respiratory viral infection. *Respiration* 1986;**49**:1–9.

59 Kumar L, Newcomb RW, Molk L. Effect of live measles vaccine on bronchial sensitivity of asthmatic children to methacholine. *J Allergy* 1970;**45**:104.

60 Pauwels R. Mediators and non-specific hyperreactivity. *Eur J Respir Dis* 1983;**64**(Suppl.129):95–111.

61 Busse WW, Cooper W, Warshaver DM, Dick EC, Wallow IHL, Albrecht R. Impairment of isoproterenol, H_2 histamine, and prostaglandin E1 response of human granulocytes after incubation *in vitro* with live influenza vaccines. *Am Rev Respir Dis* 1979;**119**:561–9.

62 Ida S, Hooks JJ, Siraganian RP. Notkins A. Enhancement of IgE-mediated

histamine release from human basophils by viruses; role of interferon. *J Exp Med* 1977;**145**:892–906.

63 Chretien J, Holland W, Macklem P, Murray J, Woolcock A. Acute respiratory infections in children; a global public-health problem. *N Engl J Med* 1984;**310**:982–84.

64 Acute respiratory infections in under-fives; 15 million deaths a year. *Lancet* 1985;ii:699–701.

65 Cookson JB. Prevalence rates of asthma in developing countries and their comparison with those in Europe and North America. *Chest* 1987;**91**:97S-103S.

66 Anderson HR. The epidemiological and allergic features of asthma in the New Guinea Highlands. *Clin Allergy* 1984;**4**:171–83.

67 Colley JRT, Reid DD. Urban and social origins of childhood bronchitis in England and Wales. *Br Med J* 1970;**2**:213–7.

68 Taylor B, Wadsworth J, Goldring J, Butler N. Breast-feeding, bronchitis, and admissions for lower-respiratory illness and gastroenteritis during the first five years. *Lancet* 1982;i:1227–9.

69 Office of Population and Consensus Studies. Child health; a collection of studies. *Studies on medical and population subjects*, No. 31. London: HMSO 1976.

70 Anderson HR, Bland JM, Patel S, Peckham C. The natural history of asthma in childhood. *J Epidemiol Community Health* 1986;**40**:121–9.

71 Anderson HR. Is the prevalence of asthma changing? *Arch Dis Child Health* 1989;**4**:172–5.

72 Burney PGJ. Asthma mortality in England and Wales; evidence for a further increase 1974–84. *Lancet* 1986;ii:323–6.

73 Khot A, Burn R, Evans N, Lenney C, Lenney W. Seasonal variation and time trends in childhood asthma in England and Wales 1975–81. *Br Med J* 1984;**289**:235–7.

74 Medical Research Council, subcommittee on respiratory syncytial virus. Respiratory syncytial virus infection; admissions to hospital in industrial, urban and rural areas. *Br Med J* 1978;**2**:796–8.

75 Asthma and the weather (editorial). *Lancet* 1985;i:1079–80.

76 Anderson HR, Bailey PA, Bland JM. The effect of birth month on asthma, eczema, hayfever, respiratory symptoms, lung function, and hospital admissions for asthma. *Int J Epidemiol* 1981;**10**:45–51.

77 Bland JM, Holland WW, Elliot A. Development of respiratory symptoms in cohort of Kent schoolchildren. *Bull Eur Physiopathol Resp* 1984;**10**:69–71.

78 Burrow B, Knudson RJ, Lebowitz MD. The relationship of childhood respiratory illness to adult obstructive airways disease. *Am Rev Respir Dis* 1977;**115**:751–60.

79 Holland WW, Bailey P, Bland JM. Long term consequences of respiratory disease in infancy. *J Epidemiol Community Health* 1978;**32**:256–9.

80 Rooney JC, Williams HE. The relationship between proved viral bronchiolitis and subsequent wheezing. *J Pediatr* 1971;**79**:744–7.

81 Sims DG, Downham MAPS, Gardner PS, Webb JKG, Weightman D. Study of 8-year-old children with a history of respiratory syncytial virus bronchiolitis in infancy. *Br Med J* 1978;i:11–4.

82 Pullan CR, Hey EN. Wheezing, asthma and pulmonary dysfunction 10 years after infection with respiratory syncytial virus in infancy. *Br Med J* 1982;**284**:1665–9.

83 Mok JY, Simpson H. Outcome of acute lower respiratory tract infection in infants; preliminary report of seven-year follow-up study. *Br Med J* 1982;**285**:333–7.

84 Mok JYQ, Simpson H. Symptoms, atopy, and bronchial reactivity after lower respiratory infection in infancy. *Arch Dis Child* 1984;**59**:299–305.

85 Johnson IDA, Bland JM, Ingram D, Anderson HR, Warner JO, Lambert HP. Effect of whooping cough in infancy on subsequent lung function and bronchial reactivity. *Am Rev Respir Dis* 1986;**134**:270–5.

86 Johnson IDA, Anderson HR, Lambert HP. Patel S. Respiratory morbity and lung function after whooping cough. *Lancet* 1983;ii:1104–8.

87 Swansea Research Unit of the Royal College of General Practitioners. Respiratory sequelae of whooping cough. *Br Med J* 1985;**290**:1937–40.

88 Sims DG, Gardner PS, Weightman D, Turner MW, Soothill JF. Atopy does not predispose to RSV bronchiolitis or postbronchiolitic wheezing. *Br Med J* 1901;**282**:2086–8.

89 Cogswell JJ, Halliday DF, Alexander JR. Respiratory infections in the first year of life in children at risk of developing atopy. *Br Med J* 1982;**284**:1011–3.

90 Schrenk HH, Heimann H, Clayton GD, Gafafer WM, Wexler H. Air pollution in Donora, Pennsylvania: epidemiology of the unusual smog episode of October 1948. *Public Health Bulletin* 1949:306.

91 Firket J. Sur les causes des accidents survenus dans la vallée de la Meuse, lors des brouillards de Decembre. *Bull Acad R Med Belge* 1931;2:683.

92 Fry J. Effects of severe fog on a general practice. *Lancet* 1953;i:235–6.

93 Huber TE, Sheldon WJ, Knoblock E, Redfearn PL, Karakawa JA. New environmental respiratory disease. *Arch Indstr Hyg* 1954;**10**:399–408.

94 Phelps HW, Koike S. Tokyo-Yokohama asthma. *Am Rev Respir Dis* 1962;**86**:55–63.

95 Sponitz M. The significance of Yokohama asthma. *Am Rev Respir Dis* 1965;**92**:371–5.

96 Oshima Y, Ishizaki T, Miyamoto T, Kabe J, Makino S. A study of Tokyo-Yokohama asthma among Japanese. *Am Rev Respir Dis* 1964;**90**:632–4.

97 Anto JM, Sunyer J. A point source asthma outbreak. *Lancet* 1986;i:900–3.

98 Goldstein IF, Weinstein AL. Air pollution and asthma; effects of exposure to short-term sulphur dioxide peaks. *Environ Res* 1986;**40**:332–45.

99 Bates DV, Sizto R. Relationship between air pollutant levels and hospital admissions in Southern Ontario, Canada. *J Public Health* 1983;**74**:117–22.

100 Wittemore AS, Korn EL. Asthma and air pollution in the Los Angeles area. *Am J Public Health* 1980;**70**:687–96.

101 Charpin D, Kleisbauer JP, Fondarai J, Graland B, Viala A, Govezo F. Respiratory symptoms and air pollution changes in children; the Gardanne Coal-Basin Study. *Arch Envir Health* 1988;**43**:22–7.

102 Vedal S, Schenker MB, Munoz A, Samet JM, Batterman S, Speizer FE. Daily air pollution effects on children's respiratory symptoms and peak expiratory flow. *Am J Public Health* 1987;**77**:694–8.

103 Kagamimori S, Katsh T, Naruse Y, Watanabe M, Kasuya M, Shinkai J. The changing prevalence of respiratory symptoms in atopic children in response to air pollution. *Clin Allergy* 1986;**16**:299–308.

104 Hunt TB, Holman CDJ. Asthma hospitalisation in relation to sulphur dioxide atmospheric contamination in the Kwinana industrial area of Western Australia. *Community Health Studies* 1987;**11**:197–201.

105 Schenker MB, Vedal S, Batterman S, Samet J, Speizer F. Health effects of air pollution due to coal combustion in the Chestnut Ridge region of Pennsylvania; cross-section survey in children. *Arch Environ Health* 1986;**41**:104–8.

106 Anderson HR. Respiratory abnormalities in Papua New Guinea children; the effects of locality and domestic wood smoke pollution. *Int J Epidemiol* 1978;**7**:63–72.

107 Chan-Yeung M, Lam S. Occupational asthma state of the art. *Am Rev Respir Dis* 1986;**133**:686–703.

108 Lam S, Wong R, Chan-Yeung M. Nonspecific bronchial reactivity in occupational asthma. *J Allergy Clin Immunol* 1979;**63**:28–34.

109 Chan-Yeung M, Grzybowski S. Prognosis in occupational asthma (editorial). *Thorax* 1985;**40**:241–3.

110 Lam S, Chan H, Le Riche J, Chan-Yeung M. Cellular and protein changes in bronchial lavage fluid following late asthmatic reaction in patients with red cedar asthma. *J Allergy Clin Immunol* 1987;**80**:44–50.

111 Boschetto P, Zocca E, Milani GF *et al.* Bronchoalveolar neutrophilia during late but not early asthmatic reactions induced by toluene diisocyanate (TDI). *J Allergy Clin Immunol* 1986;**77**:244.

112 Gordon T, Sheppard D, McDonald D, Scypinski L, Distefano S. Airway responsiveness and inflammation induced by toluene diisocyanate in guinea pigs. *Am Rev Respir Dis* 1985;**132**:1106–12.

113 Chan-Yeung M, Vesal S, Kus J *et al.* Symptoms, pulmonary function, atopy and bronchial reactivity in western red cedar workers compared to office workers. *Am Rev Respir Dis* 1984;**130**:1038–41.

114 Johnson A, Chan-Yeung M, MacLean L, Atkins E, Chen F, Enarson D. Respiratory abnormalities among workers in an iron and steel foundry in Vancouver. *Br J Ind Med* 1985;**42**:94–100.

115 Enarson DA, Vedal S, Chan-Yeung M. Asthma, asthma-like symptoms and bronchial hyperresponsiveness in epidemiologic occupational surveys. *Am Rev Respir Dis* 1987;**136**:613–7.

116 Brooks SM, Weiss MA, Bernstein IL. Reactive airways dysfunction syndrome (RADS); persistent airways hyperreactivity after high level irritant exposure. *Chest* 1985;**88**:376–84.

117 Zetterstrom O, Osterman K, Machado L, Johansson SGO. Another smoking hazard; raised serum IgE concentration and increased risk of occupational allergy. *Br Med J* 1981;**283**:1215–7.

118 Venables KM, Topping MD, Howe W, Luzynuska CM, Hawkins R, Newman Taylor AJ. Interaction of smoking and atopy in producing specific IgE antibody against a hapten protein conjugate. *Br Med J* 1985;**290**:201–4.

119 Zetterstrom O, Nordrall SL, Bjorksten B, Ahlstedt S, Stelander M. Increased IgE antibody responses in rats exposed to tobacco smoke. *J Allergy Clin Immunol* 1985;**75**:594–8.

120 Holt PG. Immune and inflammatory function in cigarette smokers. *Thorax* 1987;**42**:241–9.

121 Magnusson CP. Maternal smoking influences cord serum IgE and IgD levels and increases the risk of subsequent infant allergy. *J Allergy Clin Immunol* 1986;**78**:898–904.

122 Paganelli R, Ramadas D, Layward L, Harvey BAM, Southill JF. Maternal smoking and cord blood immunity functions. *Clin Exp Immunol* 1979;**36**:256–9.

123 Ramsdell JW, Nachtwey FJ, Moser KM. Bronchial hyperreactivity in chronic obstruction bronchitis. *Am Rev Respir Dis* 1982;**126**:829–32.

124 Bahous J, Cartier A, Ouimet G, Ineau L, Malo JL. Non-allergic bronchial hyperexcitability in chronic bronchitis. *Am Rev Respir Dis* 1984;**129**:216–20.

125 Ramsdale EH, Morris MM, Roberts RS, Hargreave FE. Bronchial responsiveness to methacholine in chronic bronchitis; relationship to airflow obstruction and cold air responsiveness. *Thorax* 1984;**39**:912–8.

126 Taylor RG, Joyce H, Gross E, Holland F, Pride NB. Bronchial reactivity to inhaled histamine and annual rate of decline in FEV_1 in male smokers and ex-smokers. *Thorax* 1985;**40**:9–15.

127 Yan K, Salome CM, Woolcock AJ. Prevalence and nature of bronchial hyperresponsiveness in subjects with chronic obstructive pulmonary disease. *Am Rev Respir Dis* 1985;**132**:25–9.

128 Mullen JBM, Wiggs BR, Wright JL, Hogg JC, Pare PD. Nonspecific airway reactivity in cigarette smokers. Relationship to airway pathology and baseline lung function. *Am Rev Respir Dis* 1986;**133**:120–5.

129 Cockcroft DW, Berscheid BA, Murdock KY. Bronchial response to inhaled histamine in asymptomatic young smokers. *Eur J Respir Dis* 1983;**64**:207–11.

130 Gerrard JW, Cockcroft DW, Mink JT, Cotton DJ, Poonawala R, Dosman JA. Increased nonspecific bronchial reactivity in cigarette smokers with normal lung function. *Am Rev Respir Dis* 1980;**122**:577–581.

131 Buckzo G, Day A, van der Doelen JL, Boucher R, Zamel N. Effects of cigarette smoking and short-term smoking cessation on airway responsiveness to inhaled methacholine. *Am Rev Respir Dis* 1984;**129**:12–14.

132 Brown NE, McFadden ER, Ingram RH. Airway responses to inhaled histamine in asymptomatic smokers and nonsmokers. *J Appl Physiol; Respirat Environ Exercise Physiol* 1977;**42**:508–13.

133 Higenbottom TW, Hamilton D, Clark TJH. Changes in airway size and bronchial response to inhaled histamine in smokers and non-smokers (abstract). *Clin Sci* 1978;**54**:11P.

134 Malo JL, Filiatrault S, Martin RR. Bronchial responsiveness to inhaled methacholine in young asymptomatic smokers. *J Appl Physiol; Respirat Environ Exercise Physiol* 1982;**52**:1464–70.

135 Taylor RG, Clarke SW. Bronchial reactivity to histamine in young male smokers. *Eur J Respir Dis* 1985;**66**:320–6.

136 Casale TB, Rhodes BJ, Donnelly AL, Weiler JM. Airway responses to methacholine in asymptomatic non-atopic cigarette smokers. *J Appl Physiol* 1987;**62**:1888–92.

137 Van der Lende R, Visser BF, Wever-Hess J, de Vries K, Orie NGM. Distribution of histamine threshold values in a random population. *Rev Inst Hyg Mines (Hasselt)* 1973;**28**:186–90.

138 Rijcken B, Schouten JP, Weiss ST, Speizer FE, Van der Lende R. The relationship of nonspecific bronchial responsiveness to respiratory symptoms in a random population sample. *Am Rev Respir Dis* 1987;**136**:62–8.

139 Rijcken B, Schouten JP, Weiss ST, Speizer FE, Van der Lende R. The relationship between airway responsiveness to histamine and pulmonary function level in a random population sample. *Am Rev Respir Dis* 1988;**137**:826–32.

140 Burney PGJ, Britton JR, Chinn S *et al*. Descriptive epidemiology of bronchial reactivity in an adult population; results from a community study. *Thorax* 1987;**42**:38–44.

141 Woolcock AJ, Peak JK, Salome CM *et al*. Prevalence of bronchial hyper-responsiveness and asthma in a rural adult population. *Thorax* 1987;**42**:361–8.

142 Cerveri I, Bruschi C, Zoia MC *et al*. Distribution of bronchial nonspecific reactivity in the general population. *Chest* 1988;**93**:26–30.

143 Kabiraj MU, Simonsson BG, Groth S, Bjorklund A, Bulow K, Lindell SE. Bronchial reactivity, smoking and alpha₁–antitrypsin. A population based study of middle-aged men. *Am Rev Respir Dis* 1982;**126**:864–9.

144 Sparrow D, O'Connor G, Colton T, Barry CL, Weiss ST. The relationship of nonspecific bronchial responsiveness to the occurrence of respiratory symptoms and decreased levels of pulmonary function. *Am Rev Respir Dis* 1987;**135**:1255–60.

145 Medici TC, Chodosh S. The reticulo-endothelial system in chronic bronchitis. I. Quantitative sputum cell population during stable, acute bacterial infection, and recovery phases. *Am Rev Respir Dis* 1972;**105**:792–804.

146 Hunninghake CW, Crystal RG. Cigarette smoking and lung destruction. Accumulation of neutrophils in the lungs of cigarette smokers. *Am Rev Respir Dis* 1983;**128**:833–8.

147 Chan-Yeung M, Dy Buncio A. Leukocyte count, smoking and lung function. *Am J Med* 1984;**76**:31–7.

148 Corre F, Lellouch J, Schwartz D. Smoking and leucocyte counts. *Lancet* 1971;ii:632–4.

149 Sparrow D, Glynn RJ, Cohen M, Weiss ST. The relationship of the peripheral leukocyte count and cigarette smoking to pulmonary function among adult men. *Chest* 1984;**86**:383–6.

150 Taylor RG, Gross E, Joyce H, Holland F, Pride NB. Smoking, allergy and the differential white blood cell count. *Thorax* 1985;**40**:17–22.

151 Kraan J, Koeter GH, Van der Mark ThW *et al*. Dosage and time effects of

inhaled budesonide on bronchial hyperactivity. *Am Rev Respir Dis* 1988;**137**:44–8.

152 Jenkins CR, Woolcock AJ. Effect of prednisone and beclomethasone dipropionate on airway responsiveness in asthma; a comprehensive study. *Thorax* 1988;**43**:378–84.

153 Watson A, Lim TK, Joyce H, Pride NB. Trial of inhaled corticosteroids on bronchoconstrictor and bronchodilator responsiveness in middle-aged smokers. *Thorax* 1988;**43**:231P.

154 Engle T, Heinig JH, Konar A, Madsen O, Weeka ER. Airway reactivity of smokers with chronic bronchitis; double-blind placebo controlled study of inhaled budesonide (abstract). *J Allergy Clin Immunol* 1986;**77**:153.

155 Simonsson BG, Rolf C. Bronchial reactivity to methacholine in 10 non-obstructive heavy smokers before and up to one year after cessation of smoking. *Eur J Respir Dis* 1982;**63**:526–34.

156 Lim TK, Taylor RG, Watson A, Joyce H, Pride NB. Changes in bronchial responsiveness to inhaled histamine over four years in middle-aged male smokers and ex-smokers. *Thorax* 1983;**43**:599–604.

157 Wright JL, Lawson LM, Pare PD, Wiggs BJ, Kennedy S, Hogg JC. Morphology of peripheral airways in current smokers and ex-smokers. *Am Rev Respir Dis* 1983;**127**:474–7.

158 Fletcher C, Peto R, Tinker C, Speizer FE. *The natural history of chronic bronchitis and emphysema.* Oxford: Oxford University Press 1976.

159 O'Neill S, Prichard JS. Elastolytic activity of alveolar macrophages in chronic bronchitis; comparison of current and former smokers. *Thorax* 1983;**38**:356–9.

160 Burrows B, Halonen M, Barbee RA, Lebowitz MD. The relationship of serum immunoglobulin E to cigarette smoking. *Am Rev Respir Dis* 1981;**124**:523–5.

161 Burrows B, Hasan RM, Barbee RA, Halonen M, Lebowitz. Epidemiologic observations on eosinophilia and its relation to respiratory disorders. *Am Rev Respir Dis* 1980;**122**:708–19.

162 Burrows B, Knudson RJ, Cline MG, Lebowitz MD. A re-examination of risk factors for ventilatory impairment. *Am Rev Respir Dis* 1988;**138**:829–36.

163 Glynn AA, Michaels L. Bronchial biopsy in chronic bronchitis and asthma. *Thorax* 1960;**15**:142–53.

164 Fennerty AG, Banks J, Ebden P, Bevan C. The effect of cigarette withdrawal on asthmatics who smoke. *Eur J Respir Dis* 1987;**71**:395–9.

165 Higenbottom TW, Feyerabend C, Clark TJ. Cigarette smoking in asthma. *Br J Dis Chest* 1980;**74**:279–84.

166 Vesterinen E, Kaprio J, Koskenvuo M. Prospective study of asthma in relation to smoking habits among 14 729 adults. *Thorax* 1988;**43**:534–9.

167 Hillerdahl G, Rylander R. Asthma and cessation of smoking. *Clin Allergy* 1984;**14**:45–7.

168 Nadel JA, Comroe JH. Acute effects of inhalation of cigarette smoke on airway conductance. *J Appl Physiol* 1961;**16**:713–6.

169 Guyatt AR, Berry G, Alpers JH, Bramley AC, Fletcher CM. Relation of airway conductance and its immediate change on smoking to smoking habits and symptoms of chronic bronchitis. *Am Rev Respir Dis* 1970;**101**:44–54.

170 Wiedmann HE, Mahler DA, Loke J, Virgulto JA, Snyder P, Matthay RA. Acute effects of passive smoking on lung function and airway reactivity in asthmatic subjects. *Chest* 1986;**89**:180–5.

171 Knight A, Breslin ABX. Passive cigarette smoking and patients with asthma. *Med J Aust* 1985;**142**:194–5.

172 Murray AB, Morrison BJ. The effect of cigarette smoke from the mother on bronchial responsiveness and severity of symptoms in children with asthma. *J Allergy Clin Immunol* 1986;**77**:575–81.

173 O'Connor GT, Weiss ST, Tager IB, Speizer FE. The effect of passive smoking on pulmonary function and non-specific bronchial responsiveness in a population based sample of children and young adults. *Am Rev Respir Dis* 1987;**135**:800–4.

174 Martinez FD, Antognoni G, Macri F *et al.* Parental smoking enhances bronchial responsiveness in nine-year-old children. *Am Rev Respir Dis* 1988;**138**:518–23.

Index